● **Jill Black Lattanzi**, PT, EdD
Adjunct Professor
Widener University Institute of Physical Therapy
Chester, PA

PTA Program Coordinator
Delaware Technical & Community College
Wilmington, DE

Manager of Allied Health Education Programs
Christiana Care Health System
Newark, DE

● **Larry D. Purnell**, PhD, RN, FAAN
Professor
College of Health and Nursing Sciences
University of Delaware
Newark, DE

Developing Cultural Competence in Physical Therapy Practice

F. A. Davis Company
1915 Arch Street
Philadelphia, PA 19103
www.fadavis.com

Printed in the United States of America

Last digit indicates print number: 10 9 8 7 6 5 4 3 2 1

Acquisitions Editor: Margaret M. Biblis
Developmental Editor: Jennifer Pine
Manager of Art & Design: Carolyn O'Brien

As new scientific information becomes available through basic and clinical research, recommended treatments and drug therapies undergo changes. The author(s) and publisher have done everything possible to make this book accurate, up to date, and in accord with accepted standards at the time of publication. The author(s), editors, and publisher are not responsible for errors or omissions or for consequences from application of the book, and make no warranty, expressed or implied, in regard to the contents of the book. Any practice described in this book should be applied by the reader in accordance with professional standards of care used in regard to the unique circumstances that may apply in each situation. The reader is advised always to check product information (package inserts) for changes and new information regarding dose and contraindications before administering any drug. Caution is especially urged when using new or infrequently ordered drugs.

Library of Congress Cataloging-in-Publication Data

Lattanzi, Jill Black.
Developing cultural competence in physical therapy practice / Jill Black Lattanzi, Larry D. Purnell.
p. ; cm.
Includes bibliographical references and index.
ISBN-13: 978-0-8036-1195-5 (alk. paper)
ISBN-10: 0-8036-1195-1 (alk. paper)
1. Physical therapy–Practice. 2. Culture–Social aspects.
[DNLM: 1. Physical Therapy (Specialty)–methods. 2. Cultural Diversity. 3. Culture. 4. Population Groups.
5. Professional-Patient Relations. WB 460 L364d 2006] I. Purnell, Larry D. II. Title.
RM705.L38 2006
362.17'8–dc22   2005022371

Dedication

We would like to dedicate this work to the many patients and healthcare providers who have broadened our understanding of culture throughout various parts of the United States and the world, and to the students and physical therapists who have chosen to be part of the cultural learning experience by venturing beyond their comfort zone to serve and care for patients of cultures different from their own.

Jill Black Lattanzi
Larry D. Purnell

The Editors

*J*ill *Black Lattanzi,* PT, MS, EdD, is an adjunct professor at the Widener University Institute of Physical Therapy Education in Chester, Pennsylvania, and regularly guest lectures for the University of Delaware Physical Therapy Program and the Delaware Technical and Community College Physical Therapist Assistant Program. She also serves as the Manager of Allied Health Education Programs for the Christiana Care Health System of Newark, Delaware. She received her physical therapy degree from the University of Delaware as well as a master's in Exercise Physiology. She also earned her EdD from the University of Delaware, where she focused on multicultural education for the physical therapy student. Dr. Lattanzi's doctoral dissertation was a qualitative research project conducted at a Salvation Army homeless shelter where Thomas Jefferson physical therapy students conduct a service-learning clinic. The Journal of Physical Therapy Education awarded Dr. Lattanzi the Stanford award in 2002 for her article summarizing her findings. Dr. Lattanzi has also been conducting volunteer physical therapy mission trips to rural southern Mexico since 1991, as well as other parts of Central and South America and the Caribbean. She has taken over 30 trips and hosted more than 100 students and physical therapy professionals in these cross-cultural service-learning experiences.

Larry D. Purnell, PhD, RN, FAAN, is a professor in the College of Health Sciences at the University of Delaware, where he heads the master's program in Nursing and Health Services Administration and teaches transcultural healthcare in several departments. He is also on the faculty at the University of Panama, an Excelsior College. He is a Fellow of the American Academy of Nursing, a Virginia Henderson Fellow, and a Distinguished Lecturer for Sigma Theta Tau International. Dr. Purnell has authored 5 books, over 50 book chapters, and 100 refereed articles. His textbook *Transcultural Health Care: A Culturally Competent Approach* won the prestigious Brandon Hill Book award two years in a row. In addition, he has made more than 150 presentations on culture, globalization, and health-related topics in the United States, Finland, Sweden, Denmark, Spain, England, Scotland, China, Hong Kong, Panama, Turkey, and Belize. Additionally, he has grants exceeding one million dollars. Dr. Purnell's current research, "Hispanic Health Beliefs and the Meaning of Respect Afforded Them by Health Care Providers" includes participants from all countries in Central America and Mexico, and their cohort groups in the United States.

Contributing Authors

Kim Nixon-Cave, PhD, PT, PCS, is an associate professor, acting Chair of the Department of Physical Therapy, and director of the DPT program in the Department of Physical Therapy at Temple University. Dr. Nixon-Cave is also the Academic Coordinator of Clinical Education and has a research agenda related to her interest in cultural, racial, and ethnic influences on physical therapy care, especially for children and families. Her dissertation examined the influence of family, environment, and evaluation issues in pediatric care. She has given lectures locally and nationally on the topic of recruitment, retention, and graduation of persons from racial/ethnic and minority groups as well as on cultural issues in pediatrics. Dr. Nixon-Cave completed her physical therapy education at the University of Pittsburgh, received an MS in Physical Therapy at Temple University, and a PhD in Special Education from Temple University. She is also a Pediatric Certified Specialist.

Theresa J. Kraemer, PhD, PT, ATC, is an assistant professor of physical therapy at A.T. Still–University–Arizona School of Health Sciences in Mesa, Arizona. Dr. Kraemer received both her Bachelor of Arts in Psychology and her Bachelor of Science in Physical Therapy from the University of New Mexico, her Master's of Science degree in Health Sciences and Health Education from San Francisco State University, and her Doctorate in Education, with a double emphasis in Educational Leadership and Research, from Virginia Commonwealth University. Dr. Kraemer has published and presented both nationally and internationally in the areas of cultural understanding. She is currently completing several fully funded grants and cross–cultural research projects.

Florence Thillet-Bice, PT, DPT, MA, PCS, is a pediatric certified physical therapy specialist who received her PT degree from the University of Puerto Rico Medical Sciences Campus in 1973, her MA degree in Adult and Higher Education from the University of Texas in San Antonio in 1992, and her doctorate in Physical Therapy in 2003 from the University of Central Arkansas. She is currently enrolled in the Doctor in Science Studies at Rocky Mountain University of Health Professions. Her professional interest has focused on working with children and families in underserved inner-city and rural areas and on health issues of Hispanic families. She is currently in private practice in Ringgold, Louisiana, where she works in the local school system and early intervention program. She is also a clinical assistant professor at the University of Louisiana Medical Sciences Center in Shreveport, Louisiana.

Teresa M. Cochran, PT, DPT, GCS, MA, is an assistant professor in the Department of Physical Therapy at Creighton University Medical Center. She is also co-director of the Office of Interprofessional Service and Scholarship and Education at Creighton. Dr. Cochran earned a BA in Psychology and an MA in Developmental Psychology from the University of Nebraska, and a DPT from Creighton University. Dr. Cochran serves as a consulting physical therapist at the Carl T. Curtis Health Education Center within the Omaha Nation in Macy, Nebraska, as well as at the United States Public Health Service / Indian Health Service Hospital serving the Winnebago Nation of Winnebago, Nebraska. Dr. Cochran has lectured and published extensively in the area of culturally appropriate healthcare delivery to American Indians. Her research interests include the role of rehabilitation in American Indian healthcare and cross-cultural practice.

Patrick S. Cross, PT, DPT, is Director of Rehabilitation for Carl T. Curtis Health Education Center. Dr. Cross also acts as a clinic and community physical therapist at the Carl T. Curtis Health Education Center serving the Omaha Nation, as well as the United States Public Health Service / Indian Health Service Hospital serving the Winnebago Nation of Winnebago, Nebraska. His research interests and publications include topics related to service learning, rural health, cross-cultural physical therapy, and community physical therapy.

Elizabeth Dean, PT, PhD, is on the faculty of the School of Rehabilitation Sciences at the University of British Columbia in Canada. Her academic and clinical career and experiences have spanned the "corners of the globe," with invitations to Australia, Belgium, Brazil, China, Greece, Hong Kong, Japan, Kuwait, Monaco, the Netherlands, New Zealand, Pakistan, Saudi Arabia, Singapore, Switzerland, and the United Kingdom, as well as the United States and at home in Canada. Her research has focused on integrating knowledge of culture relativism and diversity in promoting health and wellness worldwide with an emphasis on the translation of evidence-based physical therapy practice in the prevention, management, and cure of diseases, such as heart disease, hypertension, stroke, diabetes, and cancer, which are prevalent worldwide. Dr. Dean is also the Coordinator of the UBC postpolio clinic. Her work through the UBC Post Polio Clinic has taken her to Pakistan on an Asia Pacific University Scholar's Award. She spent a year as Senior of the Cardiovascular/Cardiorespiratory Team on the Kuwait Dalhousie Project in Kuwait, and a year as a visiting professor at the Hong Kong Polytechnic University in Hong Kong.

Surreya Mahomed, PT, DEd, is a lecturer in the Department of Physical Therapy at Kuwait University in Kuwait.

Aisha Omar Maulana, MPH, is the HIV/AIDS coordinator for the Kenya Red Cross Society in Nairobi, Kenya.

Ronnie Leavitt, PhD, MPH, PT, has served as an associate professor at the University of Connecticut School of Allied Health since 1979. She received her BS in physical therapy from Boston University, her master's in public health from Columbia University, and her PhD in medical anthropology from the University of Connecticut. She has taken innumerable physical therapy trips to developing countries and has conducted extensive research of community-based rehabilitation in Jamaica. She is also well published in the area of cultural competence and international rehabilitation. Dr. Leavitt has been a pioneer in the area of cultural competency development for the physical therapist as founder and president of the APTA Cross-Cultural Special Interest Group as well as serving on the APTA Committee for the Promotion of Cultural Competence.

Stephanie Beaman, MPT, graduated from the University of Delaware with a master's in physical therapy in 1999 and has worked as a staff physical therapist at the Veterans Administration Medical Center in Elsmere, DE.

Peter C. Glover, DPT, received his military commission from the United States Military Academy at West Point in 1988. He currently holds the rank of captain in the Army Medical Specialist Corps of the United States Army Reserve. Dr. Glover's civilian education includes a BS in mechanical engineering from West Point, and an MS and DPT in physical therapy from the University of Miami School of Medicine. Presently, Dr. Glover is a Staff Physical Therapist at the 2290th United States Army Hospital, Walter Reed Medical Center, in Washington, DC, as well as the Senior Physical Therapist for the Veterans Administration Medical Center at Perry Point, Maryland.

Robin L. Dole, PT, EdD, PCS, is the department chair of the Physical Therapy Program at Widener University's Institute for Physical Therapy Education. Dr. Dole completed her BS in physical therapy at Ithaca College, her MS in physical therapy with an emphasis in pediatrics at the University of Indianapolis, and her EdD in child and youth studies at Nova Southeastern University. She is a Pediatric Certified Specialist and has lectured extensively in the area of pediatrics and community health. She has been instrumental in initiating service-learning projects at Widener University's Institute for Physical Therapy Education and has demonstrated a commitment to culturally competent care in pediatrics.

Reviewer List

Nicceta Davis
Associate Professor of Physical Therapy
School of Allied Health Professions
Loma Linda University
Loma Linda, CA

Beverly D. Fein, PT, EdD
Associate Professor of Physical Therapy
Sacred Heart University
Fairfield, CT

Moni Fricke, BMR (PT), MSc
Instructor, School of Medical Rehabilitation
University of Manitoba
Winnipeg, Manitoba
Canada

Donald L. Gabard, PT, PhD
Associate Professor of Physical Therapy
Chapman University
Los Angeles, CA

Patricia A. Hageman, PhD, PT
Director and Associate Professor of Physical
    Therapy Education
University of Nebraska Medical Center
Omaha, NE

Rebecca Henson Pearson, PT, EdD
Associate Professor of Physical Therapy
University of Mississippi Medical Center
Jackson, MS

Kathy Hummel-Berry, PT, MEd
Director and Associate Professor of Physical
    Therapy
University of Washington at Puget Sound
Tacoma, WA

Lisa Ann Steinkamp, PT, MS, MBA
Director, Department of Physical Therapy
University of Wisconsin
Madison, WI

Denise Wise, PT, PhD
Chair and Assistant Professor of Physical
    Therapy
The College of St. Scholastica
Duluth, MN

Antonio Valenzuela, PTA, EdD
Assistant Professor of Physical Therapy
School of Allied Health Professions
Loma Linda University
Loma Linda, CA

Preface

The physical therapy profession has recognized the importance of considering a patient's culture in physical therapy evaluation and intervention, as evidenced by the American Physical Therapy Association's vision statement, the *Guide to Physical Therapist Practice,* the Commission for the Accreditation of Physical Therapy Education's criteria for education of PT and PTA students, and the normative models for PT and PTA education. To date, however, a text of cultural considerations specific to physical therapists and physical therapist assistants has not existed.

Dr. Jill Lattanzi, a physical therapist who did her doctoral study in multicultural education for the physical therapy student and who has facilitated cultural international physical therapy training for 14 years, teamed with Dr. Larry Purnell, author of "The Purnell Model for Cultural Competence" in the best-selling text *Transcultural Healthcare: A Culturally Competent Approach,* and the handbook *Guide to Culturally Competent Health Care.* Together, Dr. Lattanzi and Dr. Purnell have pooled an excellent group of contributing authors, all physical therapists with firsthand knowledge of specific cultural groups and expertise in culture, diversity, and physical therapy. This unique combination provides an invaluable perspective on specific cultural groups. The main goal of this text is to provide a framework for cultural self-exploration, information about general cultural differences, and a selection of culture-specific information for consideration.

The text is divided into five sections. The first begins with an introduction to the study of culture and presents the Purnell Model of Cultural Competence, which is used throughout the text as an organizing framework.

The second section provides a self-exploration of culture. The editors hope that physical therapist students will work through this section to gain a better understanding of themselves and their own cultures and how they affect the practitioner-patient interaction. Understanding one's own culture is the first and most important step to the development of cultural competency. The student should always begin here.

Throughout the text, the editors and contributing authors have included "reflective exercises" for the reader to consider. These reflective exercises can also be used for class discussions. Cultural self-assessment exercises are included at the end of each of these early chapters to facilitate learning and to aid in understanding oneself. A vignette at the beginning of each chapter provides a basis for questions throughout the chapter and at the end. Each chapter concludes with a comprehensive case study. The case studies are meant to stimulate thought and discussion. The readings do not supply all the answers to the case studies, but instead allow the student to begin the process of cultural exploration. Greater understanding may arise as the student further studies the text. We recommend that students revisit the case studies to enhance learning.

The third and fourth sections provide information for specific cultural groups that physical therapists may encounter. The editors chose the various ethnic cultures presented on the basis of lengthy classifications of groups of people as well as the contributing authors' areas of knowledge and expertise. The special population groups were chosen according to the areas of practice for the contributing authors as well as populations presenting with unique physical therapy needs. Perhaps a future work can include additional ethnic and special population groups. Intercultural and well as intracultural variations exist within all groups according to the primary and secondary characteristics of culture that constitute a person's worldview. Thus, physical therapists need both culture-general and culture-specific knowledge about the groups with whom they interact. The chapters are meant to be only a starting point for cultural considerations. To claim that each person adheres to the characteristics of one culture would be to stereotype and introduce grave error. Instead, the reader should consider each chapter a reflection of some generalities that may facilitate additional questions or explorations of a patient's culture. These chapters also include reflective exercises as well as an initial vignette and concluding case study.

The fifth section focuses on strategies and resources for physical therapy students, physical therapy professionals, physical therapy practices, and physical therapy educators toward the development of greater cultural understandings and outreach to people of diverse groups. It should be noted that the text is equally valuable to the physical therapist and the physical therapist assistant. To simplify the reading of the text, "physical therapist" is used throughout, but the reader should understand that this could just as easily read "physical therapist assistant," as the interaction skills and understandings are equally important for all physical therapist and physical therapist assistant licensed professionals.

The text can be used as a classroom guide to the study of culture and cultural encounters in physical therapy as well as a resource for the physical therapy professional, educator, researcher, or administrator. The text will have value to the student in the classroom and will be something the student will want to save as a resource for his or her professional practice. The editors hope that readers will learn a lot more about themselves as well as how to better understand the patients and communities of patients that they serve.

Given the increasing diversity of clients and healthcare professionals, cultural competence is a necessity, not a luxury. Knowing about clients' cultures and individual beliefs is as important as knowing about the impairments and functional limitations of the client; without such knowledge on the part of the physical therapy professional, the client may not understand or follow through with recommended physical therapy interventions. The editors hope you use, value, and enjoy the book.

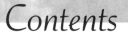

Contents

Culture: Exploration and Discovery

1

SECTION

What Is Culture and How Do I Grow in Cultural Competence?

Chapter 1

Introducing Cultural Concepts

- Jill Black Lattanzi, PT, EdD
- Larry D. Purnell, PhD, RN

The Need for Culturally Competent Healthcare in Physical Therapy

Vignette

Vera Morozov, a Russian Jew, and her daughter, Olga, were in a limousine accident on their way from the airport to the home of Vera's brother. Mother and daughter are Jewish and are from Russia. They had come to the United States to visit family for 3 weeks. Seventy-two-year-old Vera suffered broken ribs and a fractured right ulna and right femur. Forty-two-year-old Olga suffered a head trauma and multiple soft-tissue contusions. Both are taken to a nearby Catholic hospital, where they are treated in the Emergency Department and admitted to the hospital. Although Vera speaks very little English, Olga had just completed a 6-week course in conversational English before their arrival in the United States.

The nurse caring for Vera and Olga in the Emergency Department, Mr. de Estrada, was born in the United States. His parents are from Colombia. The physician in the Emergency Room, Dr. Patel, is from Pakistan. The nurse on the inpatient unit, Mrs. Choi, is from Taiwan. The patient care assistant on the inpatient unit, Miss Lawrie, is from Haiti. The physical therapist, Melissa Dougherty, was born in the United States and is unsure of her ancestry. Mr. Rami Tambouz is the physical therapist assistant, and he immigrated to the United States with his parents from Jordan when he was 7 years old. The occupational therapist, Ms. Bernice Jones, was born in the United States. Her distant ancestors were forced to immigrate as slaves in the early 1800s. The transporter, Mr. Patrick Hardie, is from Northern Ireland and has been in the United States for 16 months. The rehabilitation unit secretary, Ms. Patricia Kozlowski, was born in the United States and grew up in a Polish ethnic enclave. Her grandparents emigrated from Poland in the early 1900s.

Scenarios similar to the above vignette, with clients and staff coming from multiple countries and various ethnic and cultural backgrounds, are becoming more common in today's healthcare organizations, resulting in a diverse clientele and workforce needing to understand and respect each other's perspectives on health and illness. Accordingly, multicultural diversity has emerged as a major issue for healthcare, businesses, and educational organizations. The U.S. government, accrediting bodies,[1] the mass media, professional organizations,[2-4] and employers have addressed the need for individuals to understand and strive for cultural competence (Fig. 1-1).

The United States is a sea of people on the move. Visit an international airport, and you will see a host of people from many ethnic and cultural backgrounds boarding airplanes for a variety of reasons. Some are visiting relatives, some are on educational pursuits, and others are on vacation or work assignments. Unfortunately, a few will need healthcare while they are away from their home country. The United States is also an amalgamation of cultures and ethnicities, having received and integrated immigrants from all parts of the world since its founding. Whether people are Native Americans, recent immigrants, older immigrants, children of immigrants, refugees, vacationers, or sojourners, they all have the right to expect physical therapists to respect their personal beliefs and healthcare practices. They will need culturally sensitive and culturally competent healthcare.

Diversity is not always as apparent as in the introductory vignette. People may wear the same brand and style of clothes, eat at the same restaurants, enjoy the same recreational activities, and watch the same television shows but still be worlds apart in the cultural and ethnic backgrounds that define their basic heritage and values. The more dissimilar in appearance individuals are, the easier it becomes for others to realize that they may have differing beliefs, attitudes, and ideologies. Unfortunately, this observation does not necessarily lead to better acceptance of individual differences. The increased similarity in the appearance of culturally diverse individuals challenges others to be more consciously aware of the differences underlying ethnocultural diversity.[5] The physical therapist must recognize and respect clients' nonharmful cultural beliefs and practices and integrate them into the plan of care (Fig. 1-2).

Physical therapists provide care to people of diverse cultures in skilled nursing facilities, acute-care facilities, rehabilitation centers, outpatient clinics, school systems, and clients' homes. Although physical therapists, physicians, nurses, nutritionists, technicians, morticians, home health aides, and other caregivers need similar culturally specific information, the manner in which the information is used may differ significantly based on the discipline, individual experiences, and specific circumstances of the client. Each discipline has its own unique knowledge base to support its ways of knowing, techniques, roles, norms, values, ideologies, attitudes, and beliefs, which interlock to make a reinforced and supportive system within its defined practice. For instance, physical therapists must closely examine ethnocultural diversity and its potential impact on evaluation, plans of care, and interventions.[6-10] This text is written to assist the physical therapist in the development of greater cultural understanding

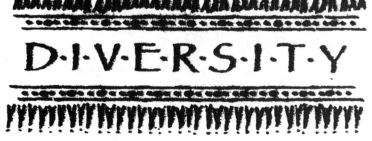

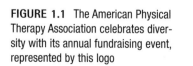
FIGURE 1.1 The American Physical Therapy Association celebrates diversity with its annual fundraising event, represented by this logo

and skill in the practice of culturally congruent physical therapy.

Reflective Exercise

• What cultural groups have you encountered in your workplace, school, or professional practice?
• What cultural beliefs regarding physical therapy do you hold? • What other cultural beliefs have you encountered?

The physical therapy profession has acknowledged the importance of cultural diversity recognition and understandings in many ways. Included in the American Physical Therapy Association's (APTA) vision statement is a sentence that reads, "They (physical therapists) will provide culturally sensitive care distinguished by trust, respect, and an appreciation for individual differences."[11] Within the APTA, two groups exist to promote cultural competency. The Committee on Cultural Competence was established specifically to develop a strategic plan for the APTA to promote cultural competence in physical therapy. The committee reviews core APTA documents and monitors related education, practice, and research endeavors to ensure cultural sensitivity and adherence to principles of cultural competence. Second, the Cross-Cultural and International Special Interest Group (CCISIG) within the Section on Health Policy and Administration of the APTA serves to promote cultural competency with its activities.[10]

The Normative Models of Physical Therapist Professional Education[12] and Physical Therapist Assistant Education[13] identify professional practice expectations related to cultural competence. The precise educational outcomes defined by each model are presented in Tables 1-1 and 1-2.

In addition, the Commission on Accreditation in Physical Therapy Education (CAPTE) lists standards related to culturally congruent practice.[10] Under the evaluative criteria for the physical therapist and physical therapist assistant, CAPTE standards indicate that the professional should "recognize individual and cultural differences and respond appropriately in all aspects of physical therapy services."[14] Additionally, the Centers for Medicare and Medicaid Services (CMS) mandate quality-of-care standards for Medicare and Medicaid recipients. In June 2000, CMS required organizations to ensure that services are provided in a culturally competent manner to all enrollees, including those with limited English proficiency or reading skill and those with diverse cultural and ethnic backgrounds.[15]

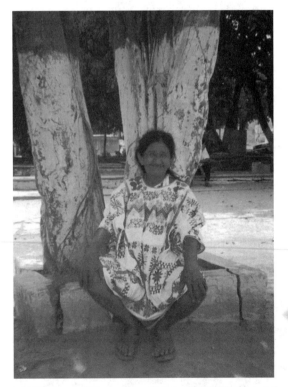

FIGURE 1.2 Culture encompasses more than differences in dress or customs. Differences in culture are not always as apparent as they might be with this woman, who is from an indigenous tribe in Mexico.

Reflective Exercise

• What adaptations have you made in your clinical practice or educational program to accommodate cultural diversity? • What does your organization or institution do to ensure that culturally competent physical therapy services are provided or taught to all patients or students (Fig. 1-3)?

Organizations, institutions, and individuals who understand their clients' cultural values, beliefs, and practices are in a better position to be co-participants with their clients and provide culturally acceptable and safe care. Accordingly, there will be improved opportunities for health promotion, impairment and disability, and health maintenance and rehabilitation. To this end, physical therapists need not only culture-general knowledge, but also culture-specific knowledge about the group(s) to whom they provide care so that they know which questions to ask.[5] For example, if the therapist is not aware that some cultures value interdependence rather than the traditional U.S. value of independence, a miscommunication or misjudgment may occur within the physical therapy program as a result of the cultural misalignment of values.[7]

The aim of this text is twofold. First, the text endeavors to assist the physical therapist in identifying his or her own culture in order to begin to understand how a cultural misalignment might occur within the interaction or administration of physical therapy programs. Second, the text

TABLE 1.1

Professional Practice Expectation 7: Cultural Competence

Definition: *Cultural and linguistic competence* is a set of congruent behaviors, attitudes, and policies that come together in a system, agency, or among professionals that enables effective work in cross-cultural situations.[a]

Culture refers to integrated patterns of human behavior that include the language, thoughts, communications, actions, customs, beliefs, values, and institutions of racial, ethnic, religious, or social groups.[a]

Competence implies having the capacity to function effectively as an individual and an organization within the context of the cultural beliefs, behaviors, and needs presented by consumers and their communities.[a]

7.1 Identify, respect, and act with consideration for patients'/clients' differences, values, preferences, and expressed needs in all professional activities.

Educational Outcomes

The graduate:

- Recognizes individual and cultural differences and adapts behavior accordingly in all aspects of physical therapy services.
- Displays sensitivity by considering differences in race/ethnicity, religion, gender, age, national origin, sexual orientation, and disability or health status in making clinical decisions.
- Recognizes aspects of behavior and care affected by individual needs and cultural differences.
- Discovers, respects, and values individual differences, preferences, values, life issues, and emotional needs within and among cultures.

- Promotes representation of individual and cultural differences in practice, research, and education.
- Incorporates an understanding of the implications of individual and cultural differences in the management and delivery of physical therapy services.
- Values the sociocultural, psychological, and economic influences on patients/clients and responds accordingly.
- Is aware of and suspends own social and cultural biases.
- Understands and applies principles of cultural competence.
- Provides care in a nonjudgmental manner when the patients'/clients' beliefs and values conflict with the individual's belief system.
- Demonstrates respect for patient's/client's privacy.
- Values the dignity of patients/clients as individuals.

[b] Working definition adapted from *Assuring Cultural Competence in Health Care: Recommendations for National Standards and an Outcomes-Focused Research Agenda,* Office of Minority Health, Public Health Service, U S Department of Health and Human Services; 1999.

From A Normative Model of Physical Therapist Professional Education: Version 2004. American Physical Therapy Association, Alexandria, Va, 2004. Used with permission.

TABLE 1.2

Performance Expectation Theme 2: Individual and Cultural Differences

2.1 Demonstrates sensitivity to Individual and cultural differences in all aspects of physical therapy services.

Educational Outcomes

The graduate will:

- demonstrate an understanding of the major differences between individuals and cultures.
- promote representation of individual and cultural differences in practice, research, and education.
- engage in continuing education opportunities that facilitate and enhance understanding of cultural and individual differences.
- be guided at all times by concern for the dignity and welfare of the patients entrusted to his/her care.
- adapt interactions and services in response to individual and cultural differences.

From A Normative Model of Physical Therapist Assistant Education: Version 99. American Physical Therapy Association, Alexandria, Va, 1999. Used with permission.

strives to provide both culture-general and culture-specific information to assist the physical therapist from the United States to perform culturally competent evaluations and assessments, to develop culturally appropriate plans of care, and to conduct culturally congruent interactions and interventions.

Diversity in the World and in the United States

The world's population reached 6.1 billion people in the year 2000 and is expected to approach 7.6 billion by 2020. By the year 2050, the estimated population will be 9.3 billion, an increase of 3.2 billion, or approximately a 30% increase from the present day. Asia has a population of 3.6 billion, Africa has a population of 770 million, Europe and Latin America each have a population of 507 million, and North America has a population of 301 million, with most of these living in the United States. A significant number of immigrants to the United States and Canada come from the world's most populous countries: China, India, Indonesia, Brazil, Russia, Pakistan, Bangladesh, Japan, Nigeria, Mexico, Germany, the Philippines, Vietnam, Egypt, Turkey, Iran, Ethiopia, Thailand, and the United Kingdom[16] (Fig. 1-4).

Between 1990 and 2000, the U.S. population increased from 248.7 million to 281.4 million. U.S. population growth varied significantly in the last decade, with higher rates in the West (19.7%) and South (17.3%).[17] Of the people included in this census, 75.1% were white, 12.5% were Spanish/Hispanic/Latino (of any race), 12.3% were black or African American, 0.9% were American Indian or Alaskan Native, 3.6% were

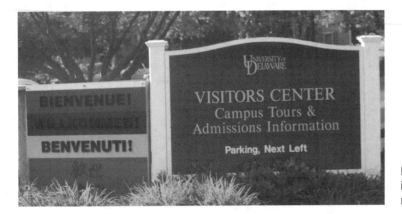

FIGURE 1.3 An educational institution welcomes students in multiple languages.

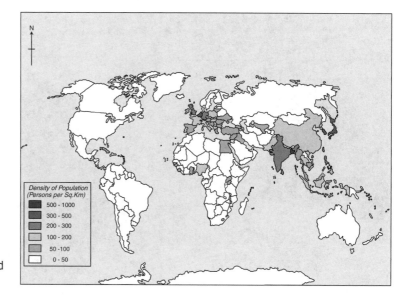

FIGURE 1.4 A map of the world showing population density.

Asian, 0.1% were Native Hawaiian or other Pacific Islander, 5.5% were some other race, and 2.4% were of two or more races[17] (Fig. 1-5). Note that these figures total more than 100% because the federal government considers race and Hispanic origin to be two separate and distinct categories. The U.S. census has changed its classification of race and ethnicity every decade since 1860, when it considered only three groups: white, black, and mulatto. It was not until 1970 that Hispanics became a category.[18] Thus, comparisons with previous census data are not appropriate.

Diversity in the United States has emerged in many ways. Early diversity existed when European immigrants first came to the New World and encountered Native Americans. African American culture initially emerged secondary to the forced emigration of Africans from their homeland. The New World of opportunity and dreams coupled with the potato famine and drought of the mid-1800s brought a new wave of immigrants from Ireland, Italy, Poland, and other countries. Most recently, immigrants have arrived from Asian countries and Central and South America. Recent advances in technology and ease of international travel have led to a wave of travelers coming to the United States for a variety of reasons (see Chapter 3).

In contrast to the statistics depicting the growing diversity of the United States, the statistics on the ethnicities of recent physical therapy graduates demonstrate greater homogeneity. According to CAPTE,[14] the ethnicities of the 2003–2004 graduates of physical therapy programs are as follows: 80.9% Caucasian, 6.1% Asian, 4.5% Hispanic/Latino, 5.2% African American, 0.5% American Indian, 1.7% other, and 1.1% unknown (Fig. 1-6).

Reflective Exercise

• How diverse was your physical therapy class?
• How did the diversity contribute or detract from learning in the classroom? • How does that diversity contribute or detract from the value of the profession?

Native Americans, immigrants, and their descendants have transformed the United States into the world's most powerful nation. Moreover, North America is increasingly becoming a mosaic of many cultures, reflecting a mixture of ideologies, beliefs, and healthcare practices. As society

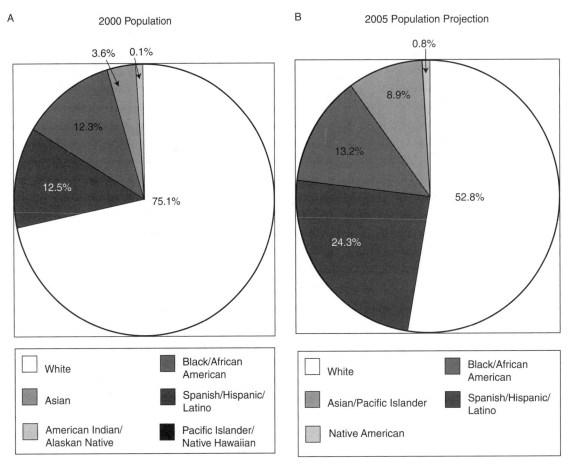

A   2000 Population

3.6%   0.1%

12.3%

12.5%

75.1%

□ White	■ Black/African American
■ Asian	■ Spanish/Hispanic/ Latino
■ American Indian/ Alaskan Native	■ Pacific Islander/ Native Hawaiian

B   2005 Population Projection

0.8%

8.9%

13.2%

52.8%

24.3%

□ White	■ Black/African American
■ Asian/Pacific Islander	■ Spanish/Hispanic/ Latino
■ Native American	

FIGURE 1.5 U.S. population by ethnicity as reported in the 2000 U.S. Census. (Data from U.S. Census Bureau.)

has become more diverse, learning about and developing an awareness of cultural and ethnic differences are more important than ever for physical therapists, who are less likely to have encountered a wide range of cultural differences among their classmates or faculty.

Reflective Exercise

• From where have your ancestors come? • What contributions have they made to the mosaic of U.S. culture?

Cultural Concepts and Essential Terminology

Anthropologists, sociologists, and others have proposed many definitions of culture. For the purposes of this book, **culture** is defined as

The totality of socially transmitted behavioral patterns, arts, beliefs, values, customs, lifeways, and all other products of human work and thought characteristics of a population of people that guide their worldview and decision making.[5]

Ethnicities of 2001 PT graduates

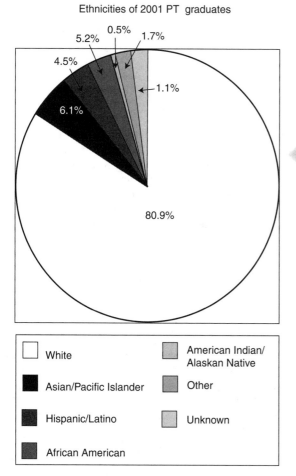

FIGURE 1.6 Ethnicities of 2003/2004 graduates of physical therapy programs according to CAPTE (2003).

These patterns may be explicit or implicit, are primarily learned and transmitted within the family, are shared by most members of the culture, and are emergent phenomena that change in response to global events. Thus, in essence, culture is a set of guidelines and standards for existing in society. As we well know, not everyone in society agrees with or adheres to the same guidelines and standards, and the same is true for culture. Not everyone in a representative culture follows the expected cultural characteristics prescribed by the majority. Moreover, expected be-

haviors are context dependent and change with the setting. For example, wearing a miniskirt for a night on the town dancing may be appropriate dress; however, a miniskirt is not acceptable dress when caring for patients in an inpatient setting. Likewise, a traditional Muslim woman may dress differently at home than in public.[19,20] Culture is largely unconscious and has powerful influences on health and illness.

Reflective Exercise

• Who in your family was the primary person who taught you your cultural values and practices?
• What cultural practices and rituals that you observed as a child do you no longer practice?

People from a given racial group may, but do not necessarily, share a common culture. Furthermore, racial terms are confusing at best. For example, most people who identify with the African American culture have black skin. However, the term *African American* denotes a cultural heritage, not race. A person who self-identifies as African American could have white skin. Another example follows: John and Jane Smith, both third-generation white Americans of English heritage, adopted a Korean infant, Shin, at birth. Shin may belong to the "Asian" race, but Shin's cultural heritage, practices, and values will primarily be the dominant American cultural values, assuming he is raised in the dominant American society.

A well-recognized fact is that some professionals do not like to use the word *race*, preferring other terms.[21] The Human Genome Project provides evidence that all human beings share a genetic code that is over 99% identical.[22] Although there is less than 1% difference in the genetic makeup of humans, this difference may still heavily influence one's culture and one's health profile. **Race** is genetic in origin and includes physical characteristics that are similar among members of the group, such as skin color, blood type, and hair and eye color.[5] Race sometimes determines differences in drug metabolism or predisposition to certain diseases. Likewise, given that the U.S. government uses the classification of race rather than ethnicity to collect data, it is essential for healthcare providers to be cognizant of race when researching data on cultural groups. The term *racial and ethnic disparities* is heavily used in the literature to address differences in healthcare. Race categories used in the 2000 census are listed in Box 1-1.[23]

BOX 1.1

Race Categories Used in U.S. Census 2000

1. *White* refers to people having origins in any of the original peoples of Europe, the Near East, and the Middle East, or North Africa. This category includes Irish, German, Italian, Lebanese, Turkish, Arab, and Polish.
2. *Black* or *African American* refers to people having origins in any of the black racial groups of Africa, and includes Nigerians and Haitians or any person who self-designated this category regardless of origin.
3. *American Indian* and *Alaskan Native* refer to people having origins in any of the original peoples of North, South, or Central America and who maintain tribal affiliation or community attachment.
4. *Asian* refers to people having origins in any of the original peoples of the Far East, Southeast Asia, or the Indian subcontinent. This category includes the terms *Asian Indian, Chinese, Filipino, Korean, Japanese, Vietnamese, Burmese, Hmong, Pakistani,* and *Thai.*
5. *Native Hawaiian and other Pacific Islander* refers to people having origins in any of the original peoples of Hawaii, Guam, Samoa, Tahiti, the Mariana Islands, and Chuuk.
6. "Some other race" was included for people who are unable to identify with the other categories. Additionally, the respondent could identify, as a write-in, with two races.[23]

Reflective Exercise

• What are your personal beliefs about the term *race?* • Do you prefer another word? • Why? • Why not? • Do you know the ethnic/racial/cultural composition of the community in which you live and/or work?

Primary and Secondary Characteristics of Culture

Major influences that shape people's worldview and the degree to which they identify with their cultural group of origin are called the primary and secondary characteristics of culture.[5] The **primary characteristics** are nationality, race, color, gender, age, and religious affiliation. In essence, each of these primary characteristics forms a subculture; for example, teenagers (age) form their own subculture. Take two people—one a 72-year-old devout white Muslim woman from Iran, and the other a 21-year-old black African American fundamentalist Baptist man from Louisiana. Obviously, the two do not look alike, and they probably have very different worldviews and beliefs. The primary characteristics represent what one generally regards as *culture*. With the exception of religious affiliation, they are largely unchangeable and shape one's worldview from an early age. One is born into a particular nationality, race, color, or gender[5] (Table 1-3).

Reflective Exercise

• What are your primary characteristics of culture? • How has each one influenced you and your worldview? • How have they changed or not changed over time? • How has your worldview changed as your primary characteristics have changed?

  Secondary characteristics encompass more of life's circumstances and experiences as one grows and develops. They may change throughout one's lifetime. The secondary characteristics include educational status, socioeconomic status, occupation, military experience, political beliefs,

TABLE 1.3

Primary and Secondary Characteristics of Culture

Primary Characteristics

Nationality
Race
Color
Gender
Age
Religious affiliation

Secondary Characteristics

Educational status
Socioeconomic status
Occupation
Military experience
Political beliefs
Urban versus rural residence
Enclave identity
Marital status
Parental status
Physical characteristics
Sexual orientation
Gender issues
Reason for migration (sojourner, immigrant, or
    undocumented status)
Length of time away from the country of origin

potential subculture, as will be discussed in the next section.

Reflective Exercise

• What are your secondary characteristics of culture?
• How has each one influenced you and your worldview? • have they changed or not changed over time?
• How has your worldview changed as your secondary characteristics have changed?

Subcultures

Within all cultures are subcultures and ethnic groups that may not hold all the values of the dominant culture. Subcultures, ethnic groups, or ethnocultural populations are groups of people who have experiences different from those of the dominant culture. These differences may include socioeconomic status, ethnic background, residence, religion, education, or other primary or secondary characteristics of culture that functionally unify the group and act collectively on each member with a conscious awareness of these differences.

Subcultures differ from the dominant ethnic group and share beliefs according to the primary and secondary characteristics of culture. For example, a second-generation Asian American woman may hold cultural values and beliefs different from those of her first-generation parents, who immigrated when she was an infant. Both share the primary characteristic of culture of an Asian heritage, but the young woman differs in her length of time away from the country of origin (a secondary characteristic of culture) (Fig. 1-7). Another example of a distinction in subculture is an African American who embraces the Catholic faith and another who embraces the Muslim religion. The two share the same African heritage but espouse different religions, thus identifying with different subcultures and creating variation within the larger cultural group.

Subcultures may cross primary cultural distinctions when shared experiences, mutual ideologies, and other unifying commonalities (secondary characteristics) bond them. Homeless persons, breast cancer survivors, and members of

urban versus rural residence, enclave identity, marital status, parental status, physical characteristics, sexual orientation, gender issues, reason for migration (sojourner, immigrant, or undocumented status), and length of time away from the country of origin.[5] Variations in secondary characteristics will lead to variations in one's culture. For example, a single female urban lesbian business executive will most likely have a different worldview from a married (heterosexual) female rural waitress who has two teenagers. In another case, a migrant farm worker from the highlands of El Salvador who has an undocumented status will have a different perspective from that of an immigrant from the Dominican Republic who has lived in Washington, DC, for 10 years. In essence, shared secondary characteristics may form a

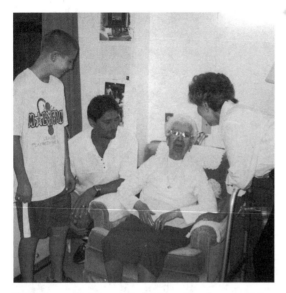

FIGURE 1.7 First-, second-, third-, and fourth-generation Italian Americans, each with different cultural characteristics. The matron of the family emigrated from Italy in 1934.

political and social groups are all examples of subcultures that may traverse dominant primary characteristics. The common secondary characteristics may unite a group representing a wide array of primary characteristics. Other examples might include unionized electricians, servicemen or -women who have seen combat, and parents of autistic children.

Reflective Exercise

• How is each of the above examples a "subculture"? • What primary or secondary characteristics unite the individuals and may promote cohesion across traditional cultural boundaries?

Reflective Exercise

• With what subcultures do you personally identify? • How has your identification with various subcultures changed over time? • How has your identification with various subcultures changed your worldview?

Reflective Exercise

• What subcultures do you encounter in your physical therapy practice? • How much do you know about these subcultures? • How might you gain better understanding of these subcultures?

Similarly, physical therapy professionals constitute a subculture of their own. Helman[24] refers to this as a **professional subculture.** As they participate in their educational experience, physical therapist students undergo a socialization process that leads to the development of a professional subculture. Part of the subculture involves the acquisition of new vocabulary. Physical therapists learn to call a mat table a "plinth" and call a leg a "lower extremity" and are challenged to use the new professional vocabulary appropriately among their colleagues while adopting an appropriate vocabulary to communicate effectively with the client (Figs. 1-8 and 1-9). Another component of the physical therapist subculture relates to perspectives on health and wellness. Spector[25] notes that healthcare students move farther from their past belief systems and those of their communities and families as they gain more knowledge within their healthcare curricula. The physical therapy professional educated in the United States will generally be exposed to health and wellness perspectives based on a biomedical model where science and research ground physical therapy diagnoses and interventions.

Reflective Exercise

• What new vocabulary or terminology did you acquire as a physical therapist student? • What do you remember about first encountering those new terms? • What terms might be foreign and not understood by your physical therapy clients?

Additionally, U.S. physical therapist programs generally uphold the U.S. values of autonomy and independence. Physical therapists learn to promote client independence, which sometimes leads to conflict with cultures in which interdependence is highly valued, such as collectivist

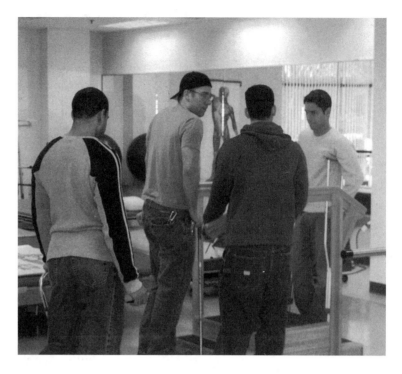

FIGURE 1.8 Physical therapist students undergo socialization into the professional subculture of physical therapy.

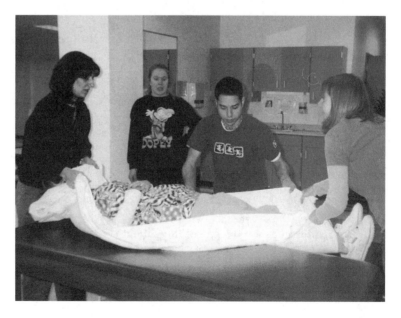

FIGURE 1.9 Physical therapy school exposes students to values, paradigms, and vocabulary particular to the physical therapy profession.

Reflection 1.1

I am from the United States and am receiving my physical therapy training in the United States. The thing I found most unusual about physical therapy school is the word *plinth*. I'll never forget when my instructor first said, "OK, let's go back to the plinths and try this technique." I remember thinking, "What is a 'plinth'? Why don't we call it a 'table' or a 'mat'? Do all medical disciplines call it a 'plinth'?" Sometimes the hardest thing about physical therapy school is learning a new language.

Will Cintron, PT student

---

cultures.[7] Thus, physical therapy professionals bring not only their personal culture, but also the culture of their profession into the interaction.

Reflective Exercise

• How has physical therapy school shaped your understandings and values? • What similarities do you share with your physical therapy classmates and colleagues?

Ethics across Cultures

The Western ethical principles of patient autonomy, self-determination, justice, do no harm, truth telling, and promise keeping are not interpreted uniformly or shared by all non-Western societies. For example, advance directives give patients the opportunity to decide about their care, and staff members are required to ask patients about this upon admission to a healthcare facility. Western ethics, with its stress on individualism, asks this question directly of the patient. However, in collectivist societies, such as among Asian Indian Hindus, the preferred person to ask may be a family member.[26-28] In most collectivist societies, a person does not stand alone but rather is defined in relation to another unit, such as the family.

Reflective Exercise

• Where or from whom have you acquired your understanding of right and wrong? • What ethical understandings did you discuss in physical therapy school? • How might those understandings differ across cultures?

Likewise, truth telling is culture bound. Even in Western cultures that espouse "complete truth telling," truth telling is sometimes tempered under a guise of civility, such as when someone asks, "How do you like my new hair color?" The socially acceptable answer may be less than truthful. However, in healthcare decision making, the provider is expected to be completely truthful.

Other cultural situations occur that raise legal issues. For instance, in Western societies, a competent person (or an alternative individual such as the spouse, if the person is married) is supposed to sign his or her own consent form for medical procedures. However, in some cultures the eldest son is expected to sign consent forms, not the spouse. In this case, both the organization and the family can be satisfied if both the spouse and the son sign the informed consent agreement.[29]

Reflective Exercise

• HIPAA is held as a high ethical principle in the United States. Is HIPAA ethically appropriate for all cultures?

As the globalization of healthcare services increases, providers must also address crucial issues such as cultural imperialism, cultural relativism, and cultural imposition.[30] **Cultural imperialism** is the practice of extending the policies and practices of one group (usually the dominant one) to disenfranchised and minority groups. An example is the U.S. government's forced migration of Native American tribes to reservations with individual allotments of lands instead of group ownership, as well as the forced attendance of children at white people's boarding schools.[31] Proponents of cultural imperialism appeal to universal human rights values and standards.

Cultural relativism is the belief that the behaviors and practices of people should be judged only from the context of their cultural system. Proponents of cultural relativism argue that issues such as abortion, euthanasia, female circumcision, and physical punishment in child rearing should be accepted as cultural values without judgment from the outside world. Opponents argue that cultural relativism undermines condemnation of human rights violations, and family violence cannot be justified or excused on a cultural basis.[30]

Reflective Exercise

• How might you as a physical therapist knowingly or unknowingly practice cultural imperialism or cultural imposition? • How might you identify cultural imperialism or cultural imposition? • How might you better understand and avoid cultural imperialism or cultural imposition? • How might you effectively intervene if you see a colleague exhibiting cultural imperialism or cultural imposition in physical therapy practice?

Cultural imposition is the intrusive application of the majority group's cultural view upon individuals and families.[32] Prescription of special diets without regard to clients' cultures and limiting visitors to immediate family, a practice of many acute-care facilities, border on cultural imposition.

Conclusion

Cultural diversity exists and will continue to exist in the United States. Sometimes obvious, sometimes not; sometimes well understood, sometimes poorly understood, the diversity permeates all aspects of physical therapy interactions and practice. Culture consists of primary and secondary characteristics and dynamically molds and shapes the communication patterns, health beliefs, health practices, and relationships of people. Subcultures, an emergent phenomenon, influence cultural understandings and experiences. This text aims to heighten the physical therapist's awareness and understanding of his or her own culture as well as provide guidance in understanding the culture of his or her client as it relates to physical therapy interactions and determinants of care. To this end, the text will cover both culture-general and culture-specific information with the hope that the physical therapist will make appropriate assessments of the interactions and applications of the material rather than negatively stereotype. The study of culture, both personal culture and the culture of others, can be an exciting and engaging endeavor, yielding more culturally congruent and therefore more effective physical therapy care.

CULTURAL SELF-ASSESSMENT EXERCISE 1

Self-Assessment of the Primary Characteristics of Culture

A. Identify your primary characteristics of culture.
   1. What is your nationality?
   2. What is your race?
   3. What sex are you?
   4. How old are you?
   5. What is your religious affiliation?

(continued)

CULTURAL SELF-ASSESSMENT EXERCISE 1 *(Continued)*

B. How has each of your primary characteristics of culture changed or not changed over your lifetime?

C. How are they similar to or different from those of your family members and close friends?

D. How does each of these primary characteristics of culture influence your view of the world, your attitudes, or your values?

CULTURAL SELF-ASSESSMENT EXERCISE 2

Self-Assessment of Secondary Characteristics of Culture

A. Identify your secondary characteristics of culture.
  1. What is your educational status?
  2. What is your socioeconomic status?
  3. What is your occupation?
  4. Do you have military experience?
  5. What are your political beliefs?
  6. Are you married?
  7. Do you have children?
  8. What are your physical characteristics?
  9. What is your sexual orientation?
  10. Were you born in this country? If not, how long have you been away from your country of origin?
  11. Are you Native American? If not, how long ago and why did your ancestors immigrate to the United States?

B. Give examples of how three of your secondary characteristics of culture influence your worldview.

C. Identify three examples of how your secondary characteristics of culture have changed in your lifetime.

D. How have each of these changed secondary characteristics altered your worldview?

CULTURAL SELF-ASSESSMENT EXERCISE 3

Self-Assessment of Subculture

A. List the subcultures with which you identify.

B. What established your association with each of the subcultures you listed?

C. Choose one of the subcultures you listed.
  1. What primary or secondary characteristics of culture do you share with others in the subculture?

2. What primary and secondary characteristics differ?

D. How has your association with each of the subcultures you listed changed your worldview?

CULTURAL SELF-ASSESSMENT EXERCISE 4

Self-Assessment of Cultural Imposition and Cultural Imperialism

A. Distinguish between the terms *cultural imposition* and *cultural imperialism*.
B. How might your physical therapy practice manifest cultural imposition?
C. How might your physical therapy practice manifest cultural imperialism?

D. How might you identify cultural imposition or cultural imperialism when it is occurring?
E. How might you avoid practicing cultural imposition or cultural imperialism?

CULTURAL SELF-ASSESSMENT EXERCISE 5

Exploring Ethics and Culture

A. Identify an ethical issue related to culture that you may encounter in your physical therapy practice.
B. Describe the ethical issue from all perspectives.

C. How might you resolve the ethical issue in an incompetent manner?
D. How might you resolve the ethical issue in a competent manner?

CULTURAL SELF-ASSESSMENT EXERCISE 6

Understanding Others

Any time one has to see a healthcare professional for an unknown illness, an anxiety-producing experience ensues. Imagine having fractured your ankle while visiting a foreign country. You do not speak the language and are unfamiliar with the healthcare system. Your traveling companion asks for help, and together you go to the local health clinic. The healthcare provider does not speak English.

A. Describe how you might feel.
B. How would you handle the situation?
C. What might be your most significant concerns?
D. How would you hope to be treated?

Vignette Questions

1. What are the primary characteristics of culture of Olga and Vera Morozov?
2. What are the secondary characteristics of culture of Olga and Vera Morozov?
3. Which of the primary characteristics of culture do you share with Olga and Vera Morozov?
4. Which of the secondary characteristics of culture do you share with Olga and Vera Morozov?
5. What is the diversity among the staff compared with Olga and Vera Morozov?
6. What potential problems related to the diversity among the staff and Olga and Vera Morozov might you anticipate?
7. How might these potential problems be averted?
8. What resources should be available to staff and the patients in this vignette to provide culturally safe and competent care?

CASE STUDY SCENARIO

*M*rs. Patel, a 65-year-old female, has a prescription for physical therapy for her lumbar pain. She arrives for her appointment accompanied by her son. Her son introduces himself as Atul Patel and explains that his mother is visiting from India for a year. She speaks very little English. Mr. Patel speaks perfect English and is dressed in a suit and appears to be in his mid-40s. Mrs. Patel is dressed in a long dress with several layers of clothing and appears to be slightly obese. Mr. Patel states that he will stay and act as interpreter, and he explains that his mother is very modest and will be uncomfortable undressing.

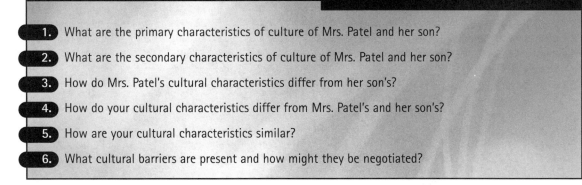

1. What are the primary characteristics of culture of Mrs. Patel and her son?

2. What are the secondary characteristics of culture of Mrs. Patel and her son?

3. How do Mrs. Patel's cultural characteristics differ from her son's?

4. How do your cultural characteristics differ from Mrs. Patel's and her son's?

5. How are your cultural characteristics similar?

6. What cultural barriers are present and how might they be negotiated?

R E F E R E N C E S

1. Office of Minority Health. Assuring cultural competence in health care. Available at: http://www.omhrc.gov/clas/indexfinal.htm. Accessed January 7, 2004.

2. American Physical Therapy Association. Cultural competence strategic plan. Available at: http://www.apta.org/Advocacy/minorityaffairs/CultCompPlan. Accessed December 17, 2003.

3. American Nurses Association. ANA Nursing World: Official web site of the American Nurses Association. Available at: http://nursingworld.org/search/vfp_search.cfm. Accessed January 7, 2004.

4. Institute of Medicine. The Committee for Guidance in Designing a National Healthcare Disparities Report. Available at: http://www.iom.edu/ search_results.asp?qs=cultural+competence. Accessed January 7, 2004.

5. Purnell L. Transcultural health care and diversity. In: Purnell L, Paulanka B, eds. *Transcultural Health Care: A Culturally Competent Approach.* 2nd ed. Philadelphia, Pa: FA Davis; 2003:1–7.

6. Black J. "Hands of Hope": A qualitative investigation of a student physical therapy clinic in a homeless shelter. *J Phys Ther Educ.* 2002;16:32–41.

7. Black J, Purnell L. Cultural competence for the physical therapy professional. *J Phys Ther Educ.* 16:3–11.

8. Black-Lattanzi J. *Overview of Cultural Competency: Considerations for Older Adults.* La Crosse, Wis: APTA; 2003:23–35.

9. Kraemer TJ. Physical therapist students' perspectives regarding preparation for providing culturally congruent cross-cultural care: A qualitative case study. *J Phys Ther Educ.* 15:36–51.

10. Leavitt R. *Developing Cultural Competence: Working with Older Adults of Hispanic Origin.* La Crosse, Wis: APTA; 2003:1–28.

11. American Physical Therapy Association. Vision statement for physical therapy 2020. Available at: http:// www.apta.org/About/aptamissiongoals/visionstatement. Accessed April 5, 2005.

12. American Physical Therapy Association. *A Normative Model of Physical Therapist Professional Education: Version 2004.* Alexandria, Va: APTA; 2004.

13. American Physical Therapy Association. *A Normative Model of Physical Therapist Assistant Education: Version 99.* Alexandria, Va: APTA; 1999.

14. Commission on Accreditation in Physical Therapy Programs (CAPTE). 2004 fact sheet: Physical therapist education programs, September 2004. Available at: http://www.apta.org/documents/Public/Accred/2004PTFactSheet.pdf. Accessed April 5, 2005.

15. Centers for Medicare and Medicaid Services. Medicare program, Aug. 15, 2001. Available at: http://www.gao.gov/decisions/majrule/d011048r.htm. Accessed January 18, 2004.

16. Family Education Network. Population statistics. Available at: http://www.infoplease.com/ipa/A0873845.html. Accessed April 5, 2005.

17. American Factfinder. U.S. Census Bureau Factfinder. Available at: http://www.factfinder.census.gov/. Accessed January 1, 2003.

18. Population Reference Bureau. Population trends. Available at: www.prb.org. Accessed January 25, 2003.

19. Hafizi H, Lipson J. People of Iranian heritage. In: Purnell L, Paulanka B, eds. *Transcultural Health Care: A Culturally Competent Approach.* 2nd ed. Philadelphia, Pa: FA Davis; 2003:177–193.

20. Kulwicki A. People of Arab ancestry. In: Purnell L, Paulanka B, eds. *Transcultural Health Care: A Culturally Competent Approach.* 2nd ed. Philadelphia, Pa: FA Davis; 2003:90–105.

21. Bhopal R, Donaldson L. White, European, Western,

Caucasian, or what? Inappropriate labeling in research on race, ethnicity, and health. *Am J Public Health.* 1998;88:1303–1307.

22. Human Genome Project. Human Genome Project information. Available at: http://www.ornl.gov/sci/techresources/Human_Genome/home.shtml. Accessed January 7, 2004.

23. Bureau of the Census. United States census 2000. Available at: http://www.census.gov/. Accessed January 1, 2003.

24. Helman CG. *Culture, Health, & Illness.* 4th ed. Oxford, UK: Butterworth-Heinemann; 2000.

25. Spector RE. *Cultural Diversity in Health & Illness.* 5th ed. East Norwalk, Conn: Appleton & Lange; 2000.

26. Doorenbos A, Nies M. The use of advanced directives in a population of Asian Indian Hindus. *J Transcult Nurs.* 2003;14:17–24.

27. Jambanathan J. Hindus [chapter on CD-ROM]. In: Purnell L, Paulanka B, eds. *Transcultural Health Care:*

A Culturally Competent Approach. 2nd ed. Philadelphia, Pa: FA Davis; 2003.

28. Uba L. Cultural barriers to health care for Southeast Asian refugees. *Public Health Rep.* 1992;107:544–548.

29. Sharts-Hopko N. People of Japanese heritage [chapter on CD-ROM]. In: Purnell L, Paulanka B, eds. *Transcultural Health Care: A Culturally Competent Approach.* 2nd ed. Philadelphia, Pa: FA Davis; 2003.

30. Purnell L. Cultural competence in a changing health-care environment. In: Chaska NL, ed. *The Nursing Profession: Tomorrow and Beyond.* Thousand Oaks, Calif: Sage; 2001:451–461.

31. Still O, Hodgins D. Navajo Indians. In: Purnell L, Paulanka B, eds. *Transcultural Health Care: A Culturally Competent Approach.* 2nd ed. Philadelphia, Pa: FA Davis; 2003:279–283.

32. Amnesty International. *Universal Declaration of Human Rights.* Available at: http://www.amnesty.org. Accessed January 1, 2003.

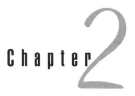

Chapter 2

Introducing Steps to Cultural Study and Cultural Competence

● Larry D. Purnell, PhD, RN
● Jill Black Lattanzi, PT, EdD

vignette

*S*ister Mary Susan is a 75-year-old woman who recently underwent a total hip replacement and is now in the rehabilitation hospital. Sister Mary Susan, a Catholic nun, comes to the physical therapy gym in her long, black dress and headpiece. The physical therapist is of the Jewish faith and has very little knowledge of the Catholic faith and its religious practices. The physical therapist does not know how he should address the patient by name and is unsure how he should manage the cumbersome garb throughout the physical therapy session. The physical therapist experiences apprehension regarding the culturally appropriate management of this patient.

The Development of Cultural Competence

When individuals of dissimilar cultural orientations meet in a work or therapeutic environment, the likelihood of their developing a mutually satisfying relationship is improved if both parties in the relationship attempt to learn about each other's culture. The literature reports many definitions for the terms *cultural awareness, cultural sensitivity,* and *cultural competence.* Sometimes these definitions are used interchangeably. However, **cultural awareness** has more to do

with an appreciation of the objective, external signs of diversity, such as the arts, music, dress, and physical characteristics. **Cultural sensitivity** has more to do with personal attitudes and not saying things that might be offensive to someone from a cultural or ethnic background different from the physical therapist's. Increasing one's consciousness of cultural diversity improves the possibilities for physical therapists to provide culturally competent care (Fig. 2-1). The components of **cultural competence,** as the term is used in this text, are listed in Box 2-1.

This text is committed to assist the physical therapist in the development of cultural compe-

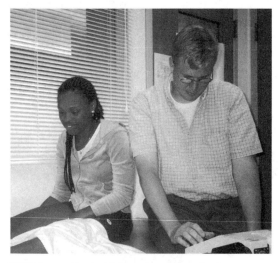

FIGURE 2.1 Physical therapy encounters often bring together patients and physical therapists of diverse cultures. Increasing awareness of diverse cultures helps the physical therapist to provide culturally competent care.

tence. The first step, cultural self-awareness, is the most important step in the development of cultural competence. Without self-awareness, cultural competence is not possible. The activities

BOX 2.1

Components of Cultural Competence

1. Developing an *awareness* of one's own existence, sensations, thoughts, and environment without letting it have an undue influence on those from other backgrounds
2. Demonstrating *knowledge and understanding* of the patient's culture, health-related needs, and meanings of health and illness
3. *Accepting and respecting* cultural differences
4. *Not assuming* that the therapist's beliefs and values are the same as the patient's
5. *Resisting judgmental* attitudes, such as "different is not as good"
6. *Being open* to cultural encounters
7. *Being comfortable* with cultural encounters
8. *Adapting care* to be congruent with the patient's culture[1]

and reflective exercises throughout the text are designed to assist the therapist in cultural self-exploration. The second step, demonstrating knowledge and understanding of the patient's culture, requires cultural study. The physical therapist can acquire a knowledge and understanding of general and specific cultural features through use of the cultural model described in this text and the culture-general and culture-specific information provided in Part 2 of this text. Throughout the text, the reader will be challenged to consider steps 3 through 8 in developing cultural competence. Figure 2-2 introduces a schematic depicting cultural competence development specifically for the physical therapist.

Reflective Exercise

• How would you describe your culture?

The development of cultural competence is a conscious process and is not necessarily linear. One progresses from unconscious incompetence (not being aware that one lacks knowledge about

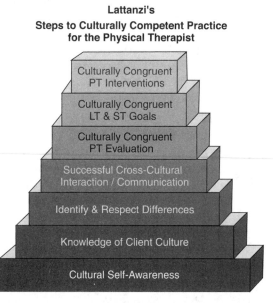

**Lattanzi's
Steps to Culturally Competent Practice
for the Physical Therapist**

Culturally Congruent
PT Interventions

Culturally Congruent
LT & ST Goals

Culturally Congruent
PT Evaluation

Successful Cross-Cultural
Interaction / Communication

Identify & Respect Differences

Knowledge of Client Culture

Cultural Self-Awareness

FIGURE 2.2 Steps toward cultural competence for the physical therapist.

another culture), to conscious incompetence (being aware that one lacks knowledge about another culture), to conscious competence (learning about the patient's culture, verifying generalizations about the patient's culture, and providing culturally specific interventions), and finally, to unconscious competence (automatically providing culturally congruent care to patients of diverse cultures). Unconscious competence is difficult to accomplish and is potentially dangerous because individual differences exist within ethnocultural groups.[2,3] Developing mutually satisfying relationships with diverse cultural groups involves good interpersonal skills and the application of knowledge and techniques learned from the physical, biological, and social sciences, as well as the humanities.

Reflective Exercise

• Where do you fall on the continuum of cultural competence (Fig. 2-3)? • Unconscious incompetence? • Conscious incompetence? • Conscious competence? • Unconscious competence? • Where were you 5 years ago? • What has happened to facilitate your growth?

An understanding of one's own culture and personal values and the ability to detach oneself from "excess baggage" associated with personal views are essential to cultural competence. Even then, traces of ethnocentrism may unconsciously pervade one's attitudes and behavior. **Ethnocentrism,** the universal tendency of human beings to think that their ways of thinking, acting, and believing are the only right, proper, and natural ways, can be a major barrier to providing culturally competent care (Figs. 2-4 and 2-5).[1]

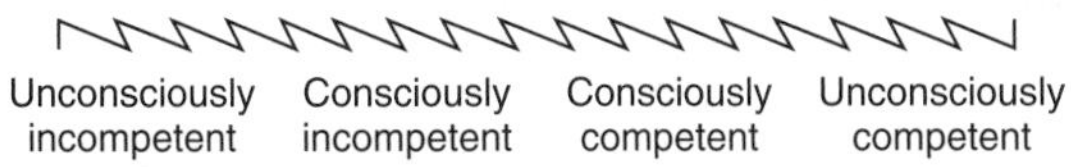

$\sim\sim\sim\sim\sim\sim\sim\sim\sim\sim\sim\sim\sim$

| Unconsciously incompetent | Consciously incompetent | Consciously competent | Unconsciously competent |

FIGURE 2.3 The process of cultural competence development. (Adapted from Purnell, L. D., & Paulanka, B. J. (1998). The Purnell Model for Cultural Competence. In L. D. Purnell & B. J. Paulanka (Eds.), *Transcultural health care: A culturally competent approach* (p. 10). Philadelphia: F.A. Davis.)

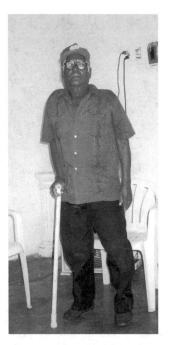

FIGURE 2.4 This gentleman from Mexico had fabricated his own cane from PVC pipe. The physical therapist demonstrating ethnocentrism might insist that a standard aluminum cane would be better, without considering the potential appropriateness of the homemade PVC pipe cane.

Ethnocentrism perpetuates the attitude that beliefs that differ greatly from one's own are strange, bizarre, or unenlightened and, therefore, wrong. Values are principles and standards that have meaning and worth to an individual, family, group, or community. The extent to which one's cultural values are internalized influences the tendency toward ethnocentrism. The more one's values are internalized, the more difficult it is to avoid the tendency toward ethnocentrism.

Reflective Exercise

• In what ways do you tend to be ethnocentric in your communication with physical therapy patients?
• How did you become aware of this ethnocentrism?
• What negative influence might the ethnocentrism have on the encounter?

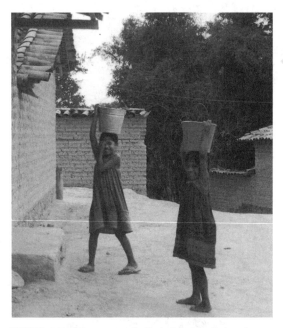

FIGURE 2.5 Many women in Central and South America learn to carry loads on their head at an early age. The physical therapist demonstrating ethnocentrism might insist that the loads be carried close to the chest, without considering that the top of the head is appropriately aligned with the lady's center of gravity.

Reflective Exercise

• In what ways do you tend to be ethnocentric in your practice of physical therapy? • What negative results might the ethnocentric practice have on the physical therapy intervention?

Any **generalization** made about the behaviors of any individual or large group of people is almost certain to be an oversimplification. We have a tendency toward generalizing in our attempt to manage the overwhelming complexity of diversity.[4] When a generalization relates less to the actual observed behavior than to the motives thought to underlie the behavior (that is, the why of the behavior), it is likely to be oversimplified. Thus, generalizations can lead to **stereotyping,** an oversimplified conception, opinion, or belief about some aspect of an individual or group of people.[1]

Reflective Exercise

• What stereotypes do you hold? • How might they hinder effective physical therapy care?

However, there is value in being able to make generalizations about cultural groups in that the therapist knows what questions to ask. Broad categories are practical for descriptive purposes and provide a starting point for inquiry. Much as the physical therapist must not assume that all patients with back pain will present in the same manner; the physical therapist must not assume that particular ethnic groups will be similar. Instead, the physical therapist conducts the evaluation, gains information, compares it with information known, and makes assessments based on prior knowledge and current findings from the evaluation.[5] The therapist must be aware of both inter-ethnic and intra-ethnic variations.

One example of a valuable broad cultural understanding is knowing if the person comes from an individualistic versus a collectivistic culture. People identifying with a **collectivist culture,** such as most Asians, are more likely to place a higher value on the family than on the individual.[6,7] However, people who identify with an **individualistic culture,** such as the dominant American or Swedish cultures, are more likely to place a higher value on the individual than on the family or the community. People from an individualistic culture primarily look after their personal and nuclear family's interests; people from a collectivist culture more typically belong to closed groups and look after their in-group and expect continuing loyalty.[1,8] Table 2-1 depicts additional differences between traditionally individualistic and collectivistic cultures.

Reflective Exercise

• Do you come from a collectivistic or an individualistic culture? • Give examples to support your answer.

TABLE 2.1

Individualistic Cultural Values versus Collectivistic Cultural Values: Cultural Considerations Relevant to Physical Therapy

INDIVIDUALISM—THE INDIVIDUAL	COLLECTIVISM—THE GROUP
Privacy	Company
Time over human interaction	Human interaction over time
Precise time	Loose time
Future–oriented	Past oriented
"Doing" or achieving (task related)	"Being" or personal growth (non–task related)
Appreciates competition	Appreciates cooperation
Human equality	Hierarchy/rank/status
Those in authority minimize position	Those in authority emphasize position
Promotes "self-help" for individuals	Understands birthright inheritance
Characterized by informality in interactions	Characterized by formality in interactions
Communication is direct (low-context)	Communication is indirect (high-context)
Practicality and efficiency	Idealism and theory
Youth	Elders
Autonomy	The group
Independence	Interdependence
Respect for individuality	Respect for authority
Individual security	Group security
Assigns individual credit and blame	Group shares credit and blame
Common sense and change	Order and tradition

Developing Self-Awareness

Developing an awareness of one's own existence, sensations, thoughts, and environment without letting it have an undue influence on those from other backgrounds is the first step in the development of cultural competence. Culture has a powerful unconscious impact on health professionals. Each physical therapist adds a new and unique dimension to the complexity of providing culturally competent care. The way physical therapists perceive themselves as competent providers is often reflected in the way they communicate with patients. Thus, it is essential for physical therapists to take time to think about themselves, their behaviors, and their communication styles in relation to their perceptions of culture. They should also examine the impact they have on others, including patients, who are culturally diverse. Before addressing the multicultural backgrounds and unique perspectives of each patient, physical therapists must address their own personal and professional knowledge, values, beliefs, ethics, and life experiences in a manner that optimizes interactions and assessment of culturally diverse patients.[5,9–11]

Reflective Exercise

• How aware are you of your cultural practices and worldviews? • Do you take them for granted on a daily basis without much thought about them?

• How aware are you of the potential impact your cultural views may have on your patient?

Many trainers of cultural competence believe that the best way to meet the various needs of individual healthcare professionals is to promote a high level of self-awareness, knowledge, and skills and a level of professional maturity that fosters the use of effective communication in diversity situations. According to Cook,[12] many of these beliefs are based on the assumption that in order to provide optimal care for others, one must first understand oneself. Self-knowledge and understanding promote strong professional perceptions that free physical therapists from prejudice and allow them to interact with others in a manner that preserves personal integrity and respects uniqueness and differences among individual patients.[13–16]

The process of professional development and diversity competence begins with self-awareness, sometimes referred to self-exploration. While the literature provides numerous definitions of self-awareness, there is minimal discussion of research integrating the concept of self-awareness with multicultural competence. Many theorists and diversity trainers imply that self-examination or awareness of personal prejudices and biases is an important step in the cognitive process of developing cultural competence;[17–19] however, discussions of the emotions elicited by this cognitive awareness are somewhat limited given the potential impact of emotions and conscious feelings on behavioral outcomes.

Self-awareness in cultural competence is defined as a deliberate and conscious cognitive and emotional process of getting to know yourself: your personality, your values, your beliefs, your professional knowledge standards, your ethics, and the impact of these factors on the various roles you play when interacting with individuals who are different from you. The ability to understand oneself sets the stage for integrating new knowledge related to cultural differences into the professional's knowledge base and perceptions of health interventions.[1]

The definition of culture includes the terms *attitude, belief,* and *ideology.* An attitude is a state of mind or feeling about some aspect of a culture. Attitudes are learned; for example, some people think that one culture is better than another culture. A belief is something that is accepted as true, especially as a tenet or a body of tenets accepted by people in an ethnocultural group. A belief among certain cultures is that if a pregnant woman craves a particular food substance—strawberries, for example—and does not satisfy the craving, the baby will be born with a birthmark in the shape of the craved food. Attitudes and beliefs do not have to be proven; they are unconsciously accepted as truths. Ideology consists of the thoughts and beliefs that reflect the social needs and aspirations of an individual or an ethnocultural group. For example, some people believe that healthcare is a right of all people, while others see healthcare as a privilege.

Reflective Exercise

• How aware are you of the stereotypes and generalizations you hold that influence your interactions and interventions with your physical therapy patients?
• Can you give any examples of these?

A Model for Cultural Competence

How comfortable are you with completing a cultural assessment? What framework do you use to ensure a complete assessment? How comfortable are you with your knowledge and understanding of the cultural practices of diverse groups such as Hispanics, Asians, Pacific Islanders, Arabs, Native Americans, Asian Indians, Irish, and Italians, to name a few? How might you obtain the culture-general and culture-specific information to use as a starting point in understanding a patient's culture?

This portion of the chapter presents an overview of the Purnell Model for Cultural Competence with an organizing framework composed of tables with questions the physical therapist can use for assessing the cultural values, beliefs, behaviors, and healthcare practices of patients. The Model does not deal with the objective (material) culture, including arts, music, literature, and the humanities, but rather addresses the subjective culture of attitudes, beliefs, values, behaviors, and practices in the context of healthcare.[3,20]

The Model can assist clinicians, managers and administrators, educators, and researchers in all physical therapy settings to provide professional, holistic, culturally competent care and interactions. Although not all components of the Model are directly applicable to physical therapists, a holistic view of the Model will assist physical therapy professionals in developing a broad understanding of culture and assist them in providing more culturally competent examinations, evaluations, diagnoses, prognoses, and interventions across a wide range of impairments, functional limitations, and disabilities.

The Purnell Model has been classified as holographic and complexity theory because it includes a model and organizing framework that can be used by all healthcare providers in various disciplines and settings. The Model (Fig. 2-6) is a

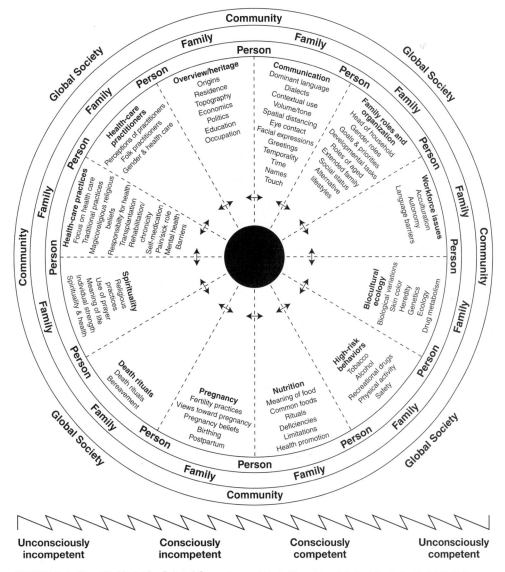

FIGURE 2.6 Purnell's Model for Cultural Competence. (Adapted from Purnell, L. D., & Paulanka, B. J. (1998). The Purnell Model for Cultural Competence. In L. D. Purnell & B. J. Paulanka (Eds.), *Transcultural health care: A culturally competent approach* (p. 10). Philadelphia: F.A. Davis.)

circle, with an outer rim representing global society, a second rim representing community, a third rim representing family, and an inner rim representing the person. The interior of the circle is divided into 12 pie-shaped wedges depicting cultural domains and their concepts. The dark center of the circle represents unknown phenomena. Along the bottom of the model is a jagged line representing the nonlinear concept of cultural consciousness. The 12 cultural domains (constructs) provide the organizing framework of the model. No one domain stands alone; they are all interconnected. Accordingly, physical therapy professionals can use these same domains to better understand and assess their own cultural beliefs, attitudes, values, practices, and behaviors. If physical therapists answer the questions related to the domains from their own perspectives,

they will better understand their own cultures and consequently will have a better understanding of patients' cultures and will be better able to assess interactions and culturally competent interventions. Assumptions upon which the Purnell Model for Cultural Competence is based are listed in Box 2-2.

Macro Aspects of the Model

The macro aspects of this interactional model include the metaparadigm concepts of a global society, community, family, person, and conscious competence. The theory and model are conceptualized from biology, anthropology, sociology, economics, geography, history, ecology, physiology, psychology, political science, pharmacology, and nutrition, as well as theories from communication, family development, and social support.

BOX 2.2

Assumptions on Which the Model Is Based

1. All healthcare professions need similar information about cultural diversity.
2. All healthcare professions share the metaparadigm concepts of global society, family, person, and health.
3. One culture is not better than another culture; the two are just different.
4. There are core similarities among all cultures.
5. There are differences within and among cultures.
6. Cultures change slowly over time.
7. The primary and secondary characteristics of culture (see Chapter 1) determine the degree to which an individual varies from the dominant culture.
8. If patients are co-participants in their care and have a choice in health-related goals, plans, and interventions, their compliance and health outcomes will be improved.
9. Culture has a powerful influence on one's interpretation of and responses to healthcare.
10. Individuals and families belong to several cultural groups.
11. Each individual has the right to be respected for his or her uniqueness and cultural heritage.

12. Caregivers need both cultural-general and cultural-specific information in order to provide culturally sensitive and culturally competent care.
13. Caregivers who can assess, plan, intervene, and evaluate in a culturally competent manner will improve the care of their patients.
14. Learning culture is an ongoing process that develops in a variety of ways, but primarily through cultural encounters.[19]
15. Prejudices and biases can be minimized through cultural understanding.
16. To be effective, healthcare must reflect an understanding of the unique values, beliefs, attitudes, lifeways, and worldviews of diverse populations and individual acculturation patterns.
17. Differences in race and culture often require adaptations to standard interventions.
18. Cultural awareness improves the caregiver's self-awareness.
19. Professions, organizations, and associations have their own culture, which can be analyzed using a grand theory of culture.[3]

Physical therapists in clinical practice, education, research, and the administration and management of healthcare services can use the Model to better understand, recognize, and address cultural issues.

Global Society

Phenomena related to a global society include world communication and politics; conflicts and warfare; natural disasters and famines; international exchanges in education, business, commerce, and information technology; advances in the health sciences; space exploration; and the expanded opportunities for people to travel around the world and interact with diverse societies. Global events that are widely disseminated by television, radio, satellite transmission, newsprint, and information technology affect all societies, either directly or indirectly. Such events create chaos while forcing people to consciously and unconsciously alter their lifeways and worldviews.

Reflective Exercise

• Think of a recent event that has affected global society, such as a conflict or war, health advances in technology, or recent travel and possible environmental exposure to health problems. How did you become aware of this event? • How has this event altered your view and other people's views of worldwide cultures?

Community

In its broadest definition, a community is a group of people having a common interest or identity. Community includes the physical, social, and symbolic characteristics that cause people to connect. Bodies of water, mountains, rural versus urban living, organizational affiliations, and even railroad tracks help people define their concept of community in physical terms. Today, however, technology and the Internet allow people to expand their community beyond physical boundaries. Economics, religion, politics, age, generation, and marital status may also delineate the social dimensions of community. Sharing a specific language or dialect, lifestyle, history, dress, art, or musical interest is a symbolic characteristic of a community. People actively and passively in-teract with the community, which necessitates adaptation and assimilation for equilibrium and homeostasis in their worldview. Individuals may willingly change certain aspects of their physical, social, and symbolic community when it no longer meets their needs.

Reflective Exercise

• How do you define your community in terms of objective and subjective cultural characteristics?
• How has your community changed over the last 5 years? • The last 10 years? • The last 15 years? • The last 20 years? • If you have changed communities, think of the community in which you were raised.

Reflective Exercise

• Do you belong to more than one community?
• How are your communities similar? • How are they different?

Family

A family is two or more people who are emotionally connected. They may, but do not necessarily, live in close proximity to each other. A family may include physically and emotionally close and distant consanguineous relatives, as well as physically and emotionally connected and distant non–blood-related significant others. Family structure and roles change according to the primary and secondary characteristics of culture (see Chapter 1), requiring each person to rethink his or her individual beliefs and lifeways.

Reflective Exercise

• Whom do you consider family? • How have they influenced your culture and worldview?

Person

A person is a biopsychosociocultural being who is constantly adapting to his or her community, even in the presence of catastrophic events such as hurricanes and earthquakes. Human beings adapt biologically and physiologically to the aging process; psychologically in the context of social relationships, stress, and relaxation; socially as they interact with the changing community; and ethnoculturally within the broader global society. In Western cultures, a person is a separate physical and unique psychological being and a singular member of society; such a culture is commonly called an individualistic society or culture. The self is separate from others. However, in other cultures, such as some Asian and Hispanic cultures, the individual is defined in relation to the family, including ancestors or some other group, rather than as a basic unit of nature; these are commonly called collectivistic societies or cultures.[5–7,21–24]

Reflective Exercise

• In what ways have you adapted (a) biologically and physiologically to the aging process, (b) psychologically in the context of social relationships, (c) socially within your community, and (d) ethnoculturally within the broader society?

Health

Health, as used in this book, is a state of wellness as defined by people within their ethnocultural group. Health generally includes physical, mental, and spiritual states because group members interact with the family, community, and global society. The concept of health, which permeates all concepts of culture, is defined globally, nationally, regionally, locally, and individually. Thus, people can speak about their personal health status or the health status of the nation or community. Health can also be subjective or objective in nature.

Reflective Exercise

• How do you define health? • Is health the absence of illness, disease, and/or disability? • How does the physical therapy profession define health? • How does your nation or community define health?

Micro Aspects of the Model

On a microlevel, the model has an organizing framework consisting of 12 domains and their concepts, which are common to all cultures. These 12 domains are interconnected and have implications for health. The utility of this organizing framework comes from its ability to be used in any setting, its applicability to a broad range of empirical experiences, and its capacity to foster inductive and deductive reasoning in the assessment of cultural characteristics. Once cultural data are analyzed, the physical therapy professional can adopt, modify, or reject interventions and treatment regimens in a manner that respects the patient's cultural differences. Such adaptations improve the quality of the patient's healthcare experiences and personal existence. The following chapters are all organized around the domains of culture as defined by the Purnell Model for Cultural Competence. The 12 domains and associated concepts essential for assessing the ethnocultural attributes of an individual, family, or group are listed in Box 2-3.

BOX 2.3

The Twelve Domains of Culture[3]

1. *Overview, inhabited localities, and topography:* Concepts include origins, residence, topography, economics, politics, education, and occupation.
2. *Communication:* Concepts include dominant language and dialects, contextual use of the language, voice volume and tone, spatial distancing practices, use of eye contact, facial expressions and gesturing, temporality, time, format for names, and use of touch.
3. *Family roles and organization:* Concepts include head of household, gender roles, family goals and priorities, roles of the aged and extended family, social status, and alternative lifestyles.

4. *Workforce issues:* Concepts include acculturation, autonomy, and language barriers.
5. *Biocultural ecology:* Concepts include biological and physiological variations, skin color, heredity and genetics, ecology, and drug metabolism.
6. *High-risk health behaviors:* Concepts include use of tobacco, alcohol, and recreational drugs; physical activity; and safety, which includes safe-sex practices and use of helmets and seatbelts.
7. *Nutrition:* Concepts include the meaning of food, common foods and food rituals, food limitations and deficiencies, and use of foods and food substances for health promotion and wellness and for illness and disease prevention.
8. *Pregnancy and childbearing practices:* Concepts include fertility practices; views toward pregnancy; and prescriptive, restrictive, and taboo practices in pregnancy, birthing, and postpartum.
9. *Death rituals:* Concepts include death rituals and bereavement practices.
10. *Spirituality:* Concepts include religious practices, use of prayer, meaning of life, sources of individual strength, and spirituality and health.
11. *Healthcare practices:* Concepts include the focus and responsibility of healthcare, traditional practices, magico-religious beliefs, rehabilitation and chronicity, self-medicating practices, pain and the sick role, views toward mental health, barriers to healthcare, organ transplantation and donation, and acceptance of blood and blood products.
12. *Healthcare practitioners:* Concepts include perceptions of healthcare practitioners, folk practitioners, and gender and healthcare.

While an understanding of all aspects of a patient's culture would be beneficial, the physical therapy program and interaction is likely to be most impacted by the domains of communication, healthcare practices, and healthcare practitioners (Fig. 2-7). The domains of overview and heritage, family roles and organization, pregnancy and childbearing practices, and workforce issues also merit serious consideration. Finally, this text touches on aspects of the domains of biocultural ecology, high-risk behaviors, nutrition, death rituals, and spirituality as these may influence physical therapy interactions and interventions. Trust and respect between the patient and physical therapist must be established for truly successful physical therapy interactions and interventions to occur (Fig. 2-8).

The following section will guide the reader through an exploration of his or her own culture using Purnell's domains as an organizing framework. Readers should also be able to begin the process of understanding others and, we hope, to develop acceptance and respect for the diverse cultures of their patients.

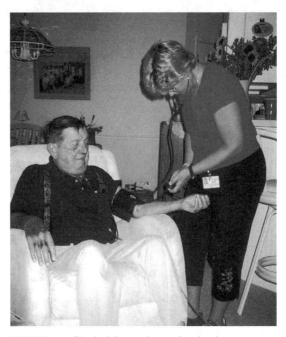

FIGURE 2.7 Physical therapy interactions involve many aspects of diversity. What aspects might be considered here?

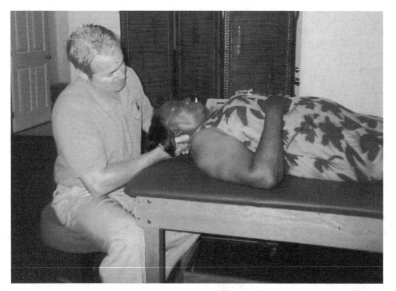

FIGURE 2.8 Physical therapy involves trust and respect between the patient and physical therapist.

CULTURAL SELF-ASSESSMENT EXERCISE 1

Assessment of Individualistic and Collectivistic Cultures

A. Look at Table 2-1. For each item listed, determine whether you are more strongly individualistic or collectivistic. Identify where you fall on the scale for each item.

Individualistic   Collectivistic

1	2	3	4	5

Add up all the numbers. If you scored 19–35 points, you are more highly individualistic. If you scored 35–75 points,

you are somewhat bicultural with regard to individualism and collectivism. If you scored 76–95 points, you are more highly collectivistic.

B. Identify three conflicts or misunderstandings that might arise in your physical therapy practice because of a misalignment of individualistic culture and collectivistic culture.

C. Describe how you would attempt to manage each of the potential conflicts you identified.

CULTURAL SELF-ASSESSMENT EXERCISE 2

Self-Assessment of Ethnocentrism

1. Define ethnocentrism.
2. Give three examples of how ethnocentrism might manifest itself in your physical therapy practice.
3. How might you address each example differently to avoid ethnocentrism?
4. What measures do you personally take to prevent ethnocentrism within yourself?
5. How would you handle a situation where you see another therapist or healthcare provider responding ethnocentrically to the detriment of patient care?

CULTURAL SELF-ASSESSMENT EXERCISE 3

Exploring Controversial Cultural Terms

1. Distinguish among the terms *cultural awareness, cultural sensitivity*, and *cultural competence*.
   a. Do you exhibit cultural awareness? How?
   b. Do you exhibit cultural sensitivity? How?
2. Distinguish between the terms *stereotyping* and *generalization*.
   a. How might each be harmful in physical therapy practice?
   b. What stereotypes or generalizations are you aware of that you hold? List at least three.
3. Distinguish between culture-general and culture-specific information.
   a. How might each be harmful in physical therapy practice?
   b. How might each be used in a positive manner in physical therapy practice?
   c. Why does the text aim to provide both culture-general and culture-specific information?
4. Distinguish between race and culture.
   a. Give an example of how race might influence your physical therapy practice.
   b. Give an example of how culture might influence your physical therapy practice.

CULTURAL SELF-ASSESSMENT EXERCISE 4

Self-Assessment of Cultural Competence Development

For each of the following steps toward the development of cultural competence, rate yourself on a scale of 1–10, with 10 being completely competent and 1 being completely incompetent. Give a rationale for each ranking.

1. How would you rate your awareness of your own existence, sensations, thoughts, and environment and your ability to avoid undue influence on others from other backgrounds?
2. How would you rate your knowledge and understanding of patients from other cultures, their health-related needs, and their cultural meanings of health and illness?
3. How would you rate yourself on your practice of accepting and respecting cultural differences?
4. How would you rate yourself on your ability to avoid assuming that your beliefs and values are the same as your patient's?
5. How would you rate yourself on your ability to resist judgmental attitudes?
6. How open are you to cultural encounters?
7. How comfortable are you with cultural encounters?
8. How competent are you in adapting care to be congruent with the patient's culture?

CULTURAL SELF-ASSESSMENT EXERCISE 5

Self-Assessment of Cultural Competence Practice

1. Give an example of your awareness of your own culture, and describe how it might have an undue influence on your physical therapy patient from another culture.
2. Identify potential healthcare beliefs or practices of another culture, and describe how they might contrast with your physical therapy beliefs or plan of care.
3. Give an example of how you have demonstrated respect and acceptance of cultural differences in your physical therapy practice.
4. Give an example of an instance where you assumed or did not assume that your beliefs and values were the same as those of your physical therapy patient.
5. Give an example of a judgmental attitude that you have resisted or should learn to resist.

6. Describe how you try or how you would like to try to be open to cultural encounters. How might you foster openness to cultural encounters?

7. Describe a situation in which you did or did not adapt the physical therapy care to be congruent with the patient's culture.

CULTURAL SELF-ASSESSMENT EXERCISE 6

Exploring the Value of Cultural Competence

A. Do you think cultural competence makes marketing sense? Why or why not?

B. Do you think cultural competence makes economic sense? Why or why not?

C. Do you think cultural competence makes health sense? Why or why not?

D. Do you think cultural competence is the right goal? Why or why not?

CULTURAL SELF-ASSESSMENT EXERCISE 7

Understanding Others

Ask the questions from Cultural Self-Assessment Exercise 6 of another physical therapist or healthcare provider. Be sure to ask for the rationale for the person's responses.

1. How are his or her responses similar to yours?

2. How are his or her responses different from yours?

3. What insights have you gained as a result of this exercise?

Vignette Questions

1. What cultural differences are evident in this scenario?
2. How might the physical therapist best manage the scenario culturally competently?
3. How might the physical therapist mismanage the scenario?
4. What would be important for the physical therapist to recognize about his or her own culture?
5. How might the physical therapist learn more about the practices and beliefs and values of Catholic nuns?

CASE STUDY SCENARIO

*A*ntonio Vargas, Angelica Vargas Diaz (his wife), their four children (ages 3, 7, 9, and 16), and Maria Diaz (Angelica's mother) have just moved to your suburban community and live next door to you. Antonio and Angelica are able to achieve basic verbal English communication skills. The two oldest children have very good language skills, and they communicate for their parents. They have seen the signage on your utility vehicle advertising physical therapy services and want to ask your advice on several issues.

a. Their 16-year-old daughter is experiencing knee pain, and they would like a female clinician to examine her.

b. They wish to know where they can find a pediatrician that understands their Mexican way of life.

c. Angelica has been watching a Spanish television station that stresses the importance of osteoporosis, and she would like to know more about this.

d. They do not like the choice of foods in the local grocery store and want to know where they can purchase more authentic Mexican foods.

1. Would you be able to advise them on each of these issues?
2. What do you know about the Mexican culture and the diversity within it? How might you go about assisting the family to meet their needs?
3. If you were to move to Mexico (or some other country), what would be the most important issues you would need to address? How might you go about getting your questions answered?

REFERENCES

1. Purnell L. Transcultural diversity and health care. In: Purnell L, Paulanka B, eds. *Transcultural Health Care: A Culturally Competent Approach.* 2nd ed. Philadelphia, Pa: FA Davis; 2003:1–7.
2. Purnell L. Workforce cultural diversity. *Surg Serv Manage.* 1996;2:26–30.
3. Purnell L. The Purnell Model for Cultural Competence. In: Purnell L, Paulanka B, eds. *Transcultural Health Care: A Culturally Competent Approach.* 2nd ed. Philadelphia, Pa: FA Davis; 2003:8–40.
4. MacLachlan M. *Culture and Health.* Chichester, UK: Wiley; 1997.
5. Leavitt R. *Developing Cultural Competence: Working with Older Adults of Hispanic Origin.* La Crosse, Wis: APTA; 2003:1–28.
6. Purnell L, Kim S. People of Korean heritage. In: Purnell L, Paulanka B, eds. *Transcultural Health Care: A Culturally Competent Approach.* 2nd ed. Philadelphia, Pa: FA Davis; 2003:249–278.
7. Wang Y. People of Chinese heritage. In: Purnell L, Paulanka B, eds. *Transcultural Health Care: A Culturally Competent Approach.* 2nd ed. Philadelphia, Pa: FA Davis; 2003:106–121.
8. Williams J. Why compare? *Int Educ.* 2003;3:26–31.
9. American Physical Therapy Association. APTA Guide for Professional Conduct. Available at: http://apta.org/rt.cfm/ PT_Practice/ethics-pt/pro_conduct. Accessed April 15, 2004.
10. Black J. "Hands of Hope": A qualitative investigation of a student physical therapy clinic in a homeless shelter. *J Phys Ther Educ.* 2002;16:32–41.
11. Leavitt RL. *Cross-Cultural Rehabilitation: An International Perspective.* Philadelphia, Pa: WB Saunders; 1999.
12. Cook S. The self in self-awareness. *Arch Psychiatr Nurs.* 1999;12:1292–1299.
13. Purnell L. Panamanians' practices for health promotion and the meaning of respect afforded them by healthcare providers. *J Transcult Nurs.* 1999;10:333–340.
14. Purnell L. Panamanian health beliefs and the meaning of respect afforded by healthcare providers. *J Multidisc Cienc Salud.* 1999;3:23–34.

15. Purnell L. Guatemalans' practices for health promotion and wellness and the meaning of respect afforded them by healthcare providers. *J Transcult Nurs.* 2000;11:40–46.

16. Purnell L. El Modelo de Purnell de competéncia cultural: Una descripción y el uso en practica, educación, administración y investigación. *J Cult Antropol.* [Alicante, Spain] 2000:46–55.

17. Anand R. *Cultural Competence in Health Care: A Guide for Trainers.* Washington, DC: National Multicultural Institute; 1997.

18. Andrews M., Boyle J. *Transcultural Concepts in Nursing.* 4th ed. Philadelphia, Pa: Lippincott.

19. Campinha-Bacote J. *The Process of Cultural Competence in the Delivery of Healthcare Services: A Culturally Competent Model of Care.* 4th ed. Cincinnati, Ohio: Transcultural C.A.R.E. Associates; 2002.

20. Purnell L. A model for cultural competence. In: Best H,

Sellers E. *International Images of Health: Perspectives, Power and Practice.* Ballarat, Victoria, Australia: University of Ballarat; 2001:131–144.

21. Ling W. *An Overview of East Asian Cultures for Physical Therapists.* La Crosse, Wis: APTA; 2003:1–27.

22. Nowak T. People of Vietnamese heritage. In: Purnell L, Paulanka B, eds. *Transcultural Health Care: A Culturally Competent Approach.* 2nd ed. Philadelphia: FA Davis; 2003:327–344.

23. Pacquiao D. People of Filipino heritage. In: Purnell L, Paulanka B, eds. *Transcultural Health Care: A Culturally Competent Approach.* 2nd ed. Philadelphia, Pa: FA Davis; 2003:138–159.

24. Sharts-Hopko N. People of Japanese heritage [chapter on CD-ROM]. In: Purnell L, Paulanka B, eds. *Transcultural Health Care: A Culturally Competent Approach.* 2nd ed. Philadelphia, Pa: FA Davis; 2003.

What Is My Culture and How Do I
Understand My Patient's Culture?

SECTION 2

Chapter 3

Exploring Cultural Heritage

● Jill Black Lattanzi, PT, EdD
● Larry D. Purnell, PhD, RN

*Geeta Choudry, age 24, immigrated to the United States after her
parents were killed in a bus accident in India. Educated in computer
technology and fluent in English, she had no difficulty getting an office
position in a physical therapy department in a large medical center in the
United States. In India, Geeta had lived in a swampy, mosquito-infested
rural village most of her life. She had been on malaria medication for
many years. Geeta is reluctant to tell her co-workers that her primary
reason for immigrating was that she was supposed to enter a marriage
arranged by her family. She felt that she should marry for love. One day
at work she began shaking and having chills. She told her co-workers
not to worry, that she occasionally had these episodes because of her
malaria.*

Knowing and understanding a different culture
includes becoming familiar with the heritage of
its people and the part of the world from which
they come. Salient historical events such as discrimination in the country of origin influence
value systems, beliefs, and explanatory frame-
works used in everyday life. Knowing and understanding a different culture's heritage must begin
with knowing and understanding your own heritage. Given the intercultural and intracultural
variations that exist within primary and secondary characteristics of culture (Table 3-1), the physical therapist must consider each client's cultural
heritage individually. One's cultural heritage

largely shapes one's cultural beliefs and values
about health and wellness.

Reflective Exercise

● What is your cultural heritage? ● How might you
learn more about it? ● What influence has your
cultural heritage had on you? ● How does your
cultural heritage influence your beliefs and values
about health and wellness?

The domain *overview, inhabited localities, and
topography* within the Purnell Model for Cultural

TABLE 3.1

Primary and Secondary Characteristics of Culture

Primary Characteristics

Nationality
Race
Color
Gender
Age
Religious affiliation

Secondary Characteristics

Educational status
Socioeconomic status
Occupation
Military experience
Political beliefs
Urban versus rural residence
Enclave identity
Marital status
Parental status
Physical characteristics
Sexual orientation
Gender issues
Reason for migration (sojourner, immigrant, or
   undocumented status)
Length of time away from the country of origin

Competence[1] includes concepts related to the country of origin, current residence, the effects of the topography of the country of origin and current residence on health, economics, politics, reasons for migration, educational status, and occupations (Fig. 3-1). These concepts are interrelated. For example, economic and political conditions may affect one's reason for migration, and educational attainment is usually interrelated with employment choices and opportunities. Sociopolitical and socioeconomic conditions influence individual behavioral responses to health and illness. In essence, this domain is an ethnohistory of the cultural group.

Immigration Status

Immigration status influences a person's worldview. For example, people who voluntarily immigrate generally **acculturate** more willingly; that is, they modify their own culture as a result of contact with another culture. Similarly, they **assimilate,** that is, gradually adopt and incorporate the characteristics of the prevailing culture, more easily than people who immigrate unwillingly or as sojourners. **Sojourners,** who immigrate with the intention of remaining in their new homeland only a short time, or **refugees,** who think they may return to their home country, may not need to acculturate or assimilate. Additionally, **undocumented individuals** (illegal aliens) may have a different worldview compared with those who have arrived legally with work visas or as "legal immigrants."

Variations within a cultural group include people who are bicultural, traditional, acculturated, or marginal. **Bicultural people** function equally well in their traditional culture and the dominant culture. **Traditional people** maintain their historical culture of origin and remain encapsulated in their new environment. **Acculturated people** have adopted most of the culture of their new country, giving up most of the culture of their county or family of origin. **Marginal people** have little to do with the dominant culture or their culture of origin. Migrant workers frequently fall in this category.[1]

Reflective Exercise

• Would you consider yourself bicultural, traditional, acculturated, or marginal? • Why? • Are your family members bicultural, traditional, acculturated, or marginal? • Why? • Are the people with whom you work bicultural, traditional, acculturated, or marginal? • Why?

Immigration Eras in U.S. History

The Open Door Era
The United States has absorbed more immigrants throughout its history than any other nation.[2] U.S. immigration policy, closely linked to immigration patterns of people, is described and organized by historians into eras.[2-5] The first era encompasses the foundation of the nation from 1776 to 1882 and is commonly labeled the "Open

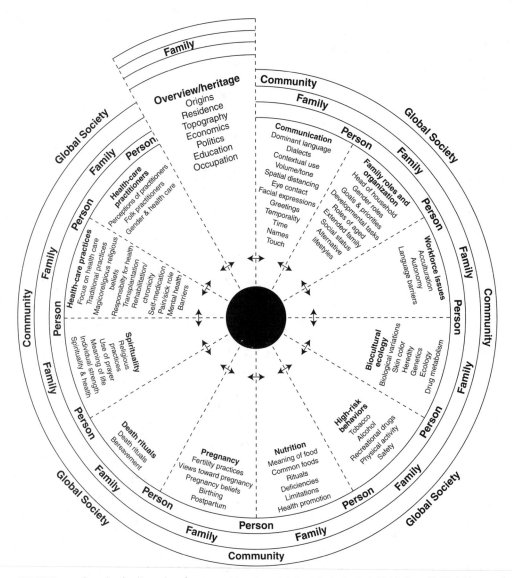

FIGURE 3.1 Overview/heritage domain. (Adapted from Purnell, L. D., & Paulanka, B. J. (1998). Purnell's Model for Cultural Competence. In L. D. Purnell & B. J. Paulanka (Eds.), *Transcultural health care: A culturally competent approach* (p. 10). Philadelphia: F.A. Davis.)

Door Era" because the United States opened its doors without restrictions to immigrants from all over the world. More than 80% of the immigrants were from western and northern Europe, predominantly Great Britain, Ireland, and Germany.[5] The new arrivals began settling in a land inhabited by over 2 million American Indians, who mostly lived in geographically isolated tribes with distinctly different cultures. Most of the early immigrants settled in the northeastern states, particularly New York and Pennsylvania.[5]

During the "Open Door Era," several important U.S. immigration policies emerged. In 1848, following the Mexican-American War, the Treaty of Guadalupe Hidalgo guaranteed U.S. citizenship to all Mexicans living in the territory ceded by Mexico. The territory became the states of New Mexico, Arizona, Texas, and California. The Homestead Act of 1862 brought a surge of immigration to the West when Congress granted up to 160 acres of land to settlers who would establish residence and develop the land for at least 5 years. The forced relocation of western Africans began in 1619 and ended with the American Civil War in 1865. In 1870, Congress enacted a law granting citizenship to people of African descent.[5] Thus, the foundation of the United States consisted of Native Americans who were not recognized as citizens, European immigrants who immigrated voluntarily, and African Americans who were forced to immigrate and were not awarded citizenship until 1870.

In 1882, the Open Door Era of immigration ended when Congress passed the Chinese Exclusion Act, barring Chinese immigrants for 10 years.[2,5,6] The Chinese began to emigrate to the United States in the 1820s and 1830s, and a number were imported for labor during the California Gold Rush of 1848 and for the construction of the western portion of the transcultural railroad.[5] Over the years, the numbers of Chinese laborers grew such that the white workers began to feel threatened and encouraged legislation that would limit the number of Chinese allowed to immigrate to the United States. The Chinese Exclusion Act was renewed every 10 years until it was rescinded in 1943, at which time China was a U.S. ally in the war against Japan.

The Era of Selective Exclusion
The immigration legislation of 1882 marked the beginning of the "Era of Selective Exclusion"[5] or the "Door-Ajar Era,"[2] which lasted through 1921. While Chinese immigrants were prohibited entry to the United States, European immigrants were permitted and arrived in great waves. The first wave consisted of 8.9 million immigrants largely from western and northern Europe and was followed by a second wave of 13.4 million from southern and eastern Europe.[5] Most passed through the Ellis Island reception station in New York, which operated from 1882 to 1952.[5] Immigrants had to prove that they were literate and healthy, and arrived from Italy, Austria-Hungary, Russia, Poland, Ireland, and Germany,[7] as well as Greece, Bulgaria, Portugal, and Romania.[5] Many of these immigrants were Catholic or Jewish. By 1930, immigrants and their children provided needed labor for rapidly growing construction, manufacturing, and other industrial jobs, leading to the formation of a white, ethnic, urban working class.[4]

Also within this time period, the Spanish-American War established U.S. control over Guam, Puerto Rico, the Philippines, and Cuba, and Hawaii was annexed. In 1917, Puerto Ricans were granted U.S. citizenship. And in 1919, Congress enacted a law granting honorably discharged Native Americans U.S. citizenship for their service in World War I.[5]

The Era of Numerical Restriction
Historical events such as World War I, World War II, and the Great Depression brought a change in U.S. immigration policy once again. In response to World War I, Congress passed the Immigration Act of 1921, imposing the first immigration quotas. The Era of Numerical Restriction,[5] or the "Pet Door Era,"[2] lasted from 1921 to 1965. During this time period, several significant events occurred within immigration policy. In 1924, Congress passed an act granting citizenship to all Native Americans, not just those who had served in the war. In 1925, Congress established the border patrol. In 1942, President Roosevelt issued executive order 9066, which led to the evacuation, relocation, and internment of all Japanese and Japanese Americans. In 1949, Congress passed the Agricultural Act, granting permission for farmers to recruit temporary workers from Mexico.[2] In 1954, Ellis Island was closed, to be reopened as a museum in 1992. Only 5.5 million immigrants entered the United States between 1930 and 1965.[2,5] Figure 3-2 depicts the annual number of immigrants to the United States historically.

The Revolving Door Era
The year 1965 marked a major change in U.S. immigration policy that has continued to impact the diversity of the United States today. A change in American attitudes toward greater tolerance, a president from an immigrant family (JFK), and a prospering economy led to a re-opening of the door to immigration.[2,5] The Immigration and

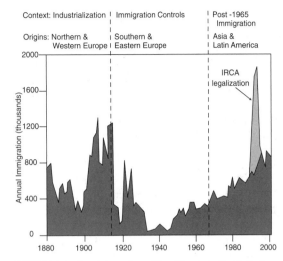

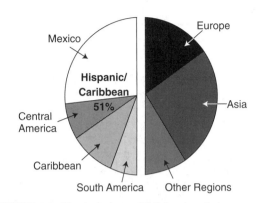

FIGURE 3.3 Pie chart of recent U.S. immigrants by ethnicity. (Data from U.S. Bureau of the Census, 2000.)

FIGURE 3.2 Annual number of immigrants to the United States historically. (Data from U.S. Immigration and Naturalization Service, 1999.)

Naturalization Act of 1965 ended the quota system, emphasized the reuniting of families, and encouraged the emigration of highly skilled laborers.[2]

Since 1965, more than 20 million immigrants have arrived with documentation and an estimated several million more have arrived without documentation.[2,3,6] Mexico accounts for the largest number of immigrants, at an estimated 4.5 million; the Caribbean, 3.4 million; other parts of Latin America, 2.4 million; and Asia, including China, the Philippines, Korea, Vietnam, and India, 6.9 million.[7] Overall, one-third of the foreign-born population are from Mexico and Central America, more than one-half are Hispanic, and one-quarter are from Asia.[3] Figures 3-3 and 3-4 illustrate the breakdown of the foreign-born in the United States by ethnicity.[3] Many of the recent immigrants reside in Los Angeles, New York, Miami, Houston, Chicago, San Francisco, and Boston.[7]

Several historical events have led to changes in immigration patterns since 1965. In 1972, Saigon fell, followed by the rest of South Vietnam, Cambodia, and Laos, leading to a migration of Asians to the United States. In 1975, Jews began fleeing the Soviet Union in large numbers and

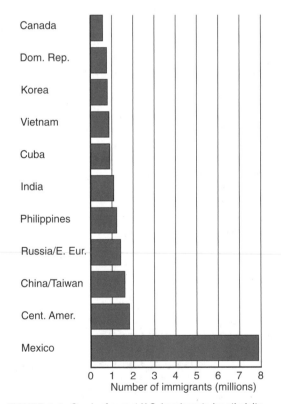

FIGURE 3.4 Graph of recent U.S. immigrants by ethnicity. (Data from U.S. Bureau of the Census, 2000.)

civil war in El Salvador resulted in refugee movement to the United States. An influx of boat people arrived from Haiti beginning in 1972 and from Vietnam and elsewhere in Southeast Asia in 1979. In response, Congress passed the Refugee Act of 1980, allowing the admission of 50,000 refugees annually.[2,5] Congress passed the Immigration and Reform Act (IRCA) in 1986, which provided amnesty and temporary resident status to all immigrants of undocumented status who had lived in the United States continuously since January 1, 1982. The Act also imposed sanctions on employers who knowingly hire undocumented immigrants and it strengthened border patrols.[2]

The immigration policy change of 1965 allowed immigrants from all parts of the world without favoritism toward or restrictions on ethnicity. The European immigrants of the 1900s were largely white and of the Jewish or Catholic religion. Today, the United States includes immigrants or descendants of immigrants of very diverse ethnicities and religions.[3] With this immigrant wave as with the last, the intertwining of this massive body of people into American society poses a massive and important challenge.

On September 11, 2001, terrorists attacked the World Trade Center and the Pentagon, bringing into question the revolving door immigration policy of the past 35 years. Subsequently, the USA Patriot Act was passed, and the Department of Homeland Security was established. In March 2003, the Immigration and Naturalization Service was abolished, and its functions and responsibilities were reorganized within the Department of Homeland Security.[2] A new era of U.S. immigration policy appears to have emerged.

Reflective Exercise

• How long have you/your ancestors been in the United States? • What aspects of your ancestors' culture are still celebrated or practiced in your family?

Reflective Exercise

• What brought you/your ancestors to the United States? • Do you have any stories about your personal or your family's immigration?

Reflective Exercise

• What immigration policies do you think the United States should have?

Reasons for Migration and Associated Economic Factors

The United States has a very large middle-class population and a small, but growing, wealthy population. Approximately 12.7% of the population live in poverty, with higher rates among children (18.9%), the elderly (19.9%), blacks (26.1%), and non-white Hispanics (27.1%).[8] The social, economic, religious, and political forces of the country of origin play an important role in the development of the ideologies and worldviews of individuals, families, and groups and are often a major motivating force for emigration. Most early immigrants to the United States came for better economic opportunities, to escape religious or political oppression, as a result of environmental disasters such as earthquakes and hurricanes, or involuntarily as slaves or indentured servants. Others have migrated for educational opportunities and personal ideologies or a combination of factors. Most people immigrate to the United States in the hope of a better life; however, the individual or group personally defines this ideology. Understanding the reason for a person's immigration, whether voluntary, sojourner, refugee, or undocumented status, may provide clues to the person's acculturation patterns.

A common practice for many immigrants is to relocate to an area that has an established population with similar ideologies that can provide initial support, serve as cultural brokers, and orient them to their new culture and healthcare system. People who live in **ethnic enclaves** and get their work, shopping, and business needs met without learning the language and customs of their host country may be more traditional than people in their home country (Figs. 3-5 and 3-6). Such was the case for an elderly Italian woman who lived in an ethnic enclave in Baltimore, Maryland. When she returned to Italy after 30 years to visit relatives, she was criticized for being

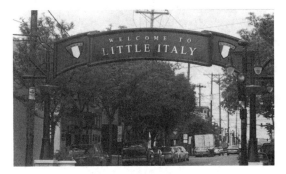

FIGURE 3.5 An Italian ethnic enclave.

too old-fashioned. Italian society had changed, while she had not. She had tenaciously held to her traditional practices.

When immigrants settle and work exclusively in predominantly ethnic communities, primary social support is enhanced, but acculturation and assimilation into the wider society may be hindered. Individuals and families without ethnic enclaves in the United States may need extra help in acculturating and adjusting to their new homeland's language, access to healthcare services, living accommodations, and employment opportunities. People who move across cultures voluntarily are likely to experience less difficulty with acculturation than people who are forced to emigrate to a new culture. Some individuals immigrate with the intention of remaining in this country only a short time, making money, and returning home, whereas others immigrate with the intention of relocating permanently. Therefore, it is imperative for physical therapists to assess the reasons behind the individual's migration to understand the implications for culturally competent care.

Reflective Exercise

• What ethnic enclaves are in your community?
• What do you know about the customs and cultures of the people in the ethnic enclaves in your community? • How often do you work with clients of the ethnic enclaves in your practice? • How might you learn more about the culture of your clients from ethnic enclaves?

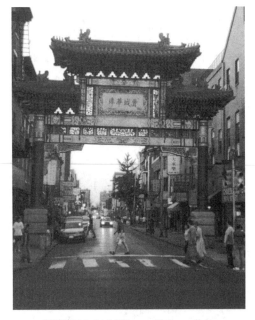

FIGURE 3.6 A Chinese ethnic enclave.

Educational Status and Occupations

The value placed on formal education differs among cultural and ethnic groups and is often related to their socioeconomic status and opportunities in their homeland, their reasons for emigrating, or their ability to emigrate. The United States places a high value on education. Some groups, however, do not stress formal education because it was not needed for employment in their homeland. Consequently, they may become engulfed in poverty, isolation, and enclave identity, which may further limit their potential for formal educational opportunities and planning for the future.

Reflective Exercise

• How strongly do you believe in the value of education? • Who in your life is responsible for instilling this value?

Theoretically, people have the freedom to choose a profession, regardless of gender and background. However, this does not always carry over into practice for many professions. Educational attainment in the United States varies by race, gender, and region of the country. Eighty-four percent of all adults age 25 years and over have completed high school, and 26% have completed a bachelor's degree or more. Among women age 25 and over, 84% have earned a high school diploma and 24% have completed a bachelor's degree or more. Proportionately, white non-Hispanics have higher educational attainment levels than other groups. High school completion levels are highest in the Midwest (87%) and lowest in the South (82%).[9]

In regard to learning styles, the Western system places a high value on the learner's ability to categorize information using linear, sequential thought processes. However, not everyone adheres to this pattern of thinking. For example, many Native Americans have spiral and circular thought patterns that move from concept to concept without being linear or sequential; therefore, they have difficulty placing information in a stepwise methodology.[10,11] When a person is unaware of the value given to such behaviors, individuals may see each other as disorganized, scattered, and faulty in their cognitive patterns, resulting in increased difficulty with written and verbal communications.

Reflective Exercise

• What is your preferred learning style? • Do you prefer to learn in groups or as a solitary activity? • Do you consider yourself to be more of a linear/ sequential learner or a random-patterned learner?

Brewer's[12] classic study supports that Native Americans learn best by observation and experiential learning in private with constant supervision and the avoidance of possible public embarrassment. Studies of Mexican Americans and collectivist cultures in general support a field-dependent orientation where learners do best in a cooperative, noncompetitive, group-oriented environment.[11,13–17] In contrast is the individualistic culture of the United States, where competition and individual goals often provide the motivation for learning and accomplishing learning activities.[1] The physical therapist professional should consider clients' learning styles and motivational patterns when establishing goals, interventions, and a plan of care for clients and when teaching staff and students.

The American educational system stresses application of content over theory. Most European educational programs emphasize theory over practical application, and Arab and Mexican education emphasizes theory, with little attention given to practical application. As a result, Arab and Mexican students are more proficient at tests requiring rote learning than at those requiring conceptualization and analysis.[18–21] Being familiar with the individual's personal educational values and learning modes allows healthcare providers, educators, and employers to adjust teaching strategies for clients, students, and employees. Educational materials and explanations must be presented at a level consistent with clients' educational capabilities and within their cultural framework and beliefs.

Reflective Exercise

• What accommodations and adaptations regarding your client's educational status and style of learning might you consider when working with your physical therapy patient?

Immigrants bring job skills from their native homelands and traditionally seek employment in the same or similar trades. Sometimes these job skills are inadequate for the available jobs in the new society; thus, immigrants are forced to take low-paying jobs and join the ranks of the working poor and economically disadvantaged. Most immigrants in America include individuals employed in a broad variety of occupations and professions; however, limited experiential, educational, and language abilities of more recent immigrants often restrict employment possibilities. More importantly, experiential backgrounds sometimes encourage employment choices that

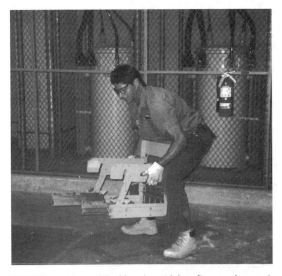

FIGURE 3.7 Low-skilled immigrant jobs often require repetitive bending and lifting or overhead tasks, leaving one prone to injury.

BOX 3.1

"Traditional" American Values

1. Individualism
2. Free speech
3. Rights of choice
4. Independence
5. Self-reliance
6. Confidence
7. "Doing" rather than "being"
8. Egalitarian relationships
9. Non-hierarchical status of individuals
10. Achievement status over ascribed status
11. Volunteerism
12. Friendliness
13. Openness
14. Future planning
15. Control of the environment
16. Material things
17. Physical comfort

are identified as high-risk for chronic conditions such as musculoskeletal overuse syndromes. Some may work in factories that require repetitive-motion assembly line tasks. Others may perform physical labor requiring repeated lifting and bending (Fig. 3-7). For some immigrant populations, the country of origin has lost many of its professional and well-educated people. These professional immigrants have difficulty finding work comparable to what they did in their homeland, resulting in a "brain drain" for the host country and underemployment in the new environment.[22]

Reflective Exercise

• What health hazards exist in your profession?
• What health hazards exist in your current position?
• What considerations should you make regarding the occupational health hazards of your physical therapy client?

The American cultural heritage includes the values of individualism, free speech, rights of choice, independence and self-reliance, and confidence. These values are not shared by all cultures around the world.[1] Other common traditional American values include "doing" rather than "being," egalitarian relationships, non-hierarchical status of individuals, achievement status over ascribed status, "volunteerism," friendliness, openness, futuristic temporality, the ability to control one's environment, and an emphasis on material things and physical comfort (Box 3-1). The following chapters will continue to examine culture and cultural differences and will allow the reader to perform cultural self-assessment.

Reflective Exercise

• Do you think there is an "American culture"? • Why or why not?

CULTURAL SELF-ASSESSMENT EXERCISE 1

Self-Assessment Exercise

A. Answer the following questions regarding the domain of *overview, inhabited localities, and topography* for yourself.
1. What is your age?
2. What is your marital status?
3. How many children do you have?
4. Who besides yourself lives in your household?
5. Where were you born? (If not in the United States, what brought you to this country?)
6. How long have you lived in the United States (if appropriate)?
7. What is your immigration status (if appropriate)?
8. In what other parts of the United States have you lived?
9. What is the ancestry of your parents?
10. Where were your parents born?
11. With what cultural group do you identify yourself?
12. How many years of schooling/ education have you completed? In what country did you go to school?
13. What is your income level (could be weekly, monthly, or yearly)?
14. Describe the neighborhood in which you live.
15. Describe the landscape or countryside where you live. Is it mountainous or swampy?
16. Were you in the military? Which branch?
17. Are there any illnesses/diseases that occur frequently in your family? Cancer? Hypertension? Diabetes? Cardiac disease?
18. In your home country, are there particular illnesses or diseases that occur frequently?
19. Have you lived other places in the United States/world?
20. What is your current occupation? If retired, what was your previous occupation?
21. Have you worked in other occupations? What were they?
22. Are there (were there) any particular health hazards associated with your job(s)?

B. After answering questions 1–22 yourself, identify how some of the answers might influence your culture or worldview.

C. Identify three ways the answers might influence your practice as a physical therapist.

D. Describe how some of your answers might conflict with those for someone of a different heritage.

CULTURAL SELF-ASSESSMENT EXERCISE 2

Understanding Others

1. Which of the preceding questions would be particularly important and appropriate to ask your physical therapy client?

2. For each question you indicate to be important, briefly describe why it is important and provide an example.

CULTURAL SELF-ASSESSMENT EXERCISE 3

Learning about Your Cultural Heritage

For this exercise, interview a parent, grandparent, or great-grandparent and ask the following questions:
1. What do you know about our ancestry?
2. When did our ancestors come to the United States?
3. Why did they come to the United States?
4. What occupations have our ancestors held?
5. What stories or memories do you have of our ancestors?
6. What special holidays do you remember?
7. What special foods are parts of our heritage?
8. What has been the health status of our family?

CULTURAL SELF-ASSESSMENT EXERCISE 4

Self-Exploration of Adherence to "Traditional" American Values

A. For each of the following, rank your level of adherence on a scale of 1 to 10, with 1 being "do not value at all" and 10 being "value very much."
   To what degree do you value:
1. Individualism
2. Free speech
3. Rights of choice
4. Independence
5. Self-reliance
6. Confidence
7. "Doing" rather than "being"
8. Egalitarian relationships
9. Non-hierarchical status of individuals

10. Achievement status over ascribed status
11. Volunteerism
12. Friendliness
13. Openness
14. Future planning
15. Control of the environment
16. Material things
17. Physical comfort

B. Answer the following questions related to the above values clarification.

1. To what degree do you hold or not hold to the "traditional" American values described above?
2. Identify three examples where a conflict in the above values might adversely affect a physical therapist's interaction or interventions with a client.
3. Describe how you might effectively manage each of the three examples of conflict you identified.

Vignette Questions

1. What do you know about the immigration patterns of Asian Indians?
2. How might you find out about the immigration patterns and health conditions of Asian Indians?
3. How difficult is it for Asian Indians to immigrate to the United States?
4. Where do most Asian Indians live in the United States?
5. How will you find out about Asian Indians' health beliefs and practices?

CASE STUDY SCENARIO

Jose Morales, a 42-year-old migrant worker from Mexico, speaks limited English. Señor Morales' parents are in Mexico. He lives with his wife and two children, his brother and his family, and his cousin. He and his brother are attempting to provide for their wives and children as well as for their aging parents back home in Mexico.

He is employed on a chicken farm, where his main job is to cut the heads off chickens. The chickens come to him hanging on an overhead line. He must pull the bird off the line, which requires both hands, hold the bird, chop off the head at the neck with a knife (he is right-handed), and rehang the bird on the right side of the line as the line continues to move from left to right. The line moves at a fixed rate, necessitating that he work at a predetermined speed. The heads are discarded into a bin on his left.

Señor Morales had been working for 8 months when he began developing pain in his right shoulder and upper arm, which was about 3 months ago. Not wanting to complain and risk losing his much-needed job, he would work through the pain and come home at night to put on his upper arm a hot herbal compress, which his wife prepared for him. The condition continued to worsen until he finally

(continued)

sought help from the plant nurse, when his productivity had dropped noticeably. The nurse sent him to the company physician, who diagnosed impingement syndrome, gave him a prescription for an anti-inflammatory, and ordered radiographs and physical therapy.

Señor Morales continues to work full-time but is allowed release time to attend physical therapy. The first day he comes with an interpreter from the company. As you take his history, he expresses that the plant is very cold and he feels that this is contributing to his condition. He will be able to come to therapy three times a week but will not always have an interpreter.

1. What cultural considerations are involved in this scenario?

2. How does your cultural heritage differ from that of Señor Morales?

3. What cultural barriers may exist as a result of the difference in cultures?

4. What barriers to therapy exist in this scenario?

5. How might these barriers be overcome?

6. What challenges does Señor Morales's work present?

7. How might these challenges be met?

8. What more would you need to know about Señor Morales's family?

9. How might you be able to obtain an interpreter for Señor Morales when one cannot accompany him to physical therapy?

10. Señor Morales is from Mexico. What do you know about Mexicans in terms of collectivist versus individualistic culture?

11. Do you think Señor Morales's wife should come with him to his physical therapy appointment? Why or why not?

12. What questions related to Señor Morales's cultural heritage would you want to ask?

REFERENCES

1. Purnell L. The Purnell Model for Cultural Competence. In: Purnell L, Paulanka B, eds. *Transcultural Health Care: A Culturally Competent Approach.* 2nd ed. Philadelphia, Pa: FA Davis; 2003:8–40.

2. LeMay MC. *U.S. Immigration: Contemporary World Issues.* Santa Barbara, Calif: ABCLIO; 2004.

3. Clark WAV. *Immigrants and the American Dream: Remaking the Middle Class.* New York, NY: Guilford Press; 2003.

4. Gerstle G, Mollenkopf J, eds. *E Pluribus Unum? Contemporary and Historical Perspectives on Immigrant and Political Incorporation.* New York, NY: Russell Sage Foundation; 2001.

5. Yang PQ. *Post-1965 Immigration to the United States: Structural Determinants.* Westport, Conn: Praeger; 1995.

6. Edmonston B, ed. *Statistics on U.S. Immigration: An Assessment of Data Needs for Future Research.* Washington, DC: National Research Council, Committee on National Statistics Committee on Population, National Academy Press; 1996.

7. Gibson C, Lennon, E. *Historical Census Statistics on the Foreign-Born Population of the United States: 1850–1990.* Washington, DC: US Bureau of the Census, Population Division; 1999. Working Paper 29.

8. US Bureau of the Census. Poverty statistics. Available at: http://www.census.gov/hhes/poverty/poverty02/r&dtable5.html. Accessed January 8, 2004.

9. US Bureau of the Census. Educational statistics. Available at: http://www.census.gov/population/www/socdemo/education/educ-sample.html. Accessed January 8, 2004

10. Crow K. Multiculturalism and pluralistic thought in nursing education: Native American world view and the nursing academic world view. *J Nurs Educ.* 1993;32:198–204.

11. Still O, Hodgins D. Navajo Indians. In: Purnell L, Paulanka B, eds. *Transcultural Health Care: A Culturally Competent Approach.* Philadelphia, Pa: FA Davis; 2003:279–284.

12. Brewer A. On Indian education. *Integr Educ.* 1977;15:21–23.

13. Dunn R, Griggs S, Price G. Learning style of Mexican-American elementary school students. *J Multicult Couns Devel.* 1993;21:237–247.

14. Gregorc A. Style as a symptom: A phenomenological perspective. *Theory Pract.* 1984;23:51–55.

15. Hudgens B. The relationship of cognitive style, planning ability, and locus of control to achievement from three ethnic groups (Anglo, African-American, Hispanic). *Dissertation Abstracts International, A53–08.* 1993: 2744.

16. Pacquiao D. Multicultural issues in nursing practice and education. *Issues Newsl Nat Counc.* 1995;16:1,4–5,11.

17. Taylor M. Learning styles. *Inquiry.* 1997;1:45–48.

18. Hafizi H, Lipson J. People of Iranian heritage. In: Purnell L, Paulanka B, eds. *Transcultural Health Care: A Culturally Competent Approach.* 2nd ed. Philadelphia, Pa: FA Davis; 2003:177–193.

19. Kulwicki A. People of Arab heritage. In: Purnell L, Paulanka B, eds. *Transcultural Health Care: A Culturally Competent Approach.* 2nd ed. Philadelphia, Pa: FA Davis; 2003:90–105.

20. Nydell M. *Understanding Arabs.* Yarmouth, Me: Intercultural Press; 1987.

21. Zoucha R, Purnell L. People of Mexican heritage. In:. Purnell L, Paulanka B, eds. *Transcultural Health Care: A Culturally Competent Approach.* 2nd ed. Philadelphia, Pa: FA Davis; 2003:264–278.

22. Purnell L. People of Brazilian heritage [chapter on CD-ROM]. In: Purnell L, Paulanka B, eds. *Transcultural Health Care: A Culturally Competent Approach.* 2nd ed. Philadelphia, Pa: FA Davis; 2003.

Chapter 4

Exploring Communication in Cultural Context

- Jill Black Lattanzi, PT, EdD
- Larry D. Purnell, PhD, RN

Park Chung Nam, age 26, relocated to the United States from Korea to assist her sister, Kim Sun, in caring for her four children. Ms. Park needs to work part-time to support herself. She has obtained a job working in the dietary department of a local hospital. As part of her pre-employment physical, they have referred her to physical therapy for evaluation of her low back pain, which Ms. Park says she has had for several years. When you ask her questions, she either nods her head or says "yes" and smiles. You ask her if she has had a back injury and she answers yes. You ask her how she injured her back and she answers yes. You ask her to undress and put on a medical exam gown and she nods her head yes. You notice that she does not look you in the eye but rather looks at your shoulder or the floor. When you return to the exam room, she has the gown over her clothes.

An effective physical therapy program cannot exist without effective communication between physical therapists and patients. Likewise, working relationships are enhanced by effective communication among colleagues, employers, employees, and other healthcare practitioners. What does effective communication entail? Communication is embedded within culture, and one must adequately understand cultural implicitness within both verbal and nonverbal communication (Fig. 4-1). The physical therapist might think he or she is communicating clearly, but the patient may misinterpret, misunderstand, or misjudge the intended communication unintentionally because he or she is hearing the message via a different cultural channel. This chapter will examine communication from a cultural context and will use the domain *communication* from the Purnell Model for Cultural Competence to guide the content (Fig. 4-2).

Reflective Exercise

- How important is effective communication to you?
- How important is it in your relationship with your colleagues, peers, and employers? • How important is it with your patient? • Can you think of an example when communication with a colleague, employer, or patient was ineffective?

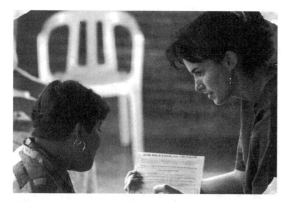

FIGURE 4.1 A successful physical therapy program cannot exist without effective verbal and nonverbal communication between clinician and client.

The communication domain is interrelated with all other domains and includes the dominant language, dialects, and the contextual use of the language; paralanguage variations such as voice volume, tone, intonations, reflections, and willingness to share thoughts and feelings; nonverbal communications such as eye contact, gesturing, and facial expressions; use of touch, body language, spatial distancing practices, and acceptable greetings; temporality in terms of past, present, or future orientation of worldview; clock versus social time; and the degree of formality in the use of names. Communication styles vary among "insiders," including family and close friends, and "outsiders," including strangers and unknown professionals such as physical therapists. Hierarchical relationships, gender, and religious beliefs affect communication. Additionally, the U.S. government's Cultural and Linguistic Standards (CLAS) identify language as the most significant barrier to accessing and receiving healthcare for people for whom English is a second language.[1] Perhaps of all domains of culture, communication is the most important one for establishing trust and promoting effectiveness of physical therapy programs.

Dominant Language and Dialects

The physical therapist must be aware of the dominant language and the difficulties that dialects may cause when communicating in the patient's native language. Dialects may pose difficulty for understanding a language, even if the physical therapist and patient speak the same language. For example, Americans speak *American English*, which differs somewhat in pronunciation, spelling, grammar, and choice of words from the English spoken in Great Britain, Scotland, Australia, and other English-speaking countries.

Although the United States has several dialects, generally the differences do not cause major concern with communications. Moreover, English dialects are not as varied as the many Spanish dialects spoken in Argentina, Mexico, Panama, Puerto Rico, Spain, and other countries. Additionally, Mexico has as many as 50 different dialects within its borders.[2–8] In such cases, dialects and choices of words vary widely, posing substantial problems for physical therapy professionals and interpreters in performing health assessments and in obtaining accurate health data, in turn increasing the difficulty of making accurate diagnoses.

Reflective Exercise

• What is your dominant language? • Do you have difficulty understanding other dialects of your dominant language? • Have you traveled abroad where you had difficulty understanding the dialect or accent?

When speaking in a nonnative language, physical therapists must select words that have relatively pure meanings, be certain of the voice intonation, and avoid the use of regional slang and jargon to avoid being misunderstood. Minor variations in pronunciation may change the entire meaning of a word or a phrase and result in inappropriate interventions. For example, in the Spanish language, there are two forms of the verb "to be" (*ser* and *estar*). Using the incorrect form can cause a miscommunication, as evidenced by the following situation. A school nurse, who spoke limited Spanish, telephoned the mother of an 8-year-old boy with diarrhea. The nurse used the phrase *es enfermo,* meaning "he is sick" (a permanent condition), instead of *esta enfermo,*

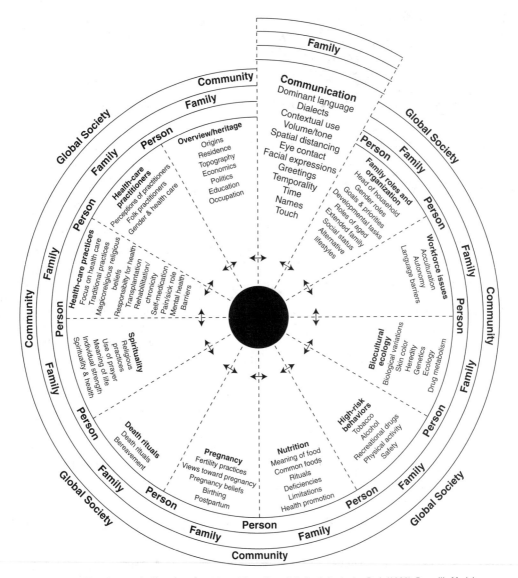

FIGURE 4.2 The communication domain. (Adapted from Purnell, L. D., & Paulanka, B. J. (1998). Purnell's Model for Cultural Competence. In L. D. Purnell & B. J. Paulanka (Eds.), *Transcultural health care: A culturally competent approach* (p. 10). Philadelphia: F.A. Davis.)

meaning "he is sick" (a temporary situation). This subtle distinction in language translation increased the mother's concern and anxiety over her child's illness and resulted in her thinking something was seriously wrong with him.

Reflective Exercise

• Can you give an example of communicating with someone whose language was different from yours that resulted in miscommunication?

Given the difficulty of obtaining the precise meaning of words in a language, it is best for physical therapists to obtain someone who can interpret the meaning and message, not just translate the individual words. Some guidelines for communicating with non–English-speaking patients are listed in Box 4-1.

Reflective Exercise

• Give some examples of problems communicating with patients who did not speak or understand English. What did you do to promote effective communication?

BOX 4.1

Guidelines for Communication with Non–English-Speaking Patients

1. Use interpreters who know the culture. Translators just restate the words from one language to another. An interpreter decodes the words and provides the meaning behind the message.
2. Use dialect-specific interpreters whenever possible.
3. Use interpreters trained in the healthcare field.
4. Give the interpreter time alone with the patient.
5. Provide time for translation and interpretation.
6. Use same-gender interpreters whenever possible.
7. Maintain eye contact with both the patient and interpreter to elicit feedback; read nonverbal cues.
8. Speak slowly without exaggerated mouthing, allow time for translation, use active rather than passive tense, wait for feedback, and restate the message. Do not rush; do not speak loudly.
9. Use as many words as possible in the patient's language and turn to nonverbal communication when you are unable to understand the language.
10. Use phrase charts and picture cards if available.
11. During the assessment, direct your questions to the patient, not to the interpreter.
12. Ask one question at a time, and allow interpretation and a response before asking another question.
13. Be aware that interpreters may affect the reporting of symptoms, insert their own ideas, or omit information.
14. Remember that patients can usually understand more than they can express; thus, they need time to think in their own language. They are alert to the healthcare provider's body language, and they may forget some or all of their English in times of stress.
15. Avoid the use of relatives, who may distort information or not be objective.
16. Avoid using children as interpreters, especially with sensitive topics.
17. Avoid idiomatic expressions and medical jargon.
18. If an interpreter is unavailable, the use of a translator may be acceptable. The difficulty with translation is omission of parts of the message; distortion of the message, including transmission of information not given by the speaker; and messages not being fully understood.
19. If possible, use an interpreter who is older than the patient.
20. Review responses with the patient and interpreter at the end of a session.
21. *Note:* Social class differences between the interpreter and the patient may result in the interpreter's not reporting information that he or she perceives as superstitious or unimportant.
22. *Note:* Take caution when using programmed computer translations. Many of these programs are context dependent, resulting in some interesting translations, especially when the sentence structure varies greatly between languages. Additionally, sometimes a word for the concept does not exist in both languages.[10]

People with limited English ability may have inadequate vocabulary and grammar skills to communicate in stressful situations or where strong or abstract levels of verbal skills are required, such as in communicating one's history of the present illness. Helpful communication techniques with diverse patients include tact, consideration, and respect; gaining trust by listening attentively; addressing the patient by his or her preferred name; and showing genuine warmth and openness to facilitate full information sharing. Asking a patient his or her preferred name demonstrates respect across all cultures. When giving directions, be explicit. Give directions in sequential, procedural steps (for example, first, second, third). Do not use complex sentences with conjunctions.[9]

Before trying to engage in more sensitive areas of the health interview, the physical therapist may need to start with social exchanges to establish trust, use an open-ended format rather than "yes" or "no" closed-response questions, elicit opinions and beliefs about health and symptom management, and focus on facts rather than feelings. An awareness of nonverbal behaviors is essential to establishing a mutually satisfying relationship.

Reflective Exercise

• What methods have you used in the past to establish a trusting relationship? • Give an example where the trust was less than satisfactory. How might the situation have been improved?

Guidelines for Cross–Cultural Communication

Considering that most people for whom English is a second language may have difficulty at times and in certain situations with English, some general guidelines are included in Box 4-2. Implementing the simple considerations listed will greatly enhance effective communication with nonnative English speakers.

Whether a language is low or high context is another important aspect of communication. In

---

BOX 4.2

Guidelines for Cross–Cultural Communication

a. Speak clearly.
b. Do not cover your mouth with your hands.
c. Speak at a moderate speed.
d. Use short, non-complex sentences.
e. Do not have more than one idea in a sentence.
f. Do not exaggerate mouthing when you speak.
g. Avoid colloquial expressions, slang, and jargon.
h. Restate important concepts and terms.
i. Gesture using body language and facial expressions.
j. Do not use contractions.
k. Ask the patient to repeat and/or demonstrate instructions to ensure understanding.[10]

---

low-contextual cultures, such as the dominant American culture, most of the message is in the verbal mode; verbal communication is more important than nonverbal communication. In such low-contextual cultures, the communication style is logical, rational, and factual, which stresses the information that is to be transmitted.[3,11,12] English, German, Swedish, and the Romance languages are low in context, and most of the message is explicit, requiring many words to express a thought.[7,13–15] Thus, people who are from low-contexted cultures, such as most English-speaking North Americans, are more likely to miss subtle nuances of nonverbal communication.

Reflective Exercise

• What is your second language? • What makes communication in your second language easier or harder for you? • How might you promote effective communication with someone whose second language is English?

In high-contexted cultures, such as the Amish (Fig. 4-3), Koreans, and Native Americans, to name a few, communication of the message occurs mostly in the nonverbal mode and is dependent on the context of the situation; the fewer words said, the better. What is communicated depends heavily on the situation, on who is communicating, and under what circumstances and with what purpose.[11,12,16–18] Chinese, Middle Eastern, Amish Deutsch, and Native American languages are highly contexted, with most of the information either in the physical context or internalized, resulting in the use of fewer words and with more emphasis on unspoken understandings.[9,17–19]

Reflective Exercise

• On a scale of 1 to 10, with 1 low and 10 high, where do you place yourself on the scale of high-contexted versus low-contexted communication? • Do you tend to use a lot of words to express your thoughts? • Do you know of friends/acquaintances/ relatives who are your opposite in terms of high- and low-contextual communication? • Does this sometimes cause concerns in communication?

Although many Finns, Chinese, Hopi, and Turks primarily speak English in the present tense and do not use the future tense, this practice should not be confused with present temporal orientation.[9,17,21] They find it difficult to use the future tense because there is no future tense in their languages. Accordingly, healthcare providers must listen for the message in context—for example, "I see the therapist tomorrow," "I see the therapist yesterday," or "I see the therapist today."

Reflective Exercise

• Do you think that biomedical language and the culture of biomedical sciences are predominantly low context or high context? • What types of problems do you see with biomedicine and communicating with someone from the opposite context?

Voice volume and tone are important paralanguage aspects of communication. Americans and people of African American and Arab heritage may be perceived as being loud and boisterous because their volume carries to those nearby. Americans, African Americans, and Arabs[22–24] generally talk loudly in comparison with the Vietnamese, Japanese, Chinese, Koreans, Hindus, and Filipinos.[8,16,25–27] A loud voice volume may be interpreted by these cultures as reflecting anger when, in fact, it is being used merely to express thoughts in a dynamic manner. In contrast, Westerners witnessing impassioned communication among Arabs may interpret the excited speech pattern and shouting as anger, but emotional communication is part of the Arab culture and is usually unrelated to anger.[19,24] Thus, physical therapists must be cautious about voice tones when interacting with diverse cultural groups so that their intentions are not misunderstood. Likewise, the speed at which people speak varies by region; for example, in parts of Appalachia and the South, people speak more slowly than do people in the northeastern part of the United States.[10]

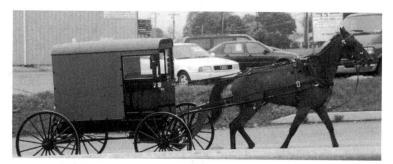

FIGURE 4.3 The Amish are an example of a highly contextual culture. They emigrated from Germany and Switzerland in the late 1600s and early 1700s. Shunning modern advances for religious reasons, the Amish continue to travel by horse and buggy rather than using motorized vehicles.

Reflective Exercise

- Do you tend to speak faster, slower, or at about the same rate as the people around you? • What happens when you meet someone who speaks much more rapidly or more slowly than you do? • In what situations does your voice volume vary? • What associations do you have with voice volume?

Cultural Communication Patterns

Communication includes the willingness of individuals to share their thoughts and feelings. Some cultural groups, such as Americans, are usually willing to disclose personal information about themselves on such topics as sex, drugs, and family problems. In fact, personal sharing is encouraged for a wide variety of topics. In the United States, having well-developed verbal skills is seen as important, whereas in Japan, the person who has very highly developed verbal skills is seen as circumspect.[4,28] Similarly, among many Appalachians, the person who has well-developed verbal skills may be seen as a "smooth talker," and therefore his or her actions may be suspect.[29]

Reflective Exercise

- How willing are you to share personal information about yourself? • How does it differ with family, friends, or strangers?

In many Asian cultures, individuals are expected to be shy, withdrawn, and diffident—at least in public—whereas in other cultures, such as Jewish and Italian, individuals are expected to be more flamboyant and expressive in their communications.[30,31] Most Appalachians as well as Mexicans and other Hispanic groups willingly share their thoughts and feelings among family members and close friends, but may not easily share thoughts, feelings, and health information with "outside" physical therapists until they get to know them. By engaging in small talk and inquiring about family members before addressing the patient's health concerns, physical therapists can help establish trust and, in turn, encourage more open communication and sharing of important health information.[8,29,32]

Nonverbal Communications

Touch, a method of nonverbal communication, has substantial variations in meaning among cultures. For the most part, North America, except for Mexico, is a low-touch society, a condition that has recently been reinforced by sexual harassment guidelines and policies. For many, even casual touching may be seen as a sexual overture and should be avoided whenever possible. People of the same gender (especially men) or of opposite genders do not generally touch each other even if they are close friends.[10,33,34] However, among most Asian cultures, two people of the same gender can touch each other without it having a sexual connotation.[9,16,28,35] Among traditional Egyptians,[36] Hindus,[26] and Orthodox Jews,[31] touch between opposite sexes is accepted in private and only between husband and wife, parents and children, and adult brothers and sisters; it is less readily accepted from strangers. Mexicans, even though they frequently touch family members and friends, tend to be modest during health examinations by members of the opposite gender. Being aware of individual practices regarding touch is essential for effective health assessments (Fig. 4-4).

Physical touch carries various meanings, positive and negative, depending upon one's life experiences. Some people, those alone or isolated, may be unaccustomed to regular physical touch and either may be uncomfortable with or may crave human touch. Others may have experienced harmful touch and therefore fear or resist human touch (Fig. 4-5).

Physical therapist professionals undergo a socialization process with physical touch as part of their professional education. Students practice palpation, massage, and manual skills on each other and potentially move from discomfort to comfort with these practices. Clinicians must remember that their familiarity and comfort with professional physical therapy touch may not be

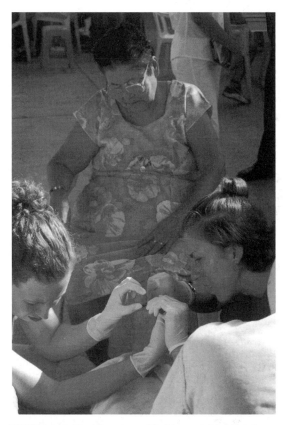

FIGURE 4.4 Wound care may involve a painful yet professionally appropriate physical touch.

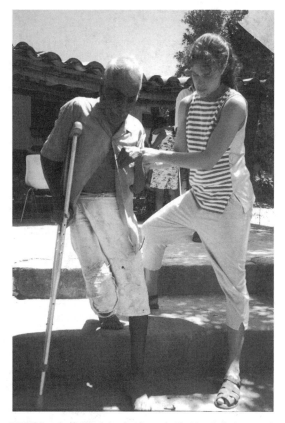

FIGURE 4.5 Gait training involves physical touch that may not be acceptable between opposite genders in certain cultures.

reciprocated by their patients. One should always ask permission before touching a patient as well as provide a full explanation of the purpose and what the patient might expect. Professional, appropriate, and respectful touch when performed with the patient's consent is effective and builds trust (Figs. 4-6 and 4-7).

Reflective Exercise

• How comfortable are you with being touched on the arm or shoulder by friends? • By people you do not know well? • Do you consider yourself to be a "person who touches" frequently, or do you rarely touch friends? • How has your comfort level with touch changed since you became a physical therapist?

Personal space needs to be respected in work with multicultural patients and staff. American, Canadian, and British conversers tend to place at least 18 inches of space between themselves and the person with whom they are talking.[3,10,37] Arabs require less personal space when talking with each other.[19,23,24] They are more comfortable standing close to each other than are the British; in fact, they interpret physical proximity as a valued sign of emotional closeness. Middle Eastern patients, who often stand very close and stare during a conversation, may offend physical therapists. These patients may interpret American physical therapists as being cold because they stand so far away. To Germans, who view space as sacred, even the distance maintained between pieces of furniture does not make for an easy

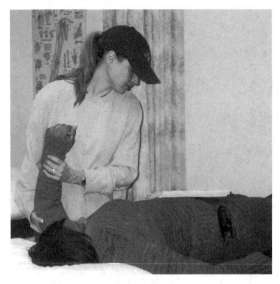

FIGURE 4.6 Physical therapist assistant students practice passive range of motion (PROM) on one another.

conversation, because people must raise their voice level to be heard. Doors are used to protect privacy and require a knock and an invitation before entering. In fact, even looking into the room can be perceived as an intrusion of privacy by Germans.[4,14] An understanding of personal space and distancing characteristics can enhance the quality of communication among individuals (Fig. 4-8).

Reflective Exercise

• What are your spatial distancing practices? • How close do you stand to family? • Friends? • Strangers? • Does this distancing remain the same with the same or with the opposite gender?

Regardless of the class or social standing of the conversers, Americans maintain direct eye contact without staring. A person who does not

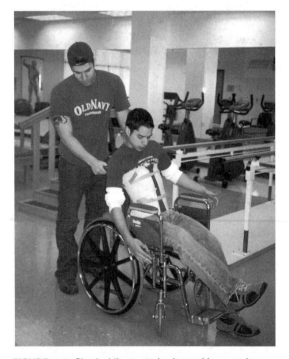

FIGURE 4.7 Physical therapy schools provide an environment where students grow accustomed to physical touch and physical handling.

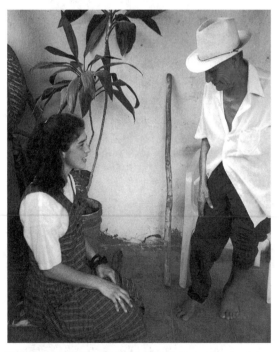

FIGURE 4.8 Different cultures dictate appropriate spatial distancing practices. The challenge arises when two people with different spatial comfort zones interact.

maintain eye contact may be perceived as not listening, not being trustworthy, not caring, or being less than truthful. Among traditional Mexicans, Cubans, Puerto Ricans, Iranians, Egyptians, Italians, and Greeks, sustained eye contact between a child and an older adult is thought to cause the illness "evil eye" or "bad eye"[8,23,30,32,36,38] (Fig. 4-9). In many Asian cultures, a person of lower social class or status should avoid eye contact with superiors or those with a higher educational status. For others—for example, among some Asian and Pacific Islander cultures—direct eye contact may be seen as sexual flirtation.[27] Thus, eye contact must be interpreted within its cultural context to optimize relationships and health assessments (Fig. 4-10).

Reflective Exercise

• Do you maintain eye contact when speaking with people? • Is it intense? • Does it vary when you speak with people of status or gender different from your own? • What does it mean to you when people do not maintain eye contact with you while speaking?

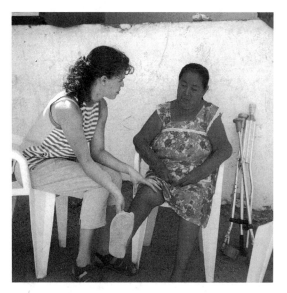

FIGURE 4.10 Often indirect eye contact is a sign of respect.

Gesturing and facial expressions vary among cultures and among people within the same cultural group. Most Americans gesture moderately when conversing and smile easily as a sign of pleasantness or happiness, although one can also smile as a sign of sarcasm. A lack of gesturing can mean that the person is too stiff, too formal, or too polite. However, when gesturing to make,

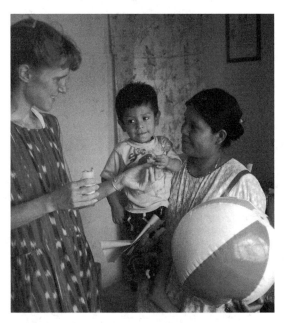

FIGURE 4.9 Eye contact carries various meanings in different cultures.

Reflection 4.1

I am from Serbia Montenegro and I am in the United States studying to be a PTA. When I first came to this country, I noticed a big difference in eye contact practices. In my country, direct, sustained eye contact can be considered rude and among strangers of the opposite sex, can be considered a sexual advance. It took me a little while to become accustomed to the direct eye contact practiced here in the United States.

Nenad Miljkovic, PTA student

emphasize, or clarify a point, one should not raise his or her elbows above the head unless saying hello or goodbye. Japanese, Filipinos, and Chinese may smile as a form of embarrassment, confusion, or failure to understand. Additionally, for them, happiness hides behind a straight face. If you truly are happy, you do not need to smile.[9,27,28]

Reflective Exercise

• Do you tend to use your hands a lot when speaking or making a point? • Can people tell your emotional state by your facial expressions?

Preferred greeting practices and acceptable body language also vary among cultural groups. An expected practice for American males and women in business is to extend the right hand when greeting someone for the first time. In northern European countries, it is considered impolite to converse with one's hands in the pockets. In the United States, confidence and competence are associated with a relaxed posture; however, in Korea[16] and Japan,[28] confidence and competence are more closely associated with slightly tense postures.[39] More elaborate greeting rituals may occur in Asian, Arab, and Latin American countries.

Reflective Exercise

• How do you prefer to be addressed and greeted?
• Does this change with the situation? • How do you normally address and greet people? • Does it change with the situation?

Although many people consider it impolite or offensive to point with one's finger, many Americans do so, and do not see it as impolite. In Iran, one beckons by waving the fingers with the palm down, whereas extending the thumb, as in a thumbs-up, is considered a vulgar sign.[23] Among the Vietnamese, signaling for someone to come by using an upturned finger is a provocation, usually done to a dog.[25] Among the Navajo it is considered rude to point; rather, the Navajo shift their lips toward the desired direction.[17]

Temporal Relationships

Temporal relationships, people's worldview in terms of past, present, and future orientation, vary. In the future-oriented American culture, people are expected to embrace change and are encouraged to sacrifice for today and work to save and invest in the future. The future is important in that people are seen as being able to influence it. Americans generally see fatalism, the belief that powers greater than humans are in control, as negative; but to many others, it is seen as a fact of life not to be judged. The German and British cultures are regarded as past-oriented societies, where laying a proper foundation by providing historical background information can enhance communication.[14,37] Most people of Central American and Caribbean heritage (and many people of low socioeconomic status) are more present oriented, placing greater importance on the here and now, not something that may occur in the future or has occurred in the past. However, for people in many societies, temporality is balanced among past, present, and future in the sense of respecting the past, valuing and enjoying the present, and saving for the future.

Reflective Exercise

• Do you consider yourself to be more past, present, or future oriented? • Give examples of being each.

North Americans see time as a highly valued resource and do not like to be delayed or encounter inefficiencies because it "wastes time."[10] When visiting friends or meeting for strictly social engagements, punctuality is less important, but one is still expected to appear within a reasonable time frame. For many Hispanics, punctuality, especially in social situations, is not taken seriously.[8,32,40] In the healthcare setting, if an appointment is made for 10 A.M., the person is expected to be there slightly before that time so that he or she is ready for the appointment and does not delay the physical therapist. Some organizations refuse to see a patient who is more than 15 to 30 minutes late for an appointment, and a few charge a fee, even though the patient was not seen. In other cultures, the patients are seen whenever they arrive. For immigrants from rural settings, time may be even less important. Some people may not even own a timepiece or be able to tell time; their day begins with sunrise and ends when the sun goes down. However, even people with a more relaxed time framework will be on time for buses and trains. Expectations for punctuality can cause conflicts between physical therapists and patients, even if one is cognizant of these differences. These details must be carefully explained to individuals when such situations occur. Being late for appointments should not be misconstrued as a sign of irresponsibility or not valuing one's health.[10]

Reflective Exercise

• Are you usually punctual for professional appointments? • Do you expect your patients to be punctual? • Are you punctual in your social engagements? • Do you expect others to be punctual with social engagements when you are involved? • How might you handle a patient's chronic tardiness?

Format for Names

Names are important to individuals, and their format differs among cultures. The American name David Thomas Jones denotes a man whose first name is David, whose middle name is Thomas, and whose family surname is Jones. Friends would call him by his first name, David. In the formal setting, he would be called Mr. Jones. Koreans use the opposite order in sequencing names. For example, the name Kim Susie denotes a woman whose last name is Kim and whose first name is Susie. Friends would address her as Susie. In a formal situation, she would be addressed as Mrs. Kim.[16]

Hispanics may have a more complex system for denoting their full names. For example, a married woman may take her husband's surname while maintaining both of her parents' last names, resulting in an extended name such as La Señora Angelica Estrada de Portillo y Sanchez. In this example, Mrs. Estrada has the first name of Angelica, her husband's surname Estrada, her mother's maiden name Sanchez, and her father's

---

> ### Reflection 4.2
>
> My name is Young Boom Kim. I am a nurse from South Korea and came to the United States in 1991. I found that people were easily confused by my name. My last name is "Kim" but Americans use it as a first name. My first name is "Young" but Americans use it as a last name. I finally decided to change my name to "Kim Bell" (Bell is my husband's last name) for Americans' convenience.
>
> *Kim Bell, RN*

---

surname Portillo. Friends would address her as Angelica, whereas in the formal setting she would be called Mrs. Estrada. This extended name format may become even more confusing because one's last name can be, for example, de la Caza. Therefore, a single woman's name might be Elena (first name) Flora (middle name) de la Caza (family name) y de la Cruz (mother's maiden name). She may choose any name she wants for legal purposes.[8,32,34,40] However, this practice varies somewhat in different Spanish-speaking cultures. When in doubt, the physical therapy professional needs to ask which name the person prefers for record keeping and which name he or she prefers to be called. Such extensive naming formats can create a challenge for physical therapists keeping medical records when they are unaware of differences in the ethnic recording of names.

Conclusion

Communication is both transmitted and understood within one's cultural framework. Communication includes language and dialects but also encompasses all manner of nonverbal communication such as eye contact, spatial distance, facial expressions, gestures, and greetings. This chapter also considers differences in the format of names, understandings of time, and time orientation as components of communication. Many of the cultural misalignments and misunderstandings that occur within healthcare interactions are a result of miscommunication.[41]

The culturally competent physical therapist will seek to understand his or her own cultural communication patterns as well as those of the individual with whom he or she is interacting. Attention to potential miscommunications resulting from cultural misalignments will promote effective communication and ultimately lead to more effective physical therapy care.

CULTURAL SELF-ASSESSMENT EXERCISE 1

Self-Assessment Exercise

Answer the following questions related to the communication domain for yourself.
1. What is your primary language? Do you speak a second or third language?
2. Do you speak a specific dialect of your language? How would you describe your accent?
3. In what language do you prefer getting written material?
4. Do you find it difficult to share your thoughts, feelings, and ideas with family? Friends? Healthcare providers?
5. Are you comfortable being touched by friends? Strangers? Physical therapy professionals?
6. Do you usually maintain eye contact with family members, friends, elders, strangers?
7. What does intense eye contact mean to you?
8. What does it mean to you if someone does not maintain eye contact with you?
9. How important is a smile to you? What does it mean if someone is not smiling?
10. What is your full name? What is your legal name?
11. By what name do you prefer to be addressed?
12. How do wish to be greeted? Handshake? Nod of the head? Other?
13. Are you usually on time for appointments?
14. Are you usually on time for social engagements?

CULTURAL SELF-ASSESSMENT EXERCISE 2

Understanding Others / Recognizing Potential Barriers

1. Answers to which of the above questions would be important to understand about your patient?
2. Identify three potential miscommunications or misunderstandings that might result if the above questions are not understood.
3. Describe how you would try to avoid each of the miscommunications or misunderstandings.
4. Describe how you would manage each of the miscommunications after they happened.

CULTURAL SELF-ASSESSMENT EXERCISE 3

Interaction: Developing Sensitivity and Awareness

1. How might you determine if your patient is used to low-context communication or high-context communication? What clues might you obtain through observation of the patient's communication?
   a. What considerations might you make when communicating with someone of a low contextual style?
   b. What considerations might you make when communicating with someone of a high contextual style?
2. How might you determine your patient's level of comfort with physical touch?
   a. What considerations should you remember and practice before physically touching someone?
   b. How can you ensure that you are using physical touch respectfully and therapeutically? How can you communicate this to your patient verbally and nonverbally?
   c. How might the physical touch be offensive to the patient?
   d. How should you *not* touch a patient?
3. How might you determine your patient's spatial distancing preferences?
   a. What happens when the spatial distancing preferences are different between the physical therapist and the patient?
   b. What responsibility does the physical therapist have in respecting the patient's spatial distancing preferences?
4. How might you determine your patient's understanding and beliefs regarding eye contact?
   a. How might you determine whether lack of eye contact denotes respect, disrespect, or disinterest?
   b. How might your eye contact practices be offensive to your patient?
   c. How might you determine if your eye contact practices are offensive to or misinterpreted by your patient?

Vignette Questions

1. What do you know about the Korean language?
2. What do you know about the name format among Koreans?
3. Why does Ms. Park nod and/or answer "yes" to every question? Is it because she does not understand English?
4. Why does she not maintain eye contact?
5. If you needed an interpreter, whom would you get?
6. Why did Ms. Park put the gown over her clothes rather than disrobing?

CASE STUDY SCENARIO I

*T*ommy Begay, a 17-year-old Navajo Indian, injured his right shoulder in a recreational lacrosse game. His physical therapist, Mr. Brad Barnett, had a difficult time trying to obtain a medical history. Tommy does not maintain eye contact and is slow to answer his questions. Brad rephrases each question several times, thinking that Tommy does not understand. In an attempt to "break the ice" and make Tommy more comfortable, Brad tells a joke about Tommy's collision with the other lacrosse player and gives him a hearty slap on his non-injured shoulder. Tommy recoils and gives only a weak smile. When Tommy does answer Brad's questions, it is only after a period of silence, and his responses are short and nondescriptive.

1. Identify the aspects of communication that are evident.

2. Identify Tommy's (the patient's) communication patterns.

3. Identify Brad's (the physical therapist's) communication patterns.

4. What misunderstandings are occurring in this situation?

5. Do you think Tommy understands the physical therapist? Why or why not?

6. How might Brad recognize the cultural differences in communication?

7. What might Brad do to lessen these cultural communication differences?

8. Consider what Tommy might be thinking. How do you think Tommy is regarding the interaction?

9. If Tommy is a traditional Navajo, how should the physical therapist greet him?

(For more information on Native Americans, see Chapter 13.)

CASE STUDY SCENARIO II

*M*r. Petrozowski is a 64-year-old male with chronic neck and upper back pain. He is a retired plumber and is coming for physical therapy. His parents emigrated from Poland and he is bilingual. The physical therapist, Wanda Diehm, is a 24-year-old female who recently graduated from physical therapy school. She is of German ancestry and grew up as an only child. She struggled in physical therapy schools with the labs because she was unaccustomed to the degree of physical touch required. She grew to be comfortable with touching others in a therapeutic manner but never quite became comfortable with strangers touching her.

Case Study Scenario II Continued

Mr. Petrozowski is 6 foot 3 inches tall and weighs over 250 pounds. Wanda enters the exam room and closes the door for privacy. Mr. Petrozowski stands to greet Wanda and gives her a very firm handshake with his strong and large hands. Wanda indicates that Mr. Petrozowski may sit, but he does not seem to hear her as he launches into his account of the pain in his neck and upper back. He maintains a very close spatial distance to Wanda, and Wanda automatically takes a step back. Mr. Petrozowski continues to describe his pain with a loud voice volume and takes a step toward Wanda as she retreats. He begins to tell her specifically where his pain is and spontaneously reaches to her mid-back and applies fingertip pressure to her back to show her where it hurts. Wanda recoils and excuses herself from the room.

1. Identify the aspects of communication that are evident.

2. Identify Mr. Petrozowski's cultural communication style.

3. Identify Wanda's communication style.

4. What miscommunications are occurring?

5. How might Wanda recognize the cultural misalignments?

6. How might Wanda's recognition of the cultural misalignments help her in the interaction?

7. How might Wanda handle the cultural misalignments so that she might have an effective interaction with her patient without compromising her own comfort or offending her patient?

REFERENCES

1. Office of Minority Health. CLAS standards. Available at: http://www.omhrc.gov/clas/. Accessed January 9, 2004.
2. Althen G. *American Ways: A Guide for Foreigners in the United States.* Yarmouth, Me: Intercultural Press; 1988.
3. Hall E. *The Silent Language.* New York, NY: Doubleday; 1959.
4. Hill R. *We Europeans.* Brussels: Europublications; 1995.
5. Kohls RR. *Learning to Think Korean: A Guide to Living and Working in Korea.* Yarmouth, Me: Intercultural Press; 2001.
6. Kras E. *Management in Two Cultures: Bridging the Gap between the U.S. and Mexican Managers.* Yarmouth, Me: Intercultural Press; 1989.
7. Stephenson S. *Understanding Spanish-Speaking South Americans.* Yarmouth, Me: Intercultural Press; 2003.
8. Zoucha R, Purnell L. People of Mexican heritage. In: Purnell L, Paulanka B, eds. *Transcultural Health Care: A Culturally Competent Approach.* 2nd ed. Philadelphia, Pa: FA Davis; 2003:264–278.
9. Wang Y. People of Chinese ancestry. In: Purnell L, Paulanka B, eds. *Transcultural Health Care: A Culturally Competent Approach.* 2nd ed. Philadelphia, Pa: FA Davis; 2003:106–121.
10. Purnell L. The Purnell Model for Cultural Competence. In: Purnell L, Paulanka B, eds. *Transcultural Health Care: A Culturally Competent Approach.* 2nd ed. Philadelphia, Pa: FA Davis; 2003:8–40.
11. Hall E. *The Hidden Dimension.* Yarmouth, Me: Intercultural Press; 1966.
12. Wolfgang A. *Everybody's Guide to People Watching.* Yarmouth, Me: Intercultural Press; 1995.
13. Hall E, Hall M. *Understanding Cultural Differences: Germans, French, and Americans.* Yarmouth, Me: Intercultural Press; 1990.
14. Steckler J. People of German heritage [chapter on CD-ROM]. In: Purnell L, Paulanka B, eds. *Transcultural Health Care: A Culturally Competent Approach.* 2nd ed. Philadelphia, Pa: FA Davis; 2003.
15. Wilson S. People of Irish heritage. In: Purnell L, Paulanka B, eds. *Transcultural Health Care: A Culturally*

Competent Approach. 2nd ed. Philadelphia, Pa: FA Davis; 2003:54–72.

16. Purnell L, Kim S. People of Korean heritage. In: Purnell L, Paulanka B, eds. *Transcultural Health Care: A Culturally Competent Approach.* 2nd ed. Philadelphia, Pa: FA Davis; 2003:249–263.

17. Still O, Hodgins D. Navajo Indians. In: Purnell L, Paulanka B, eds. *Transcultural Health Care: A Culturally Competent Approach.* 2nd ed. Philadelphia, Pa: FA Davis; 2003:279–283.

18. Wenger AF, Wenger M. The Amish. In: Purnell L, Paulanka B, eds. *Transcultural Health Care: A Culturally Competent Approach.* 2nd ed. Philadelphia, Pa: FA Davis; 2003:54–72.

19. Kulwicki A. People of Arab heritage. In: Purnell L, Paulanka B, eds. *Transcultural Health Care: A Culturally Competent Approach.* 2nd ed. Philadelphia, Pa: FA Davis; 2003:90–105.

20. Kraybill D. *The riddle of the Amish culture.* Baltimore, Md: Johns Hopkins University Press; 2001.

21. Towle C, Arslanoglu T. People of Turkish heritage [chapter on CD-ROM]. In: Purnell L, Paulanka B, eds. *Transcultural Health Care: A Culturally Competent Approach.* 2nd ed. Philadelphia, Pa: FA Davis; 2003.

22. Glanville C. People of African American heritage. In: Purnell L, Paulanka B, eds. *Transcultural Health Care: A Culturally Competent Approach.* 2nd ed. Philadelphia, Pa: FA Davis; 2003:40–53.

23. Haifizi H, Lipson J. People of Iranian heritage. In: Purnell L, Paulanka B, eds. *Transcultural Health Care: A Culturally Competent Approach.* 2nd ed. Philadelphia, Pa: FA Davis; 2003:177–193.

24. Nydell M. *Understanding Arabs.* Yarmouth, Me: Intercultural Press; 1987.

25. Nowak T. People of Vietnamese heritage. In: Purnell L, Paulanka B, eds. *Transcultural Health Care: A Culturally Competent Approach.* 2nd ed. Philadelphia, Pa: FA Davis; 2003:327–344.

26. Jambanathan J. People of Hindu heritage [chapter on CD-ROM]. In: Purnell L, Paulanka B, eds. *Transcultural Health Care: A Culturally Competent Approach.* 2nd ed. Philadelphia, Pa: FA Davis; 2003.

27. Pacquiao D. People of Filipino heritage. In: Purnell L, Paulanka B, eds. *Transcultural Health Care: A Culturally Competent Approach.* 2nd ed. Philadelphia, Pa: FA Davis; 2003:138–159.

28. Sharts-Hopko N. People of Japanese heritage. In: Purnell L, Paulanka B, eds. *Transcultural Health Care: A Culturally Competent Approach.* 2nd ed. Philadelphia, Pa: FA Davis; 2003:218–233.

29. Purnell L. (2003). People of Appalachian heritage. In: Purnell L, Paulanka B, eds. *Transcultural Health Care: A Culturally Competent Approach.* 2nd ed. Philadelphia, Pa: FA Davis; 2003:73–89.

30. Hillman S. People of Italian heritage. In: Purnell L, Paulanka B, eds. *Transcultural Health Care: A Culturally Competent Approach.* 2nd ed. Philadelphia, Pa: FA Davis; 2003:205–217.

31. Selekman J. People of Jewish heritage. In: Purnell L, Paulanka B, eds. *Transcultural Health Care: A Culturally Competent Approach.* 2nd ed. Philadelphia, Pa: FA Davis; 2003:234–248..

32. Juarbe T. People of Puerto Rican heritage. In: Purnell L, Paulanka B, eds. *Transcultural Health Care: A Culturally Competent Approach.* 2nd ed. Philadelphia, Pa: FA Davis; 2003:307–326.

33. Datesman M, Crandall J, Kearney E. *The American Ways.* White Plains, NY: Prentice-Hall; 1997.

34. Purnell L. Panamanians' practices for health promotion and the meaning of respect afforded them by healthcare providers. *J Transcult Nurs.* 1999;10:333–340.

35. Zahn L. *Asian Americans.* Sudbury, Mass: Jones and Bartlett; 2003.

36. Purnell L. People of Egyptian heritage [chapter on CD-ROM]. In: Purnell L, Paulanka B, eds. *Transcultural Health Care: A Culturally Competent Approach.* 2nd ed. Philadelphia, Pa: FA Davis; 2003.

37. Paxman J. *The English: A Portrait of the People.* New York, NY: Penguin Books; 1999.

38. Purnell L, Papadopoulos I. People of Greek heritage [chapter on CD-ROM]. In: Purnell L, Paulanka B, eds. *Transcultural Health Care: A Culturally Competent Approach.* 2nd ed. Philadelphia, Pa: FA Davis; 2003.

39. Krebs G, Kunimoto Y. *Effective Communication in Multicultural Health Care Settings.* Thousand Oaks, Calif: Intercultural Press; 1994.

40. Purnell L. People of Cuban heritage. In: Purnell L, Paulanka B, eds. *Transcultural Health Care: A Culturally Competent Approach.* 2nd ed. Philadelphia, Pa: FA Davis; 2003:122–137.

41. Levinson W. Physician-patient communication: A key to malpractice prevention. *JAMA.* 1994;272:1619–1620.

Exploring Family Roles and Organization within Culture

- Larry D. Purnell, PhD, RN
- Jill Black Lattanzi, PT, EdD

*M*r. Mazzetti is an 86-year-old, first-generation Italian immigrant. He fell and broke his hip and is now receiving home physical therapy. His daughter, Maria, cares for him morning and night and also is present to assist with translation when the physical therapist is there. Mr. Mazzetti speaks very little English, having lived in an Italian enclave in a big city. The physical therapist notices that Maria does everything to meet her father's needs, including activities in which the physical therapist has been trying to encourage independence.

Family Roles and Organization

Physical therapists work with individual patients and bring health beliefs and interaction styles they obtained from their own families. Physical therapy patients have relationships with family members who will influence care either positively, negatively, or neutrally. Often the family is the support system for the patient, and the physical therapist needs to instruct family members in aspects of the physical therapy program. Sometimes the physical therapist must work around family members, as they may frequent the physical therapy gym more than desired or offer the patient help in areas in which the physical therapist is working for the patient's independence. In any case, it is integral that the physical therapist be attentive to the family, the family dynamics, and the expectations of the patient and family if the physical therapy intervention is to be optimally effective (Fig. 5-1).

The domain *family roles and organization* culturally prescribes relationships among insiders and outsiders. This domain includes concepts related to the head of the household, gender roles (a product of biology and culture), family goals and priorities, developmental tasks of children and adolescents, roles of the aged and extended family, individual and family social status in the community, and acceptance of alternative lifestyles, such as single parenting, nontraditional sexual orientations, childless marriages, and divorce (Fig. 5-2). Family structure in the context of the larger society determines acceptable roles, priorities, and behavioral norms for its members.

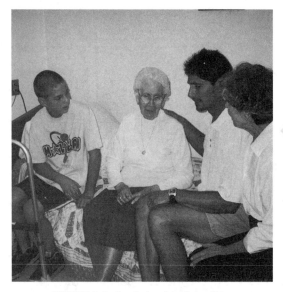

FIGURE 5.1 Family in a hospital setting.

Head of Household and Gender Roles
An awareness of family dominance patterns (i.e., patriarchal, matriarchal, or egalitarian) is important for determining with whom to speak when healthcare decisions have to be made or physical therapy instructions need to be given. Among many cultures, it is acceptable for women to have a career and for men to assist with child care and household domestic chores. Both parents work outside the home in many families, necessitating children's placement in child care facilities.

Reflective Exercise

• How would you classify the decision-making process in your family—patriarchal, matriarchal, or egalitarian? • Does it vary by what decision has to be made? • Are gender roles prescribed in your family? • How do they differ from your family unit when you were a child or teenager? • Who makes decisions with regard to physical health?

In some cultures, fathers are responsible for deciding when to seek healthcare for family members, but mothers may have significant in-

fluence on the final decisions. Among many Hispanics, the decisions may be egalitarian, but it is the role of the male in the family to be the spokesperson.[1,2] When speaking with parents about a child's condition, the physical therapist should maintain eye contact and direct questions to both parents.

Reflective Exercise

• How might HIPAA be culturally inappropriate and offensive to families?

Prescriptive, Restrictive, and Taboo Behaviors for Children and Adolescents
Every society has prescriptive, restrictive, and taboo practices for children and adolescents. Prescriptive practices are things that children or teenagers *should do* to achieve harmony with the family and a good outcome in society, such as being well behaved, following parents' and elders' advice, and studying hard in school to make good grades. Restrictive practices are things that children and teenagers *should not do* in order to create a positive outcome, such as smoking tobacco and not following proper dress codes. Taboo practices are those things that, if done, are likely to cause significant concern or negative outcomes for the child, teenager, family, or community at large, such as engaging in premarital sex and experimenting with recreational drugs.[3] What is considered a restrictive practice in some cultures or families may be a taboo practice in other cultures or families.

Family values vary among the European American individualistic culture and the collectivist cultures of many other groups, such as most Asians, Hispanics, and Native Americans. Individualistic cultures value individualism and privacy, whereas collectivist cultures emphasize the value of family as a group.[4–12] For most individualistic societies, a child's individual achievement is valued over the family's financial status. However, in many non-Western collectivistic cultures, attachment to family is more important and the need for children to excel individually is not as important. In most middle- and upper-socioeconomic-class American families, children

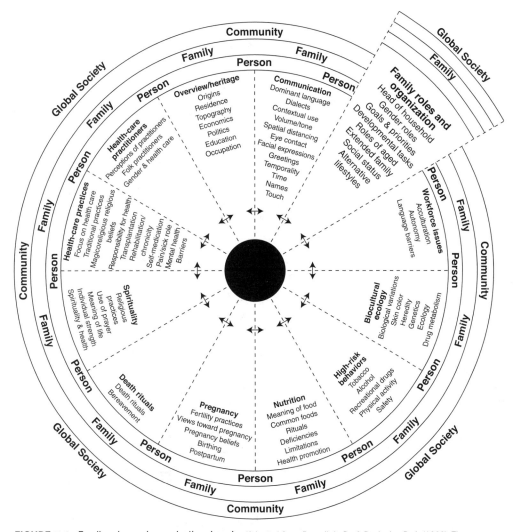

FIGURE 5.2 Family roles and organization domain. (Adapted from Purnell, L. D., & Paulanka, B. J. (1998). The Purnell Model for Cultural Competence. In L. D. Purnell & B. J. Paulanka (Eds.), *Transcultural health care: A culturally competent approach* (p. 10). Philadelphia: F.A. Davis.)

have their own room, television, and telephone, and in many homes, their own computer. At younger ages, each child has his or her own toys and is taught to share them with others rather than having group toys. Most European American and Western cultures encourage autonomy in children, and after completing homework assignments children are expected to contribute to the family by doing chores such as taking out the garbage, washing dishes, cleaning their rooms, feeding and caring for pets, and helping with cooking.[3,13–16] However, in middle-class urban Panamanian families, children are not expected to participate in household chores or to have summer jobs. Childhood years are a time for children to "be children."[2]

In European American cultures, children are allowed and encouraged to make their own choices, including managing their own allowance of money and deciding who their friends will be, although parents may gently suggest that one friend might be a better choice than another. Prescriptive behaviors for children and teenagers include having friends of the same and of the opposite gender and being well behaved, especially in public. They are taught to stand in line—first come, first served—and wait their turns. As they reach the teenage years, restrictive and taboo behaviors include refraining from premarital sex, smoking, recreational drug use, and alcohol consumption until they leave the home. However, they are not always deterred, and teenage use of these substances remains high. The teenage years are also seen as a time of natural rebellion.[3,13,16,17]

Reflective Exercise

• Were you encouraged to live independently upon becoming an adult, or were you encouraged to continue to reside with the family? • Were you taught to be independent and autonomous, or were you taught to respect and depend upon the family?

Reflective Exercise

• In your family, was there a greater emphasis on the individual or on the group?

Reflective Exercise

• How might a child or a young adult's independence or interdependence affect a physical therapy program?

In most European American cultures, when a young adult becomes age 18 or completes his or her education, he or she usually moves out of the parents' home (unless attending college) and lives independently or shares living arrangements with non–family members. In the United States, more single males (59%) than single females (48%) over the age of 18 years elect to live with their parents.[18] If the young adult chooses to remain in the parents' home, then he or she might be expected to pay room and board. However, young adults are generally allowed to return home when necessary for financial or other purposes. Individuals over the age of 18 are expected to be self-reliant and independent, qualities seen as virtues in European American cultures.[3,6,14,15,19] This is in opposition to other cultures, such as the Japanese, Italian, and some Hispanic cultures, where even adults are expected to live at home with their parents until they marry; interdependence, not independence, is the virtue.[8,12,20,21]

Reflective Exercise

• What were prescriptive behaviors for you as a child? • As a teenager? • As a young adult? • What are the prescriptive behaviors for your children or your expectations of children if you do not have children?

Reflective Exercise

• What were restrictive behaviors for you as a child? • As a teenager? • As a young adult? • What are the restrictive behaviors for your children or your expectations of children if you do not have children?

Reflective Exercise

• What were taboo behaviors for you as a child? • As a teenager? • As a young adult? • What are the taboo behaviors for your children or your expectations of children if you do not have children?

Adolescents have their own subculture, with its own values, beliefs, and practices, which may not be in harmony with those of their dominant ethnic group. It may be especially important for adolescents to be in harmony with peers and conform to the prevailing choices in music, clothing, hairstyles, and adornment. Moreover, role conflicts can become considerable sources of family strain among many cultures and among more traditional families, who may not agree with the American values of individuality, independence, self-assertion, and egalitarian relationships. Thus, many teens may experience a cultural dilemma with exposure outside the home and family.[3,15]

Family Goals and Priorities

American family goals and priorities center on raising and educating children. During this stage in the American culture, young adults make a personal commitment to a spouse or significant other and seek satisfaction through productivity in career, family, and civic interests. It is a cultural universal to place a high value on children, and many laws have been enacted to protect children, who are seen as the "future of society." Physical punishment is seen as abuse. In most Asian cultures, children are desirable and highly valued as a source of family strength, and family members are expected to care for each other more than in the American culture.[9,11,14,22]

The United States has seen an explosion in its elderly population during the 20th century, up from 3.1 million in 1900 to 34.6 million in 1999; or, stated differently, the population has gone from 1 in 25 to 1 in 8 people being over the age of 65 years. The elderly population is expected to further increase by 74% over the next 20 years. In 1990, among those over the age of 100 years, 7,901 were males and 29,003 were females.[18] The definition of aging varies among cultures and can be defined by age in years, by functional abilities, or by social mores. In the Korean culture, individuals are considered old and expected to retire at the age of 60, regardless of their health status, because they have completed the 60 cycles of the lunar calendar.[9] Within Brazilian American society, the aged live with one of their children, are included in family activities, and usually accompany their child's family on vacation.[23]

The American culture's emphasis on youth and "thinness" is not desired by all cultures. The high value placed on independence and productivity contributes to some societal views of the aged as less important members of society. A contrasting view among some Americans emphasizes the importance of the elderly in society. Filipino, Korean, and Appalachian cultures have great reverence for the wisdom of the elderly, and families eagerly make space for them to live with their extended families. Children are expected to care for the elders when the elders are unable to care for themselves. A great embarrassment may occur to family members who cannot take care of their elders.[6,9,24] Helping the family to network and find social support, resources, or acceptable long-term-care facilities within the community is a useful strategy for the physical therapy professional.

Reflective Exercise

• How do you regard aging? • Do you see it as something to respect and anticipate or as something to dread?

Reflective Exercise

• How are elders regarded in your family? • How are elders regarded in your culture?

The concept of extended family membership varies among societies. Family in the United States generally reflects the nuclear family, with less emphasis on the extended family (Fig. 5-3). Although family is valued in all societies, its prominence varies by degree and intensity. The extended family is extremely important in the Appalachian, Hispanic/Latino/Spanish, Amish, and Asian Indian cultures, and healthcare decisions are often postponed until the entire family is consulted[6,8,12,25] (Fig. 5-4). The extended family may include biological relatives and nonbiological relatives who may be considered brother, sister, aunt, or uncle.[6,17] In some Asian cultures, the influence of grandparents in decision making is considered more important than that of the parents.[11,22] A practice among Filipinos is for the grandparents to raise the grandchildren so that the parents may pursue work-related goals.[24] Grandparents, aunts, and

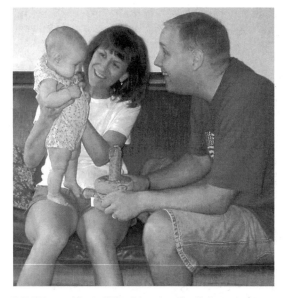

FIGURE 5.3 The traditional American family has primary emphasis on the immediate or nuclear family.

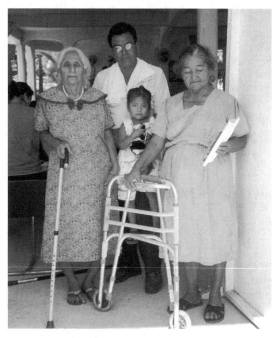

FIGURE 5.5 A multigenerational Mexican family seeking healthcare.

cousins often assume the parental role in African American families, and fellow church members are frequently considered important members of the extended family. A common practice in such cultures is for several generations of a family to live in the same household, or as near to one another as possible.[17] The physical therapist can have a significant impact on the health status of the extended family in primary, home health, acute, or long-term care by networking with the extended family when therapeutic interventions are required (Fig. 5-5).

Sometimes the high level of commitment of an extended family can lead to conflicts with visiting hours and the number of visitors allowed in a room. At times the number of family members accompanying a physical therapy patient to the gym might be overwhelming. Institutions and healthcare providers, including physical therapists, face the challenge of respecting family commitments while providing quality care.

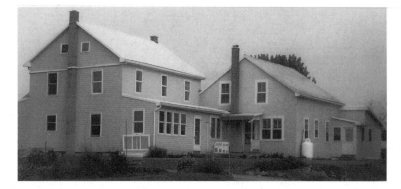

FIGURE 5.4 The Amish care for their elders by building an addition onto the farmhouse for each generation.

Reflective Exercise

- Do you consider your family nuclear or extended?
- How close are you to your extended family? • How involved are you in the healthcare concerns of your extended family?

Reflective Exercise

- How do you feel when your patient is accompanied to the physical therapy gym by numerous family members? • How might you best handle the situation?

Americans and Swedes place high value on egalitarianism, non-hierarchical relationships, and treating everyone the same, regardless of their race, color, religion, ethnicity, educational or economic status, sexual orientation, or country of origin. However, these beliefs in the United States are more theoretical and are not always seen in practice. For example, women still have a lower status than men, especially when it comes to prestigious positions and salaries. Most top-level political officials and corporate executive officers are white men. In 1951, women's earnings were 63.9% of men's; in 1998, the number was still only 73%, down from 74.2% in 1997.[18] Subtle classism exists as evidenced by comments referring to "working-class men and women." Despite the current inequities, Americans value equal opportunities for all, and progress continues.

Americans are known worldwide for their informality and for treating everyone the same. They call people by their first names, whether in the workplace, in social situations, in classrooms, in restaurants, or in places of business. In Sweden, physical therapists are encouraged to call people, regardless of age or status differences, by their first name (Ing-Marie Backman, Eskilstuna, Sweden, personal communication, November 2002). Americans readily talk with waitresses and store clerks and call them by their first names. Most Americans consider this to be respectful behavior. The English language does not have familiar and formal forms of communication as the Romance languages do; however, formality can be communicated by addressing the person with his or her last (family) name

and title, such as Mr., Mrs., Miss, Ms., or Dr. To this end, achieved status is more important than ascribed status. What one has accumulated in material possessions, where one went to school, and one's job position and title are more important than one's family background and lineage.

Reflective Exercise

- How do you prefer to be addressed?
- Does it change with younger or older people?
- Does it change with your patients?

The United States does not have a caste or class system and one can move readily from one socioeconomic position to another with hard work. Thus, most Americans identify themselves by personal achievements, not family lineage. Europeans and Asians are more attentive to status than are Americans. To many Americans, maintaining formality is seen as pompous or arrogant, and some even deride the person who is very formal.[3,6] However, formality is a sign of respect in many other cultures, and it is also valued by older Americans. Status in some cultures, such as Hindu, is connected to a specific and rigid caste system into which people are born and out of which they are unable to move, regardless of changes in their socioeconomic status.[6] However, in other societies, such as among Koreans, not as much attention is given to one's heritage; educational accomplishments give one status.[9,26] With hard work in American society, a person can climb the socioeconomic scale and gain respect; however, the person can fall from high socioeconomic status just as quickly.

Reflective Exercise

- How is status measured in your culture? • Is it ascribed, achieved, or both? • How important is money for status? • How are the elderly perceived in your culture?

Alternative Lifestyles

The traditional American family is nuclear, with a married man and woman living together with one or more of their unmarried children. However, the American family is becoming a more varied community. It includes unmarried people, men or women, living alone; single people of the same or opposite gender living together with or without children; single parents with children; and blended families consisting of two parents who have remarried, with children from their previous marriages and additional children from their current marriage. However, in many collectivist cultures, the traditional family is extended, with parents, unmarried children, married children with their children, and grandparents all sharing the same living space or at least living in close proximity, if at all possible. The number of grandchildren living with grandparents has been increasing. In some societies, divorce continues to carry a stigma. High levels of marital instability challenge norms and create new patterns of family life.[27]

In some cities in the United States, rights of traditional married couples are granted to unmarried heterosexual, homosexual, elderly, or disabled couples who share the traditional bond of the family.[18] Among more rural subcultures, same-sex couples living together may not be as accepted or recognized in the community as they are in larger cities.

Reflective Exercise

• Mary Jane, age 26, has severe lacerations to her right wrist, which she sustained while trying to open a window in her kitchen. She has undergone surgical repair of a lacerated tendon, artery, and vein. You are called to see her and evaluate her for rehabilitative exercises. As you prepare to enter her room, a medical student and nurse are talking about Mary Jane being a "pervert" and remarking that they do not understand why she wants to undergo gender reassignment surgery. How might you handle the staff's derogatory attitude toward this patient?

Social attitudes toward homosexual activity vary widely, and homosexual behavior occurs in societies that deny its presence. Homosexual behavior carries a severe stigma in some societies. To discover that a son is gay or a daughter is lesbian is akin to a catastrophic event for Egyptian Americans.[7] In Iran[4] and in some provinces of China,[11] a lesbian or gay individual may be killed. In February 2001, a judge in Somalia sentenced two Somali lesbians to death for "exercising unnatural behavior."[28] For more information on gay, lesbian, bisexual, and transgendered cultures, which is beyond the scope of this text, the reader is referred to a monograph published by the American Physical Therapy Association.[8]

When the physical therapist needs to provide assistance and make a referral for a person who is gay, lesbian, bisexual, or transsexual, a number of options are available. There are some local referral agencies, as well as others that are national, with local or regional chapters. Many are ethnically or religiously specific. Some national groups that have links to local and regional organizations are listed in Box 5-1.

Reflective Exercise

• What are your personal views of two people of the same gender living together in a physical relationship? • What about heterosexual couples living together before marriage? • How are your views similar to or different from those of your parents and those representative of your cultural background?

Conclusion

Consideration of family roles and organization includes understanding who is the head of the household, gender roles, family goals and priorities, developmental tasks of children and adolescents, roles of the aged and extended family, individual and family social status in the community, and acceptance of alternative lifestyles such as single parenting, nontraditional sexual orientations, childless marriages, and divorce. The physical therapist must be attentive to the family, the family dynamics, and the expectations of the patient and family if the physical therapy intervention is to be optimally effective.

List of Resources for Gay and Lesbian Patients

1. Gay, Lesbian, and Straight Education Network: www.glsen.org
2. National Latino(a) Lesbian, Gay, Bisexual, & Transgender Organization: www.lego.org
3. Parents, Families, & Friends of Lesbians & Gays: www.pflag.org
4. National Center for Lesbian Rights: info@nclrights.org
5. Log Cabin Republicans: www.lcr.org
6. National Stonewall Democratic Federation: www.stonewalldemocrats.org
7. National Youth Advocacy Coalition: www.nyacyouth.org
8. Family Pride Coalition: www.familypride.org
9. IT'S Time, America: www.gender.org
10. BINET US: www.binetUS.org
11. National Black, Lesbian, and Gay leadership Forum: www.nblglf.org

Pregnancy and Childbearing Practices

Most societies have prescriptive, restrictive, and taboo beliefs regarding maternal behaviors and the delivery of a healthy baby. Such beliefs affect lifestyle behaviors during pregnancy, birthing, and the postpartum period. Prescriptive practices are things that the mother should do to have a good outcome (a healthy baby and pregnancy). Restrictive belief practices are those things that the mother should *not* do in order to enjoy a positive outcome (healthy baby and delivery). Taboo practices are those things that, if done, are likely to harm the baby or mother (Fig. 5-6).

A prescriptive belief among European Americans is that women are expected to seek preventive care, eat a well-balanced diet, get adequate rest, and get moderate exercise in order to have a healthy pregnancy and baby (Figs. 5-7 and 5-8). The American healthcare system encourages women to breast-feed, and many places of employment have made arrangements for women to breast-feed while working. A restrictive belief among many European Americans is that pregnant women should refrain from being around loud noises for prolonged periods of time. Taboo behaviors during pregnancy include smoking, drinking alcohol, having a high caffeine intake, and taking recreational drugs, practices that may cause harm to the mother and baby.[3]

Among the Navajo a restrictive belief is that clothes should not be purchased for the infant before birth, because preparing for the infant is forbidden by Indian tradition. Thus, when an expectant woman does not prepare for the birth of her baby, it does not mean that she does not care about herself or her baby.[10] A taboo belief among some populations is that a pregnant woman should not reach over her head, because the baby may then be born with the umbilical cord around its neck. A restrictive belief among Indians in Belize and Panama is that permitting the father to be present in the delivery room and see the mother or baby before they have been cleaned can cause harm to the baby or mother (Hilda Alvaro Pitti, David, Panama, personal communication, October 1999). Because the father is absent from the delivery room or does not want to see the mother or baby immediately after birth does not mean that he does not care about them. However, in the American culture, in which the father is often encouraged to take prenatal classes with the expectant mother and provide a supportive role in the delivery process, fathers with opposing beliefs may feel guilty if they do not comply.

In the American culture, under the Family Medical Leave Program, women and men are guaranteed maternity/paternity leave of up to 90 days if their workplace employs more than 50 people. Most women, but few men, take advantage of this opportunity.[29] The woman's female relatives (mother, sisters, and aunts) provide assistance to the new mother until she is able to care for herself and her baby. Additional cultural beliefs carried over from cultural migration and American diversity are listed in Box 5-2.

In some other cultures, the postpartum

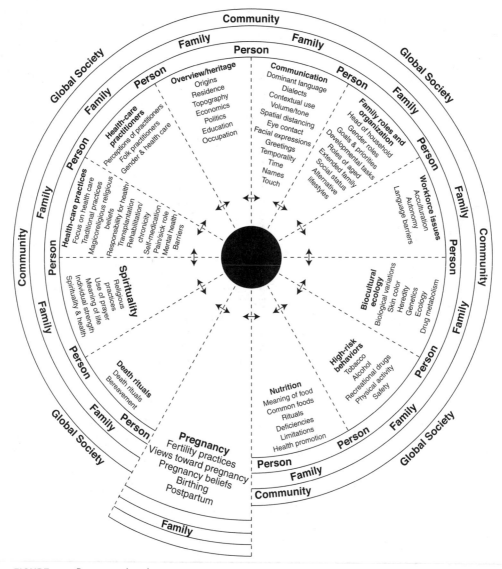

FIGURE 5.6 Pregnancy domain. (Adapted from Purnell, L. D., & Paulanka, B. J. (1998). The Purnell Model for Cultural Competence. In L. D. Purnell & B. J. Paulanka (Eds.), *Transcultural health care: A culturally competent approach* (p. 10). Philadelphia: F.A. Davis.)

woman is prescribed a prolonged period of recuperation in the hospital or at home, something that may not be feasible in the United States due to the shortened length of confinement in the hospital after delivery. Among the Vietnamese, the head is considered sacred, and it is taboo to touch the head of the mother or the infant. Even the removal of vernix, the sebaceous substance covering the infant during intrauterine life, from the infant's head can cause distress.[30]

The physical therapist must respect cultural beliefs associated with pregnancy and the birthing process when making decisions related to the healthcare of pregnant women, especially

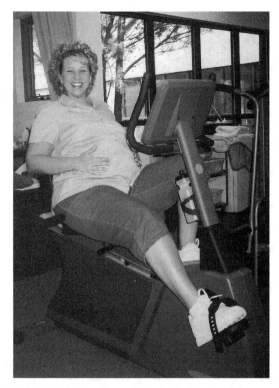

FIGURE 5.7 Pregnant woman in physical therapy.

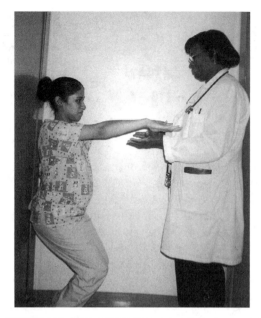

FIGURE 5.8 Some cultures encourage pregnant women to exercise and others do not.

those practices that do not cause harm to the mother or baby. Most cultural practices can be integrated into preventive teaching in a manner that promotes compliance.

Reflective Exercise

• What are your personal beliefs about prescriptive, restrictive, and taboo practices that a woman should observe in order to have a healthy pregnancy and baby? • How do these differ from your family's beliefs?

BOX 5.2

Cultural Beliefs Regarding Pregnancy and Birth

1. If you wear an opal ring during pregnancy, it will harm the baby.
2. Birthmarks are caused by eating strawberries or seeing a snake and being frightened.
3. Congenital anomalies can occur if the mother sees or experiences a tragedy during her pregnancy.
4. Nursing mothers should eat a bland diet to avoid upsetting the baby.
5. The infant should wear a band around the abdomen to prevent the umbilicus from protruding and becoming herniated.
6. Putting a coin, key, or other metal object on the umbilicus will flatten it.
7. Cutting a baby's hair before baptism can cause blindness.
8. Raising your hands over your head while pregnant may cause the cord to wrap around the baby's neck.
9. Moving heavy items can cause your "insides" to fall out.
10. If the baby is physically or mentally abnormal, God is punishing the parents.

CULTURAL SELF-ASSESSMENT EXERCISE 1

Self-Assessment

Answer the following questions related to the domain of family roles and organization for yourself.

1. Who makes most of the decisions in your house?
2. What type of decisions does the female(s) in your household make?
3. What type of decisions does the male(s) in your household make?
4. What are the duties of the women in your household?
5. What are the duties of the men in your household?
6. What should an adolescent do to make a good impression for him- or herself and for your family?
7. What should an adolescent *not* do to make a good impression for him- or herself and for your family?
8. What are adolescents forbidden to do in your family?
9. What is the most important role(s) for your family?
10. What are the priorities for your family?
11. What are the roles of the elderly in your family? Are they afforded high status?
12. Are there extended family members in your household?
13. What are the roles of extended family members in your household?
14. What gives the individual/family status in your household?
15. Is it acceptable to you for people to have children out of wedlock?
16. Is it acceptable to you for people to live together and not be married?
17. Is it acceptable to you for people not to marry?
18. Is it acceptable in your family for people to admit to being gay or lesbian?

CULTURAL SELF-ASSESSMENT EXERCISE 2

Understanding Others

1. List which of the questions above you would want to ask of your patient.
2. Identify how each question you chose would have relevance to the physical therapy program or interaction.

CULTURAL SELF-ASSESSMENT EXERCISE 3

Self-Assessment

Answer the following questions related to the domain of pregnancy and childbearing practices for yourself.

1. In your culture, what *should* women do to ensure having a healthy pregnancy and delivering a healthy baby?
2. In your culture, what should women *not* do to ensure having a healthy pregnancy and delivering a healthy baby?
3. In your culture, what things are women prohibited from doing while they are pregnant to ensure having a healthy pregnancy and delivering a healthy baby?
4. What things *should* you do and *not* do after childbirth to ensure your health and a healthy baby?
5. What things are you *prohibited from doing* after childbirth to ensure your health and a healthy baby?

CULTURAL SELF-ASSESSMENT EXERCISE 4

Understanding Others / Developing Awareness and Sensitivity

1. For both the family considerations and the pregnancy and childbearing considerations, list five potential barriers or misunderstandings that may occur between the physical therapist and the patient or the patient's family.
2. Describe how you would manage each of the conflicts you identified.

Vignette Questions

1. What cultural differences are manifested in this scenario?
2. Is the Mazzetti family more likely to value individualism or collectivism?
3. What potential conflicts or barriers might arise in this interaction?
4. What effect might the differences have on the effectiveness of the PT intervention?
5. How might the physical therapist manage this situation effectively?

CASE STUDY SCENARIO

*S*andra Yoder, a 34-year-old Amish woman with eight children, suffered head trauma in a buggy accident. Her husband, William, visits daily and always brings several children with him. William speaks little but carries an authoritative and supportive presence. The children are always well behaved and stand beside their father or their mother's bed or chair. Sandra's mother and grandmother, who live near the Yoder family, help care for the children and household chores. Other women in the community take turns preparing meals for the family, and often a meal is brought to Mrs. Yoder in the rehabilitation hospital.

Other Amish men in the community are assisting Mr. Yoder with the farm work. Mrs. Yoder seems to be uncomfortable with the nursing staff assisting her with bathing and dressing needs. Instead, her three sisters take turns assisting her with these activities of daily living (ADLs). This becomes a problem when the occupational therapist wants her to practice these ADLs.

The physical therapist has been working with Mrs. Yoder on ambulation on the parallel bars. She has poor motor control and balance. The physical therapist expects that she has significant pain as she bears weight through her casted fractured tibia, but Mrs. Yoder offers no complaint and gives no expression of pain. The rehabilitation team has begun to discuss discharge plans, and the physical therapist is recommending an electric wheelchair. The occupational therapist questions the plausibility of an electric wheelchair, as the family farm and house do not have electricity. The team begins to wonder about other discharge needs and challenges they might need to address.

1. What do you know about the Amish culture in terms of occupations, family structure, touch, and English language skills?

2. Are the Amish high or low context in terms of communication?

3. What are the roles of family and community members in the Amish community?

4. What kind of support from the family can you expect for the Yoder family?

5. What challenges does the rehabilitation team face throughout the discharge planning process?

6. Do you think that the family could accommodate an electric wheelchair?

7. From where might the Yoder family get the money for a wheelchair if they do not have the money on hand?

8. The Yoder family does not have an automobile. Do you foresee a problem with Mrs. Yoder being discharged and transported home in a buggy?

REFERENCES

1. Purnell L. Panamanians' practices for health promotion and the meaning of respect afforded them by healthcare providers. *J Transcult Nurs.* 1999;10:333–340.
2. Purnell L. Guatemalans' practices for health promotion and wellness and the meaning of respect afforded them by healthcare providers. *J Transcult Nurs.* 2000; 11:40–46.
3. Purnell L. The Purnell Model for Cultural Competence. In: Purnell L, Paulanka B, eds. *Transcultural Health Care: A Culturally Competent Approach.* 2nd ed. Philadelphia, Pa: FA Davis; 2003:8–40.
4. Hafizi H, Lipson J. People of Iranian heritage. In: Purnell L, Paulanka B, eds. *Transcultural Health Care: A Culturally Competent Approach.* 2nd ed. Philadelphia, Pa: FA Davis; 2003:177–193.
5. Juarbe T. People of Puerto Rican heritage. In: Purnell L, Paulanka B, eds. *Transcultural Health Care: A Culturally Competent Approach.* 2nd ed. Philadelphia, Pa: FA Davis; 2003:307–326.
6. Purnell L. People of Appalachian heritage. In: Purnell L, Paulanka B, eds. *Transcultural Health Care: A Culturally Competent Approach.* 2nd ed. Philadelphia, Pa: FA Davis; 2003:73–89.
7. Purnell L. People of Egyptian heritage [chapter on CD-ROM]. In: Purnell L, Paulanka B, eds. *Transcultural Health Care: A Culturally Competent Approach.* 2nd ed. Philadelphia, Pa: FA Davis; 2003.
8. Purnell L. *Cultural Competence for the Physical Therapist Working with Patients with Alternative Lifestyles.* La Crosse, Wis: APTA; 2003.
9. Purnell L, Kim S. People of Korean heritage. In: Purnell L, Paulanka B, eds. *Transcultural Health Care: A Culturally Competent Approach.* 2nd ed. Philadelphia, Pa: FA Davis; 2003:249–263.
10. Still O, Hodgins D. Navajo Indians. In: Purnell L, Paulanka B, eds. *Transcultural Health Care: A Culturally Competent Approach.* 2nd ed. Philadelphia, Pa: FA Davis; 2003:279–283.
11. Wang Y. People of Chinese heritage. In: Purnell L, Paulanka B, eds. *Transcultural Health Care: A Culturally Competent Approach.* 2nd ed. Philadelphia, Pa: FA Davis; 2003:106–121.
12. Zoucha R, Purnell L. People of Mexican heritage. In: Purnell L, Paulanka B, eds. *Transcultural Health Care: A Culturally Competent Approach.* 2nd ed. Philadelphia, Pa: FA Davis; 2003:264–278.
13. Althen G. *American Ways: A Guide for Foreigners in the United States.* Yarmouth, Me: Intercultural Press; 1988.
14. Datesman M, Crandall J, Kearney E. *The American Ways.* White Plains, NY: Prentice-Hall; 1997.
15. Kim E. *The Yin and Yang of American Culture.* Yarmouth, Me: Intercultural Press; 2001.
16. Steckler J. People of German heritage [chapter on CD-ROM]. In: Purnell L, Paulanka B, eds. *Transcultural Health Care: A Culturally Competent Approach.* 2nd ed. Philadelphia, Pa: FA Davis; 2003.
17. Glanville C. People of African American heritage. In: Purnell L, Paulanka B, eds. *Transcultural Health Care: A Culturally Competent Approach.* 2nd ed. Philadelphia, Pa: FA Davis; 2003:40–53.
18. *Time Almanac.* Boston, Mass: Time; 2001.
19. Hill R. *We Europeans.* Brussels: Europublications; 1995.
20. Hillman S. People of Italian heritage. In: Purnell L, Paulanka B, eds. *Transcultural Health Care: A Culturally Competent Approach.* 2nd ed. Philadelphia, Pa: FA Davis; 2003:205–217.
21. Sharts-Hopko N. People of Japanese heritage. In: Purnell L, Paulanka B, eds. *Transcultural Health Care: A Culturally Competent Approach.* 2nd ed. Philadelphia, Pa: FA Davis; 2003:218–233.
22. Zahn L. *Asian Americans.* Sudbury, Mass: Jones and Bartlett; 2003.
23. Purnell L. People of Cuban heritage. In: Purnell L, Paulanka B, eds. *Transcultural Health Care: A Culturally Competent Approach.* 2nd ed. Philadelphia, Pa: FA Davis; 2003:122–137.
24. Pacquiao D. People of Filipino heritage. In: Purnell L, Paulanka B, eds. *Transcultural Health Care: A Culturally Competent Approach.* 2nd ed. Philadelphia, Pa: FA Davis; 2003:138–159.
25. Jambanathan J. People of Hindu heritage [chapter on CD-ROM]. In: Purnell L, Paulanka B, eds. *Transcultural Health Care: A Culturally Competent Approach.* 2nd ed. Philadelphia, Pa: FA Davis; 2003
26. Kohls RR. *Learning to Think Korean: A Guide to Living and Working in Korea.* Yarmouth, Me: Intercultural Press; 2001.
27. Bureau of the Census. American community survey and supplementary survey noncore. Available at: http://www.census.gov/acs/www/Downloads/noncore.pdf. Accessed January 11, 2004.
28. Judge orders executions for lesbian duo. *Washington Blade.* February 23, 2001:13.
29. Office of Personnel Management. Family friendly leave policies. Available at: http://www.opm.gov/oca/leave/INDEX.asp. Accessed January 11, 2004.
30. Nowak T. People of Vietnamese heritage. In: Purnell L, Paulanka B, eds. *Transcultural Health Care: A Culturally Competent Approach.* 2nd ed. Philadelphia, Pa: FA Davis; 2003:327–344.

Chapter 6

Exploring Cultural Workforce Issues

● Larry D. Purnell, PhD, RN
● Jill Black Lattanzi, PT, EdD

*M*s. Halifizi, a 25-year-old Iranian Muslim immigrant, applies to enter physical therapy school. Her credentials are good, with a 4.0 grade point average in her undergraduate training. She expresses a strong desire to help people heal and has made application to your program. Ms. Halifizi dresses in traditional garb and is draped so that only her eyes show. You wonder how you will negotiate the requirements regarding draping and disrobing for the practice of manual techniques and how she will be able to perform on her clinical affiliations.

Culture in the Workplace

Not only must physical therapists be prepared to work with patients who are culturally different than they are, they also need to be equipped to interact effectively with co-workers and fellow students who bring their own cultures to the workplace or school. The fourth domain of the Model for Cultural Competence is workforce issues. Factors that affect these issues include language barriers, degree of assimilation and acculturation, and issues related to autonomy. Moreover, gender roles, cultural communication styles, healthcare practices of the country of origin, and selected concepts from all other domains affect workforce issues in a multicultural work or school environment (Fig. 6-1). Conflicts that occur among those in a homogeneous cul-ture in healthcare organizations or classrooms may be intensified in a multicultural workforce, even if the participants are knowledgeable about each other's culture. However, everyone has the potential to experience enrichment within a multicultural workforce or classroom (Figs. 6-2 and 6-3).

Hofstede[1] conducted extensive research for IBM on the workplace environments of more than 50 modern nations and identified five culturally related dimensions influencing organizations. The first is defined as *power/distance* and refers to the extent to which a society accepts or rejects human equality. Cultures with a high level of power/distance expect power to be distributed unequally and accept subservient roles more readily. Birth order and kinship dictate social status and power. A low–power/distance culture values human equality and is more likely to reject hierarchy and promotion based upon seniority.[1] Within organizations, power/distance is determined by the degree to which authority and leadership are centralized. A high–power/distance organization maintains a high degree of control at the upper management level, while in a low–power/distance organization subordinates participate in the decision making that will influence their work practices.[2]

Reflective Exercise

• Is your workplace or school characterized by a high power/distance or low power/distance dimension? • Which do you prefer? • What challenges or discomfort do you encounter when subjected to the opposite approach?

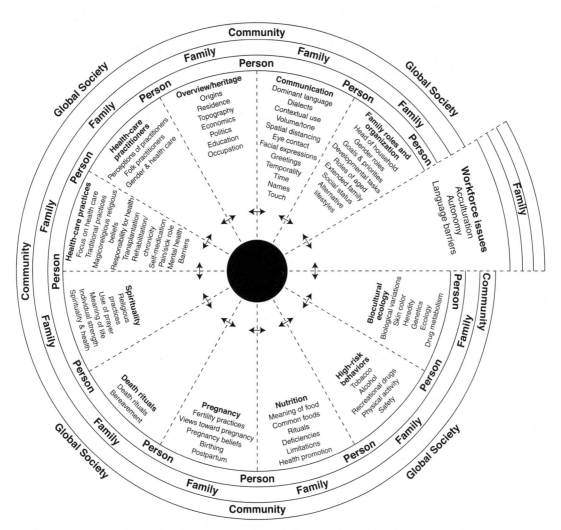

FIGURE 6.1 Workforce issues domain. (Adapted from Purnell, L. D., & Paulanka, B. J. (1998). The Purnell Model for Cultural Competence. In L. D. Purnell & B. J. Paulanka (Eds.), *Transcultural health care: A culturally competent approach* (p. 10). Philadelphia: F.A. Davis.)

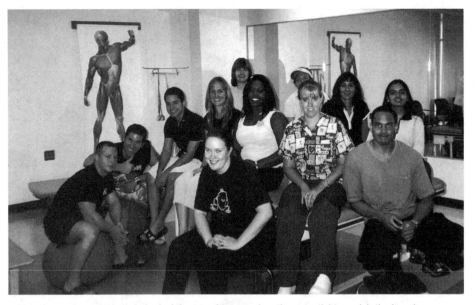

FIGURE 6.2 Diversity in the physical therapy classroom has the potential to enrich the learning environment.

The second of Hofstede's dimensions is called *uncertainty avoidance* and denotes the degree to which a culture is comfortable or uncomfortable with unstructured or unpredictable situations. Some societies socialize members into accepting

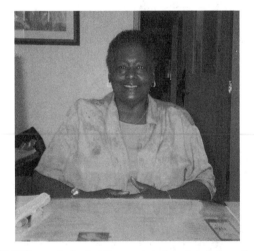

FIGURE 6.3 A physical therapy department or clinic workforce includes office staff, transporters, aides, and others in addition to the licensed clinicians.

that the future is unknown and that little can be done to alter it, and are described as weak uncertainty avoidance. Other societies teach members that the future can be influenced or controlled, and exhibit strong uncertainty avoidance. Within organizations, strong uncertainty avoidance manifests as numerous policies and procedures designed to cope with uncertainty and control the future. With weak uncertainty avoidance, organizations allow for ambiguity and individual initiative, with less emphasis on control and policy.[1,2]

Masculinity/femininity is another Hofstede dimension of workplace culture and measures the division of roles between the sexes. Masculine societies stress values such as assertiveness, acquisition of money, and disregard for others. In contrast, cooperation among people, conservation of the environment, and consideration for quality of life are values held by both sexes in a feminine society or organization.[1,2]

Finally, Hofstede identified *individualism/collectivism* as an important dimension of organizations that considers the relationships between an individual and his or her family or group. An individualistic viewpoint centers on the individual, with little regard for the extended family, group, or organization. Collectivism, on the other hand, holds the group or organization in high regard and demonstrates loyalty and commitment to the interests of the group before personal interests.[1] The consideration of individualistic and collectivistic characteristics provides a useful means of assessing and organizing cultural differences and is used in this chapter and throughout this text to describe cultural variations.

For example, individualistic cultures place high importance on timeliness and punctuality[3-7] while collectivist cultures value people and relationships more than they value timeliness.[8-11] Thus, collectivist cultures hold a loose understanding of time and timeliness in comparison with individualistic cultures. In an individualistic culture, if one is more than a minute or two late, an apology is expected, and if one is late by more than 5 or 10 minutes, a more elaborate apology is expected. When people know they are going to be late for a meeting, they are expected to call or send a message indicating that they will be late. The convener of the meeting or teacher in a classroom is expected to start and stop on time, out of respect for the other people in attendance. In contrast, in Panamanian,[12] Mexican,[11] and other collectivistic cultures, a meeting or class starts when the majority of people arrive, unless the meeting is with a high official.[13] If the meeting is with a high-ranking party, then the participants will be on time but the high official will most likely be late. However, in social situations in the United States, a person can be 15 or more minutes late, depending on the importance of the gathering. In such an instance, an apology is not really necessary or expected; however, most Americans will politely provide a reason for the tardiness.[14]

The American workforce stresses efficiency ("time is money"), operational procedures on how to get things done, accomplishing tasks, and proactive problem solving. Intuitive abilities and common sense are not valued as highly as technical abilities.[6,10] A high value is placed on the scientific method, where everything has to be proven. Americans want to know *why* more than *what,* and will search for a single factor that is the cause of the problem and the reason something is to be done in a specific way. Pragmatism is valued.

In individualistic European American cultures, "doing" is valued. In contrast, collectivistic cultures such as Chinese, Brazilian, and Latin American, to name a few,[15-18] are highly contextualized and look at workforce issues from a more holistic, introspective, and intuitive perspective, rather than relying on data. The collectivist culture values "being" rather than "doing," placing a higher emphasis on the relationships and the meanings of the task than on the accomplishment of the task.

Reflective Exercise

• Are you normally on time for work? • For meetings? • For other appointments? • Why or why not? • How do you feel when other people are late and you are on time?

Reflective Exercise

• Are you normally on time for social engagements? • Why or why not? • How do you feel when other people are late and you are on time?

In the low-context dominant U.S. culture, meetings have a predetermined agenda (although items can be added at the beginning of the meeting), and the agenda is expected to be followed. Americans vote on almost every item on an agenda, including approving the agenda itself. Communication is explicit, with little reliance on context. The verbal or written words expressed are intended to communicate the complete meaning.[14] High-context cultures assume shared knowledge and understanding based on the context, and have need of fewer words to express the thought. Someone from a high-context culture will glean much more from the context of the communication, and someone of a low-context culture will miss the cues that are being sent. Hence, interactions between persons of a high-context and a low-context culture are vulnerable to communication breakdowns. Tables 6-1 and 6-2 describe a few examples of communication breakdowns or misunderstandings.

TABLE 6.1

Common Misconceptions

Japanese can find Americans to be offensively blunt.

Americans can find Japanese to be secretive, devious, and bafflingly unforthcoming with information.

French can feel that Germans insult their intelligence by explaining the obvious.

Germans can feel that French managers provide no direction.

Source: *Differences in Cultures* (n.d.).[19]

TABLE 6.2

Some Perceptions of Americans

Europe and especially England: "Americans are stupid and unsubtle. And they are fat and bad dressers."

Finland: "Americans always want to say your name: 'That's a nice tie, Mikko. Hi, Mikko. How are you, Mikko?'"

India: "Americans are always in a hurry. Just watch the way they walk down the street."

Kenya: "Americans are distant. They are not really close to other people—even other Americans."

Turkey: "Once we were out in a rural area in the middle of nowhere and saw an American come to a stop sign. Though he could see in both directions for miles, and there was no traffic, he still stopped!"

Colombia: "In the United States, they think that life is only work."

Indonesia: "In the United States everything has to be talked about and analyzed. Even the littlest thing has to be 'Why, why, why?'"

Ethiopia: "The American is very explicit. He wants a 'yes' or 'no.' If someone tries to speak figuratively, the American is confused."

Iran: "The first time my American professor told me 'I don't know, I will have to look it up,' I was shocked. I asked myself, 'Why is he teaching me?'"

Source: *Differences in Cultures* (n.d.).[19]

Reflective Exercise

• Do you feel that everything has to be proven scientifically to be effective? • Is there room for intuitive interventions in your practice?

Reflective Exercise

• What communication barriers might occur between someone coming from a low-context culture and someone coming from a high-context culture?

Reflective Exercise

• How important is it to you to have strong verbal skills? • Do you expect your superiors to have strong verbal skills? • How do you feel about co-workers and superiors who do not have strong verbal skills or speak the English language less than "perfectly"?

Most European Americans place a high value on "fairness" and rely heavily on procedures and policies in the decision-making process; everyone is expected to have a job description.[14] However, their value for individualism, where the individual is seen as the most important element in society, favors a person's decision to further his or her own career over the interests of the employer. Therefore, people frequently demonstrate little loyalty to the organization; they leave one position to take a position with another company for better opportunities. In organizations where people generally conform out of fear of failure, there is a hierarchical order for decision making, and the person who succeeds is the one with strong verbal skills who conforms to the hierarchy's expectations. A well-liked person is one who does not stand out too much from the crowd. Frequently, others view a person with a high level of competence who stands out as a threat. Thus, to be successful in the highly technical American workforce, get the facts, control your feelings, practice precise and technical communication skills, be informal and direct, and clearly and explicitly state your conclusion.

Highly contextualized collectivistic cultures are more likely to operate from positions of hierarchy; communications tend to be more indirect and relationships more formal.[6,7,10,20]

Reflective Exercise

• In what ways might a person with a more informal and direct style of communication offend someone more accustomed to a more formal and indirect style of communication?

In the dominant U.S. culture, everything is given a time frame and deadlines are expected to be respected. In these situations, American values treat the needs of individuals as subservient to the needs of the organization. Collectivist cultures value the needs of the group, and many aspects of communication are determined by context. Hofstede[1] studied and identified an individualism index value for 50 countries and 3 regions. Nath[2] summarizes Hofstede's work as follows:

The main finding to emerge from Hofstede's work is that organizations are heavily culture bound. This not only affects people's behaviors within organizations but also influences the likelihood of successfully transporting theories of organization and management styles from one culture to another. Management and organizing are both culturally bound because they involve the manipulation of symbols that have meaning to the people involved.... Through a better understanding and awareness of a culture's values and the attitudes expressed by its members, one can better understand and interpret the behavior of organizations. (p. 28)

Gardenswartz and Rowe[21] identify four layers of diversity when considering diverse teams at work. They propose that each employee has his or her particular personality at the core; internal dimensions consisting of age, gender, sexual orientation, physical ability, ethnicity, and race as a second layer; and a third layer of external dimensions encompassing geographical location, income, personal habits, recreational habits, religion, educational background, work experience, appearance, parental status, and marital status.

These three layers closely resemble Purnell's description of primary and secondary characteristics.

Reflective Exercise

• Hofstede identifies the main organizational paradigm in the United States as "the market," in China "the family," and in Islamic countries "the pyramid." What evidence do you see in your physical therapy practice of "the market" as a driving organization force? • How might someone from another cultural organization struggle to work within the U.S. organization paradigm?

A fourth layer describes various organizational dimensions, including: functional level/classification, work content/field, division/department/unit/group, seniority, work location, union affiliation, and management status. They propose that the work culture of the individual is influenced by all four layers, and the understanding of potential differences will enhance the operation of the diverse team. Within the organization dimension, they note that work habits and practices may vary such that some place an emphasis on the task, issue or expect rewards based on individual achievement, and find intrinsic value in work. On the other hand, some place greater emphasis on relationships rather than the task, offer or expect rewards based on seniority or relationships, and regard work as a necessity of life.[21] An understanding of one's organizational dimension of culture will facilitate positive outcomes and relationships at work.

Reflective Exercise

• Give three examples of how organizational culture might affect a physical therapy practice.

Demographics of Immigrant and Minority Employment

The foreign-born workforce is now a major part of the economy in all regions of the United States.[22] Many of the recent immigrants lack a high school education, and many others immigrated with advanced educational degrees. The diversity of skills and marketability spans the diversity of the immigrants. Figure 6-4 shows the changes in the foreign-born component of the U.S. labor force by ethnic origin over the last 20 years, and Figure 6-5 illustrates the change in employment by industry.

Minority groups are underrepresented among healthcare professionals. Of physical therapists in the United States, only 0.5% are of American Indian/Alaskan Native heritage, 1.3% are of African American/black heritage, 1.9% are of Hispanic/Latino heritage, 4.1% are of Asian/

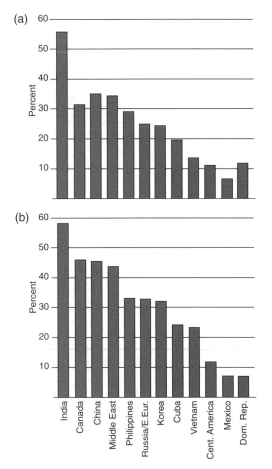

FIGURE 6.4 U.S. labor force of foreign-born by ethnic origin over the last 20 years. (Data from U.S. Bureau of the Census, Public Microdata Sample, 1980 and 1990, and Current Population Survey, 2000.)

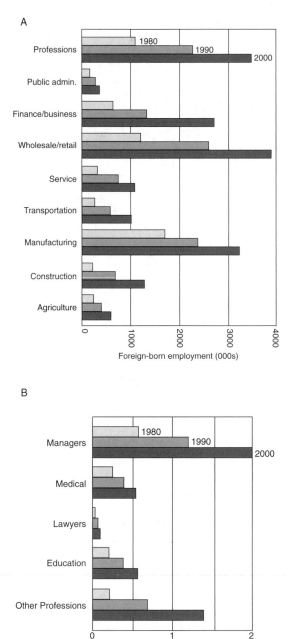

FIGURE 6.5 Changes in the employment of immigrants by industry. (*A*) Change in foreign-born employees by industry in the United States, 1980, 1990, and 2000. (*B*) Size of the immigrant labor force by professional occupation. (Data from U.S. Bureau of the Census, Public Microdata Sample, 1980 and 1990, and Current Population Survey, 2000.)

Pacific Islander heritage, and the remainder (92.2%) are white.[23] Of registered nurses (RNs) in the United States, only 0.5% are of Native American/Alaskan Native heritage, 1.6% are of Hispanic/Latino heritage, 3.4% are of Asian/Pacific Islander heritage, 4.2% are of black heritage, and the remainder (89.7%) are white.[24] Of the roughly 778,000 physicians in the United States, 65% are white, 19.4% percent are Asian/Pacific Islander, 7.9% are black, 6.9% are Hispanic, and 0.7% are Native American/Alaskan.[25] Figure 6-6 depicts the ethnic origin composition of the immigrant professional workforce in 2000.

The physical therapy profession, as practiced in the United States, carries certain expectations and requirements of its professionals. Physical therapy requires patients to disrobe to ensure accurate assessment of dysfunctions and impairments. In addition, physical touch is an essential component of palpation skills, massage, and manual techniques. Physical therapists are expected to be comfortable with physical touch and patients' disrobing while maintaining proper draping techniques. Likewise, physical therapists are expected to treat male and female patients of all cultures without discrimination.

While the physical therapy profession as a whole is quite homogeneous in composition, one of the stated goals of the American Physical Therapy Association is to increase the cultural diversity of the physical therapy workforce, academic professors, and clinical instructors (Fig. 6-7).[26] An increase in diversity brings the challenges of respecting, accepting, and working within cultural differences when they conflict with established professional work practices and expectations.

Reflective Exercise

• What is the ethnic/racial/cultural makeup of your workforce/department/class? • Is there a difference between the employees/students and the leaders/teachers? • How do you explain the difference or similarity?

The educational preparation of physical therapists in some countries is not comparable to the educational requirements of physical therapists in the United States. The variety of healthcare providers in the United States, such as physical therapists, radiologic technicians, occupational therapists, social service workers, electrocardiogram technicians, and respiratory therapists, may not exist in other countries. For example, in parts of Central America, there may be only one or two physical therapists for an entire community (S. Willaims, Belize, personal communication, January 1998). In Spain, nurses are trained to do radiology procedures and physical therapy interventions to a greater degree than they are in the United States (Roberto Gonzales, Alicante, Spain, personal communication, October 2000).

Foreign-trained physical therapists who wish to practice in the United States must prove themselves qualified for licensure. The first step involves having their physical therapy program transcript evaluated. Individuals sanctioned by the Federation of State Boards of Physical Therapy evaluate the transcripts and course syllabi for content and competencies that would be comparable with those of programs accredited in the United States. Once determined to meet the standard, the foreign-trained applicant is eligible to sit for the State Licensure Examination. Upon successful completion of the Licensure examination, the foreign-trained applicant is eligible to practice in the state as a physical therapist.

Despite the arduous credentialing process, differences may exist in philosophy, in specialization, and in communication patterns. For

Reflection 6.1

I am from Brazil and received my physical therapy training in Brazil. The thing that I found most unusual about physical therapy practice in the United States was the concept of patient confidentiality because in my country, the idea that a lawsuit could be brought against a therapist for talking about a patient and their diagnosis, etc. is unheard of.

Marcia Gahman, PT

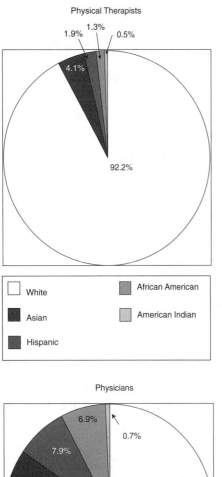

Physical Therapists

1.9% 1.3% 0.5%

4.1%

92.2%

White   African American

Asian   American Indian

Hispanic

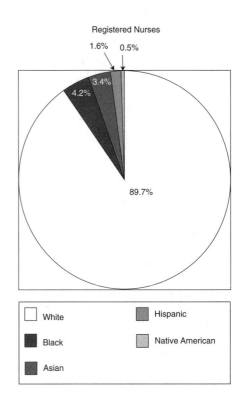

Registered Nurses

1.6% 0.5%

3.4%

4.2%

89.7%

White   Hispanic

Black   Native American

Asian

Physicians

6.9%

7.9%

0.7%

19.4%

65%

White   Hispanic

Black   Native American

Asian

FIGURE 6.6 Ethnicities of physical therapists, registered nurses, and physicians.

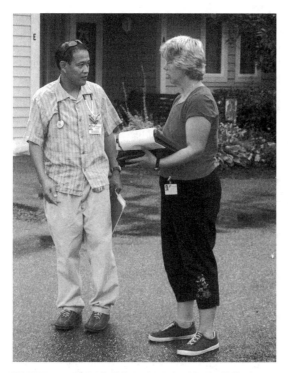

FIGURE 6.7 A physical therapist trained in the Philippines and a PTA trained in the United States confer on a home care case they share.

example, some cultures discourage students from asking questions of those in authority over them. Such questioning is regarded as disrespectful. Likewise, in work relationships with those in authority and with patients, different patterns of communication might exist.[13,27,28]

Timeliness and punctuality are two culturally based attitudes that can create serious problems in the multicultural workforce. In some situations, conflicts may arise over the issue of reporting to work on time or on an assigned day. The lack of adherence to time demands in other countries is often in direct opposition to the American ethic for punctuality. Thus, the importance of punctuality must be made clear on initial employment.

Healthcare administration and management initiatives to support a diverse work environment include (a) cultural competence and diversity workshops, (b) cultural celebrations, (c) a specific orientation to America's changing healthcare system, (d) providing cultural brokers as mentors

> ### Reflection 6.2
>
> I am from Germany and I received my PT training in Germany. The hardest adjustment I had to make to physical therapy practice in the United States was the amount of documentation required. Because of socialized healthcare and differences in the legal system, we did not have to document progress.
>
> *Christina Parsons, PT*

or preceptors to assist new immigrants in learning about the American workforce, and (e) identifying ways to work more effectively with employees of diverse backgrounds. Orientation classes may need to include topics such as (a) the difference in the length of patients' hospital stays in the United States compared with those in the employees' countries of origin, (b) the diversity in health professionals' responsibilities, (c) the influence of insurance companies in healthcare decision making, and (d) concerns related to malpractice.

Reflective Exercise

• What are the most important items to include in an orientation program for employees who are native to the U.S. workforce? • What are the most important items to include in an orientation program for employees who are not native to the U.S. workforce?

Issues Related to Autonomy

Cultural differences related to assertiveness influence how healthcare practitioners view each other. Specifically, Asian healthcare physical therapists may not be as assertive with physicians as American physical therapists.[7,9,17] The concept of the physical therapist being dependent on physicians and male administrators is inseparable from the Muslim concept of women being subject to the authority of husbands, fathers, and elder brothers.[29] These differences can pose problems in the American healthcare system.

Reflective Exercise

• In your work environment, is there a difference with assertiveness between the genders? • Between professional groups? • How do you teach employees to be assertive when they are hesitant to do so? • How would this change among diverse cultural groups? • How closely do the cultural characteristics of your profession match your personal cultural characteristics?

When people speak in their native language at work, it may become a source of contention for both patients and healthcare personnel. Negative interpretations of behaviors can be detrimental to working relationships and need to be clearly understood and communicated. The employees who speak in another language may not intend to exclude or offend others but simply find it easier to articulate ideas, feelings, and humor in their native language.

Humor is highly specific to culture, and many jokes are untranslatable. One must be careful in joking with someone from another culture, and recognize that the joke may be easily misunderstood.

Reflective Exercise

• Have you been in situations where people in the workforce/classroom spoke in a language different from yours? • How do you feel about this? • In what situations should people be permitted to speak in a foreign language in the work setting?

Organizational Self–Assessment

Few healthcare organizations exist today that do not have the need to address the language diversity of its employees, patients, and visitors. Table 6-3 lists some elements that should be in place to ensure a culturally safe organization.

TABLE 6.3

Organizational Self-Assessment

1. Written policies are in place that address the needs of non–English-speaking employees, visitors, and patients.
2. Guidelines are in place that address the need for an interpreter.
3. Guidelines exist for interpreters.
4. Directional and informational signs meet the diverse language needs of patients and visitors.
5. Discharge instructions are available in the languages of the diverse population.
6. Orientation and training programs address cultural diversity for the patient and employee population.
7. Community resources are available for the diverse population of the community.
8. Patient and staff satisfaction surveys and grievance procedures are available in the languages spoken in the community.
9. Reading materials in family and patient area are available in the languages spoken in the community.
10. Consent forms are available in the languages of the population served.
11. Ethics committees include ethnicities of the patient population, including community members.
12. The organization actively recruits bilingual staff.
13. The organization provides English classes for non-English-speaking employees and foreign language classes for employees working with diverse non-English-speaking patients and visitors.
14. The Board of Governors includes the diversity of the patient population.
15. The library has resources for cultural diversity.
16. The organization attempts to accommodate religious needs in its staffing schedules.
17. Patient education materials, including videos, are in several languages and include culturally diverse populations.
18. The mission statement incorporates the values of cultural diversity.

Conclusion

Diversity in the workplace and in the classroom has the potential to enrich and complicate the environment. Challenges may arise with language barriers; issues related to autonomy, gender roles, cultural communication styles and learning styles; and healthcare practices of the country of origin. While the diversity may lead to possible misunderstandings and cultural barriers, the culturally competent physical therapist, administrator, student, or educator will recognize the value in the diversity, will demonstrate respect for the differences, and will strive to create a flexible environment where all can learn from one another and grow.

CULTURAL SELF-ASSESSMENT EXERCISE 1

Self-Assessment

Answer the following questions regarding the workforce domain for yourself.

1. What is the gender and ethnicity of personnel in decision-making positions according to managerial level?
2. What should one do to maintain positive working relationships in your organization?
3. What should one *not* do to maintain positive working relationships in your organization?
4. What behaviors from staff would entail immediate suspension or dismissal from the organization?
5. What behaviors from managers would lead to immediate suspension or discharge in your organization?
6. What does one do to gain status in your organization?
7. How important is punctuality in your organization?
8. How important is productivity in your organization?
9. How much flexibility is permitted for policies and procedures in your organization?
10. Do staff relate differently to males versus females in hierarchical positions?
11. How assertive are you in your communications?
12. When is it acceptable to be assertive and when is it not acceptable?
13. How is physical therapy practiced differently in your home country from the way it is practiced in the United States (if appropriate)?

CULTURAL SELF-ASSESSMENT EXERCISE 2

Understanding Others / Recognizing Conflicts

1. Answers to which of the questions above would be important to learn of your employee, student, colleague, or classmate of another culture?
2. Identify three potential miscommunications or conflicts that might arise from ignorance of the other's culture.
3. Describe how you would manage each of the miscommunications or conflicts you identified.

CULTURAL SELF-ASSESSMENT EXERCISE 3

Exploring Potential Misconceptions

In the common misconception statements below, what differences in cultural context are potentially contributing to each of the beliefs?

1. Japanese can find Americans to be offensively blunt.
2. Americans can find Japanese to be secretive, devious, and bafflingly unforthcoming with information.
3. French can feel that Germans insult their intelligence by explaining the obvious.
4. Germans can feel that French managers provide no direction.

Source: *Differences in Cultures* (n.d.).

CULTURAL SELF-ASSESSMENT EXERCISE 4

Exploring Potential Perceptions of Americans

Look at the "perceptions of Americans" in Table 6–2.

1. Which ones do you see in yourself?
2. Which ones don't you see in yourself?
3. For each one, identify the cultural misunderstanding that is occurring.
4. How might each of these perceptions cause problems in the workplace or classroom?

Vignette Questions

1. What are the cultural issues?
2. How would you feel if you were Ms. Halifizi?
3. How would you feel if you were another student in the class?
4. How might the instructor negotiate the presenting issues in a culturally appropriate manner?
5. What professional expectations and requirements have been in conflict or have caused discomfort for you?

CASE STUDY SCENARIO

You have just graduated from an accredited physical therapy school in the United States, and your first job is at an outpatient orthopedic center connected with a major metropolitan hospital. Your immediate supervisor was trained in the Philippines and has been practicing in the United States for 5 years. Your other two co-workers were also trained in the Philippines and have been practicing here 2 and 3 years.

You look forward to beginning your new job and applying the orthopedic principles you learned in your school. Soon, however, you realize that your approach to physical therapy evaluation and intervention is quite different from those of your co-workers. Likewise, the interaction style that your co-workers have with their patients is much more formal than yours. It becomes awkward when several patients note the difference in interaction style as well, and acknowledge to you in secret that they would prefer to work with you. Finally, you find it difficult to get to know your co-workers. They tend to sit together to eat and speak in their own language over lunch.

1. What culture-specific challenges are you facing?

2. How should you deal with the differences in treatment philosophy?

3. What can you discern about the competency level of the foreign-trained physical therapist?

4. How should you handle the differences in interaction styles?

5. What considerations are involved in interacting with the supervisor?

6. What should you do to get to know your co-workers better?

REFERENCES

1. Hofstede G. *Culture's Consequences: Comparing Values, Behaviors, Institutions, and Organizations across Nations.* 2nd ed. Thousand Oaks, Calif: Sage; 1980.
2. Nath R. *Comparative Management: A Regional View.* Cambridge, Mass: Ballinger; 1988.
3. Althen G. *American Ways: A Guide for Foreigners in the United States.* Yarmouth, Me: Intercultural Press; 1988.
4. Datesman M, Crandall J, Kearney E. *The American Ways.* White Plains, NY: Prentice-Hall; 1997.
5. Hill R. *We Europeans.* Brussels: Europublications; 1995.
6. Kim E. *The Yin and Yang of American Culture.* Yarmouth, Me: Intercultural Press; 2001.
7. Purnell L, Kim S. People of Korean heritage. In: Purnell L, Paulanka B, eds. *Transcultural Health Care: A Culturally Competent Approach.* 2nd ed. Philadelphia, Pa: FA Davis; 2003:249–263.
8. Kohls RR. *Learning to Think Korean: A Guide to Living and Working in Korea.* Yarmouth, Me: Intercultural Press; 2001.
9. Pacquiao D. People of Filipino heritage. In: Purnell L, Paulanka B, eds. *Transcultural Health Care: A Culturally Competent Approach.* 2nd ed. Philadelphia, Pa: FA Davis; 2003:138–159.
10. Purnell L. The Purnell Model for Cultural Competence. In: Purnell L, Paulanka B, eds. *Transcultural Health Care: A Culturally Competent Approach.* 2nd ed. Philadelphia, Pa: FA Davis; 2003:8–40.
11. Zoucha R, Purnell L. People of Mexican heritage. In: Purnell L, Paulanka B, eds. *Transcultural Health Care: A Culturally Competent Approach.* 2nd ed. Philadelphia, Pa: FA Davis; 2003:264–278.
12. Purnell L. Panamanians' practices for health promotion and the meaning of respect afforded them by healthcare providers. *J Transcult Nurs.* 1999;10:333–340.
13. Still O, Hodgins D. Navajo Indians. In: Purnell L, Paulanka B, eds. *Transcultural Health Care: A Culturally Competent Approach.* 2nd ed. Philadelphia, Pa: FA Davis; 2003:279–283.
14. Stewart EC. *American Cultural Patterns: A Cross-Cultural Perspective.* Yarmouth, Me: Intercultural Press; 1972.
15. Purnell L. People of Brazilian heritage [chapter on CD-ROM]. In: Purnell L, Paulanka B, eds. *Transcultural Health Care: A Culturally Competent Approach.* 2nd ed. Philadelphia, Pa: FA Davis; 2003.
16. Stephenson S. *Understanding Spanish Speaking South Americans.* Yarmouth, Me: Intercultural Press; 2003.
17. Wang Y. People of Chinese heritage. In: Purnell L, Paulanka B, eds. *Transcultural Health Care: A Culturally Competent Approach.* 2nd ed. Philadelphia, Pa: FA Davis; 2003:106–121.
18. Zahn L. *Asian Americans.* Sudbury, Mass: Jones and Bartlett; 2003.
19. Differences in cultures. Available at: http://www.analytictech.com/mb021/cultural.htm. Accessed April 12, 2004.
20. Purnell L. People of Appalachian heritage. In: Purnell L, Paulanka B, eds. *Transcultural Health Care: A Culturally Competent Approach.* 2nd ed. Philadelphia, Pa: FA Davis; 2003:73–89.
21. Gardenswartz L, Rowe A. *Diverse Teams at Work.* Burr Ridge, Ill: Irwin; 1994.
22. Clark WAV. *Immigrants and the American Dream: Remaking the Middle Class.* New York: Guilford Press; 2003.
23. American Physical Therapy Association. Minority statistics. Available at: http://www.apta.org/About/special_interests/minorityaffairs. Accessed January 5, 2003.
24. American Nurses Association. Distribution by racial/ethnic group. Available at: http://www.nursingworld.org. Accessed August 13, 2001.
25. Total Physicians by Race Ethnicity (2003). http://www.ama-assn.org/ama/pub/category/12930.html. Accessed July 26, 2005.
26. American Physical Therapy Association. Cultural competence strategic plan. Available at: http://www.apta.org/Advocacy/minorityaffairs/CultCompPlan. Accessed December 17, 2003.
27. Hafizi H, Lipson J. People of Iranian heritage. In: Purnell L, Paulanka B, eds. *Transcultural Health Care: A Culturally Competent Approach.* 2nd ed. Philadelphia, Pa: FA Davis; 2003:177–193.
28. Kulwicki A. People of Arab heritage. In: Purnell L, Paulanka B, eds. *Transcultural Health Care: A Culturally Competent Approach.* 2nd ed. Philadelphia, Pa: FA Davis; 2003:90–105.
29. Harner R, Burns J, Marshall, P, Karmaliani R. Community-based nursing in Pakistan. *J Contin Educ Nurs.* 1994;25:130–132.

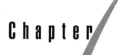

Chapter 7

Exploring High-Risk Health Behaviors, Biocultural Ecology, and Nutrition in Light of Culture

● Larry D. Purnell, PhD, RN
● Jill Black Lattanzi, PT, EdD

vignette

The Delgado family—Pedro, Rosa, and their four children ages 2, 8, 9, and 12 years—come to the physical therapy clinic in a pickup truck. Pedro, who fell from a ladder and fractured his left tibia and fibula while picking peaches, has weekly appointments for strengthening exercises and continued gait training with crutches. As the truck enters the parking lot, you notice that Pedro is driving and the older children are riding unrestrained in the open bed of the truck. As Pedro enters the clinic, he extinguishes a cigarette. Pedro is moderately obese and is not involved in a fitness program. He is 45 minutes late for his appointment.

High-Risk Health Behaviors

Cigarette Smoking

The domain *high-risk health behaviors* includes misuse of substances such as tobacco, alcohol, and recreational drugs; lack of physical activity; increased calorie consumption; nonuse of safety measures such as seatbelts, helmets, and safe driving practices; and neglecting safety measures to prevent the transmission of HIV and sexually transmitted diseases (Fig. 7-1). Although high-risk health behaviors are common to all ethnocultural groups, the interventions to decrease misuse vary among ethnocultural groups and individuals. Physical therapy programs will be impacted by a patient's use of tobacco, alcohol, and recreational drugs, as well as by a patient's obesity and/or lack of physical activity.

The incidence of cigarette smoking has been declining in the United States over the last 25 years but continues to remain steady or increase among newer immigrants (Fig. 7-2). Although

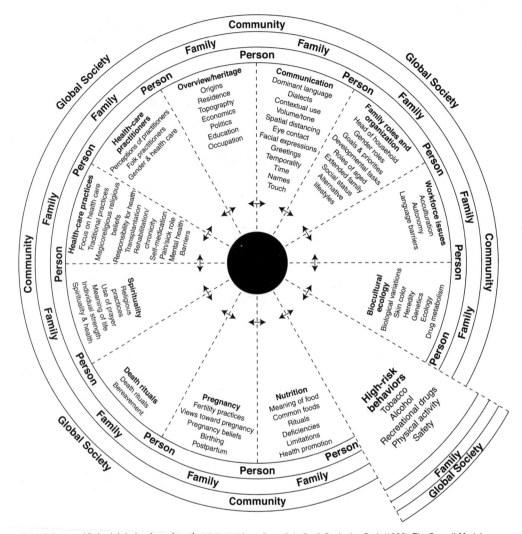

FIGURE 7.1 High-risk behaviors domain. (Adapted from Purnell, L. D., & Paulanka, B. J. (1998). The Purnell Model for Cultural Competence. In L. D. Purnell & B. J. Paulanka (Eds.), *Transcultural health care: A culturally competent approach* (p. 10). Philadelphia: F.A. Davis.)

black Americans smoke at the same rate as white Americans (28% to 34%), they (a) smoke fewer cigarettes than do white Americans, (b) take in 30% more nicotine per cigarette, and (c) take nearly 2 hours longer to clear nicotine metabolites from their bloodstream. Fewer black women than white women smoke, 22% versus 25%. The data for other ethnic groups indicate lower rates

of smoking for Asians compared with white Americans;[1] however, the data varies and is inconsistent across studies, suggesting regional variations (Fig. 7-3). Although most people are aware of the increased risk for cancer from smoking, many are not aware of the vasoconstrictive effects of tobacco, which impede the healing process.

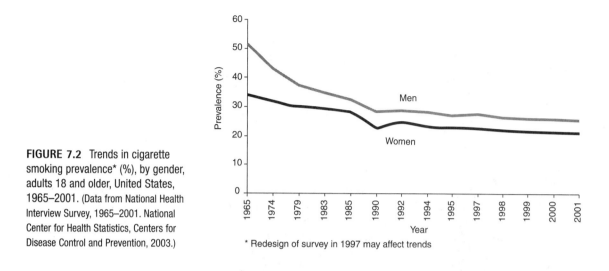

FIGURE 7.2 Trends in cigarette smoking prevalence* (%), by gender, adults 18 and older, United States, 1965–2001. (Data from National Health Interview Survey, 1965–2001. National Center for Health Statistics, Centers for Disease Control and Prevention, 2003.)

* Redesign of survey in 1997 may affect trends

Reflective Exercise

• What potential impact does smoking have on patients in a physical therapy program?

Obesity

A lack of health promotion and safety practices may be a major threat to the health of some people. Obesity falls into this category. The World Health Organization (WHO) estimated that over 300 million persons could be classified as obese as of the year 2000. This was up from 100 million as of 1995 (Fig. 7-4). In addition, WHO estimates that another 18 million children under the age of 5 are obese.[2] WHO defines overweight as a body mass index (BMI) of 25 or greater, obesity

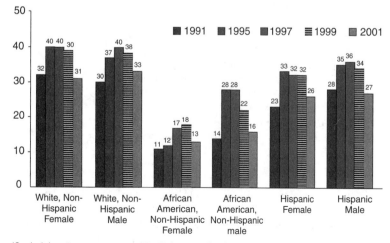

FIGURE 7.3 Current* cigarette smoking prevalence (%), by gender and race/ethnicity, high school students, United States, 1991–2001. (Data from Youth Risk Behavior Surveillance System, 1991, 1995, 1997, 1999, 2001. National Center for Chronic Disease Promotion and Health Promotion, Centers for Disease Control and Prevention, 2002.)

*Smoked cigarettes on one or more of the 30 days preceding the survey.

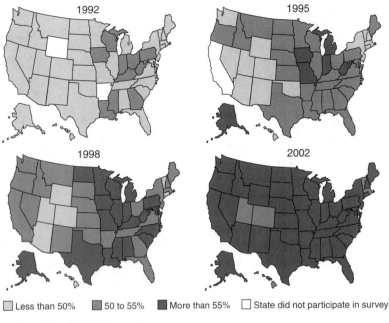

1992   1995   1998   2002

☐ Less than 50%   ■ 50 to 55%   ■ More than 55%   ☐ State did not participate in survey

*Body mass index of 25.0 kg/m² or greater

FIGURE 7.4 Trends in over-weight* prevalence (%), adults 18 and older, United States, 1992–2002. (Data from Behavioral Risk Factor Surveillance System, 1984–1995, 1998; and Public Use Data Tape, 2002. National Center for Chronic Disease Promotion and Health Promotion, Centers for Disease Control and Prevention, 1997, 2002, 2003.)

as a BMI of 30.0 or greater, and extreme obesity as a BMI of 40.0 or greater. BMI is calculated by dividing one's weight in kilograms by the square of one's height in meters. The adverse health consequences of obesity are many and include cardiovascular disease; stroke; type 2 diabetes; hypertension; cancers of the breast, endome-trium, prostate, and colon; and osteoarthritis.[3] Although the prevalence of obesity extends throughout the more developed and developing world, ethnicity also is a factor. For example, obesity is more prevalent among Amish women than among non-Amish women in Ohio.[4] Weight gain among the Amish may be related to the importance of food in the culture and the higher rates of pregnancy throughout childbear-ing years.[5,6]

The National Health and Nutrition Exam-ination Survey (NHANES) demonstrated a 64.5% prevalence of obesity in the United States. In a previous NHANES report encompassing 1988–1994, the prevalence rate had been 55.9%. Previously, from 1960 to 1980, the obesity rate

had been relatively stable (Fig. 7-5). The NHANES report categorizes subjects by three ethnic groups: non-Hispanic whites, non-Hispanic blacks, and Mexican Americans. While all ethnic groups showed an upward trend in the preva-lence of obesity between 1999 and 2000, Mexican American women were more obese than non-Hispanic white women, and non-Hispanic black women were statistically significantly more obese than Mexican American women in the United States.[7]

Reflective Exercise

• What negative impact does obesity have on health and wellness? • How does obesity impact a physical therapy program? • What role might physical therapy play in helping to control obesity?

A belief among many African Americans and people from Central America and the Caribbean is that a person who is overweight is more attrac-

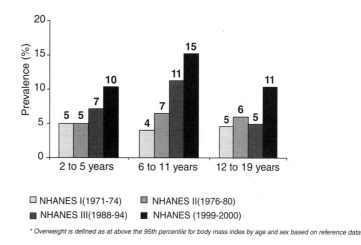

FIGURE 7.5 Trends in overweight* prevalence, children and adolescents, by age group (%), United States, 1971–2000. (Data from National Health Examination Survey, 1960–1962; National Health and Nutrition Examination Survey, 1971–1974, 1976–1980, 1988–1994, 1999–2000. National Center for Health Statistics, Centers for Disease Control and Prevention, 2002.)

☐ NHANES I(1971-74)   ▨ NHANES II(1976-80)
▪ NHANES III(1988-94)   ▪ NHANES (1999-2000)

* Overweight is defined as at above the 95th percentile for body mass index by age and sex based on reference data

tive and healthier than someone who is of "normal" weight (according to the American actuarial tables). A fat baby is a healthy baby. Obesity may affect physical therapy interventions by reducing aerobic capacity and by hindering functional activities.[8]

Reflective Exercise

• What are your personal beliefs about weight and health? • Do you agree with the dominant American belief that thinness correlates with desirability and beauty?

The cultural domain of high-risk behaviors is one area where healthcare providers can make a significant impact on patients' health status, regardless of the health discipline. High-risk health behaviors can be controlled through ethnic-specific interventions aimed at health promotion and health-risk prevention through educational programs in schools, business organizations, churches, and recreational and community centers, as well as through the use of one-on-one and family counseling techniques. Taking advantage of public communication technology can enhance participation in these programs if they are geared to the unique needs of the individual, family, or community.

Reflective Exercise

• How might a physical therapist effect a change in high-risk behaviors in a culturally competent manner? • What resources might the physical therapist use? • What venues might the physical therapist use?

Biocultural Ecology

The domain *biocultural ecology* identifies physical, biological, and physiological variations among ethnic and racial groups. These variations include skin color (the most obvious) and physical differences in body habitus; genetic, hereditary, endemic, and topographic diseases; psychological makeup of individuals; and the physiological differences that affect the way drugs are metabolized by the body (Fig. 7-6). The authors have not attempted to explain or justify the numerous and conflicting views on the genetic and environmental reasons for variations. In this chapter, observations of physical and genetic variations are identified. These observations may be more accurate with some individuals than with others. Frequently, intra-ethnic variations are greater than inter-ethnic variations, although there is no data that supports this age-old assumption. The

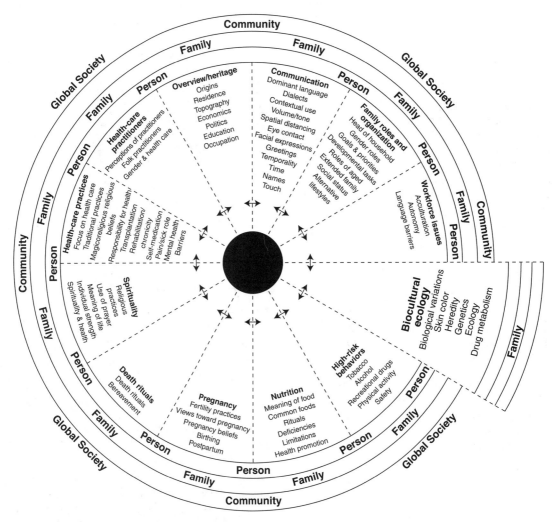

FIGURE 7.6 Biocultural ecology domain. (Adapted from Purnell, L. D., & Paulanka, B. J. (1998). The Purnell Model for Cultural Competence. In L. D. Purnell & B. J. Paulanka (Eds.), *Transcultural health care: A culturally competent approach* (p. 10). Philadelphia: F.A. Davis.)

Human Genome Project has identified 30,000 genes in human DNA and 3 billion chemical base pairs that make up human DNA; over 99% of the genetic code is shared by all racial groups.[9] Less than 1% may seem insignificant to some people, but this results in 3,000 genes and 30,000 chemical base pairs, which can be significant when it comes to assessment, interventions, and drug metabolism.

Skin Color and Other Biological Variations
Skin coloration is an important consideration for physical therapists because assessing the integumentary system requires different skills for dark-skinned people than for light-skinned people. Wounds, the healing of wounds, and scar tissue will appear different with different skin tones. To assess for oxygenation and cyanosis in dark-skinned people, the physical therapist must

examine the sclera, buccal mucosa, tongue, lips, nail beds, palms of the hands, and soles of the feet rather than rely on skin tone. Jaundice is more easily determined in Asians by assessing the sclera than by relying on the overall change in skin color. Physical therapists must establish a baseline skin color (by asking a family member or someone known to the individual), use direct sunlight if possible, observe areas with the least amount of pigmentation, palpate for rashes, and compare skin in corresponding areas. Inter-ethnic variations also occur in scar tissue formation. For example, African Americans are more likely to develop keloids, or overgrowths of connective tissue, creating a thicker, more fibrous scar.[10]

For people with fair skin, such as Appalachians,[11] Germans,[12] Polish,[13] Irish,[14] and British, to name a few, prolonged exposure to the sun places them at increased risk for skin cancer. However, this is not to say that people from other nationalities and with different skin color are not at risk for skin cancer; all people should be made aware of the harmful effects of prolonged exposure to the sun.

Reflective Exercise

• Do you have difficulty assessing wounds, rashes, and sunburn in people with darker skin?
• Do you have difficulty assessing oxygenation status and the presence of jaundice in people with dark skin?

Reflective Exercise

• What differences do you see among the ethno-cultural and racial groups with whom you work?
• Do these differences necessitate individualization for standard interventions?

Variations in body habitus occur among ethnic and racially diverse individuals. For example, the long bones of many blacks are significantly longer and narrower than those of whites,[10,15] and most Asians have narrower shoulders and wider hips compared with black and white individuals.[16] Many Vietnamese children are small by American standards and do not fall within the normal range on standardized American growth charts[16]—a trait that might be important for physical therapists determining age-appropriate physical abilities. Such biocultural data provide important information for physical therapists assessing health problems geared to the unique attributes of people of diverse cultures. Given the diverse gene pools, this type of information is often difficult to obtain.

Diseases and Health Conditions

Endemic diseases are those diseases that occur continuously in specific racial or ethnic groups. The leading causes of death in America continue to be heart disease, cancer, chronic obstructive lung diseases, unintentional injury, diabetes, and HIV. Generally speaking, all ethnic and cultural groups share these endemic illnesses and diseases, although the incidence varies somewhat among the groups. Cardiovascular disease is the leading killer of both men and women in all racial and ethnic groups in the United States. The causative factors that contribute to the development of cardiovascular disease include obesity (54.9%), lack of physical activity (27.7%), and smoking (22.9%).[17]

The leading sites of new cancer cases and deaths in the United States are listed in Figure 7-7. Although these same sites account for most cancers in non-white ethnic and racial groups, the order of occurrence differs. For example, prostate cancer is the highest reported cancer among American Indians,[18] blacks,[10] Filipinos,[19] Japanese,[20] and non-white Hispanic men.[21] In women, breast cancer incidence rates are highest in all groups except the Vietnamese, for whom cervical cancer rates rank higher. Stomach cancer appears in the top cancers for men and women in Asian populations except for Filipinos and Chinese women.[22] Cancer incidence rates and cancer death rates vary by race and ethnicity, as indicated in Figures 7-8 and 7-9. A more thorough description of the variations in the sites and incidence of cancer among racial and ethnic groups in the United States can be obtained from the National Cancer Institute.[22]

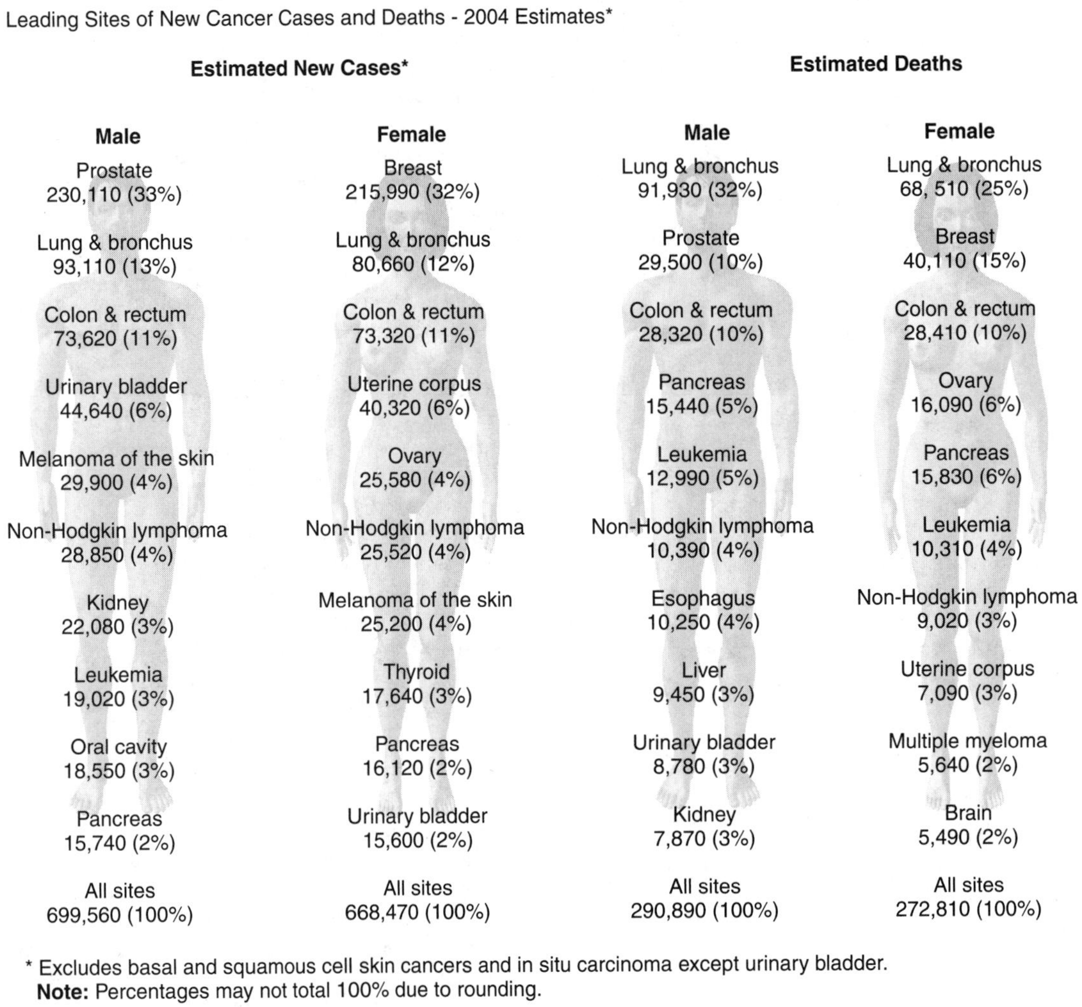

Leading Sites of New Cancer Cases and Deaths - 2004 Estimates*

Estimated New Cases*		**Estimated Deaths**	
Male	**Female**	**Male**	**Female**
Prostate 230,110 (33%)	Breast 215,990 (32%)	Lung & bronchus 91,930 (32%)	Lung & bronchus 68, 510 (25%)
Lung & bronchus 93,110 (13%)	Lung & bronchus 80,660 (12%)	Prostate 29,500 (10%)	Breast 40,110 (15%)
Colon & rectum 73,620 (11%)	Colon & rectum 73,320 (11%)	Colon & rectum 28,320 (10%)	Colon & rectum 28,410 (10%)
Urinary bladder 44,640 (6%)	Uterine corpus 40,320 (6%)	Pancreas 15,440 (5%)	Ovary 16,090 (6%)
Melanoma of the skin 29,900 (4%)	Ovary 25,580 (4%)	Leukemia 12,990 (5%)	Pancreas 15,830 (6%)
Non-Hodgkin lymphoma 28,850 (4%)	Non-Hodgkin lymphoma 25,520 (4%)	Non-Hodgkin lymphoma 10,390 (4%)	Leukemia 10,310 (4%)
Kidney 22,080 (3%)	Melanoma of the skin 25,200 (4%)	Esophagus 10,250 (4%)	Non-Hodgkin lymphoma 9,020 (3%)
Leukemia 19,020 (3%)	Thyroid 17,640 (3%)	Liver 9,450 (3%)	Uterine corpus 7,090 (3%)
Oral cavity 18,550 (3%)	Pancreas 16,120 (2%)	Urinary bladder 8,780 (3%)	Multiple myeloma 5,640 (2%)
Pancreas 15,740 (2%)	Urinary bladder 15,600 (2%)	Kidney 7,870 (3%)	Brain 5,490 (2%)
All sites 699,560 (100%)	All sites 668,470 (100%)	All sites 290,890 (100%)	All sites 272,810 (100%)

* Excludes basal and squamous cell skin cancers and in situ carcinoma except urinary bladder.
Note: Percentages may not total 100% due to rounding.

FIGURE 7.7 Leading sites of new cancer cases and deaths: 2004 estimates. (Data from American Cancer Society Surveillance Research, 2004.)

Basal cell carcinoma affects middle-aged and older white European Americans to a greater degree than it does people with dark skin. Thus, physical therapists should be on the alert and assess for this condition in their patients and make referrals as necessary. Likewise, osteoporosis affects white people more than black people, women more than men, and underweight people more than normal or overweight people. Thus, physical therapists need to assess for the possibility of osteoporosis in their patients and refer them for definitive testing.[24]

Almost 16 million Americans have been diagnosed with diabetes mellitus (DM), and there are an additional 5.4 million people in whom the disease is undiagnosed. More women than men suffer from diabetes. The prevalence of DM also varies by race and ethnicity. The prevalence of DM among non-Hispanic whites is 7.8%. However, non-Hispanic blacks are 1.7 times as

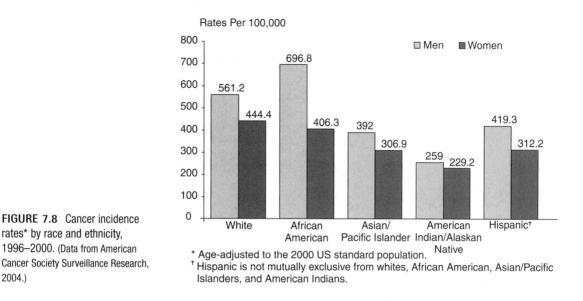

Rates Per 100,000

FIGURE 7.8 Cancer incidence rates* by race and ethnicity, 1996–2000. (Data from American Cancer Society Surveillance Research, 2004.)

* Age-adjusted to the 2000 US standard population.
† Hispanic is not mutually exclusive from whites, African American, Asian/Pacific Islanders, and American Indians.

likely to have diabetes as non-Hispanic whites, Americans of Mexican descent are 1.9 times as likely to have DM as non-Hispanic whites, and American Indians and Alaskan Natives are 2.8 times as likely to have diabetes as non-Hispanic whites. Prevalence rates for Asian and Pacific Islanders in the United States are limited, but DM prevalence among Hawaiians is twice that of white Americans in Hawaii.[25] What is unknown about the different rates of diabetes among ethnicities is how much of the difference is due to lifestyle (cultural beliefs and practices) and how

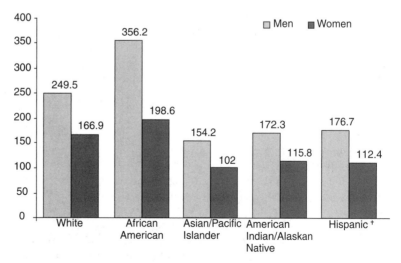

FIGURE 7.9 Cancer death rates* by race and ethnicity, 1996–2000. (Data from Surveillance, Epidemiology, and End Results Program, 1975–2000, Division of Cancer Control and Population Sciences, National Cancer Institute, 2003.)

* Per 100,000, age-adjusted to the 2000 US standard population.
† Hispanic is not mutually exclusive from whites, African American, Asian/Pacific Islanders, and American Indians

107

much is due to genetics of the individual and the race.[25]

Reflective Exercise

• What are the most common illnesses and diseases you see in your clinical setting? • Do you see differences among ethnic/racial groups?

Reflective Exercise

• What are the most common illnesses and diseases in your family? • What measures do you take to control these illnesses and conditions?

HIV continues as a pandemic trend. Over 36 million people are estimated to be living with HIV/AIDS; 16.4 million are women and 1.4 million are children under the age of 15 years. Worldwide, HIV is increasingly affecting women. The overwhelming majority of people with HIV (95%) are from developing countries.[26,27] Latin America accounts for 1.4 million people with HIV, with Brazil having the highest rate in South America. Honduras has the highest rate in Central America. Nearly 1 million people in the United States have HIV, with the highest concentration in large urban areas. The Caribbean has approximately 390,000 people with HIV, with Haiti the most affected country.[23] The WHO, the Pan American Health Organization (PAHO), the Centers for Disease Control and Prevention (CDC), and the Joint United Nations Programme on HIV/AIDS (UNAIDS) have formed a partnership for Global HIV Prevention Efforts, with specific programs for selected countries, populations, and cultural groups[28] (Table 7-1).

The diagnosis of HIV or AIDS can carry a significant stigma, not only in the community but also among family members and healthcare professionals. Thus, the physical therapist must maintain patient confidentiality and be prepared to offer emotional support and referral to mental health professionals if needed. Because of the stigma that HIV/AIDS can cause in some countries, the United States grants asylum to people diagnosed with HIV/AIDS.[29]

TABLE 7.1

Cumulative Cases by Race/Ethnicity

Estimated numbers of diagnoses of AIDS through December 2002, by race or ethnicity:

RACE OR ETHNICITY	# OF CUMULATIVE AIDS CASES
White, not Hispanic	364, 458
Black, not Hispanic	347, 491
Hispanic	163, 940
Asian/Pacific Islander	6, 924
American Indian/Alaska Native	2, 875
Unknown or multiple race	887

Variations in Drug Metabolism

Information regarding drug metabolism among racial and ethnic groups has important implications for healthcare practitioners prescribing medications. Besides the effects that (a) smoking (which accelerates drug metabolism), (b) nutritional status (malnutrition affects drug response), (c) diet (a high-fat diet increases absorption of antifungal medication, while a low-fat diet renders the drug less effective), (d) culture (attitudes and beliefs about taking medication), and (e) stress (which affects catecholamine and cortisol levels) have on drug metabolism, studies have identified some specific alterations in drug metabolism among diverse racial and ethnic groups.[30–34] For instance, the Chinese are more sensitive to the cardiovascular effects of propranolol and have increased absorption of antipsychotics, some narcotics, and antihypertensives compared with their white American counterparts. Native Americans, Eskimo Indians, and Hispanics have an increased risk of developing peripheral neuropathy while taking the drug isoniazid compared with white Americans, who inactivate the drug more rapidly.[18,21,31,35] African Americans respond better to diuretic therapy than do white ethnic groups. Moreover, African Americans are more likely to develop tardive dyskinesia than white people.[10] Hispanics and Asians metabolize dextromethorphan significantly faster than do whites.[16,21]

Among people of Greek heritage and other

groups originating from the Mediterranean, thalassemias and glucose-6-phosphate dehydrogenase (G-6-PD) deficiency are notable.[36-38] G-6-PD deficiency leads to hemolysis, which is generally well tolerated except under specific circumstances, including exercise, infections, and the presence of oxidant drugs such as primaquine, quinidine, thiazolsulfone, dapsone, furzolidone, nitrofural, naphthalene, toluidine blue, phenylhydrazine, and chloramphenicol. Even common medications such as aspirin can induce a hemolytic crisis. This threat is sufficiently severe that the WHO recommends that all hospital populations in areas with high proportions of Greeks and Greek Cypriots be screened for G-6-PD deficiency before drug therapy. Make patients aware that broad beans (fava beans) can induce hemolysis and an acute anemic crisis when ingested. Consider the possibility of G-6-PD deficiency in Greeks and patients with a Mediterranean heritage who have unconjugated jaundice.

Thalassemia is an inherited genetic disorder manifested by slow production of or failure to synthesize hemoglobin A or B chains. Two main types are commonly known: thalassemia major (sometimes known as Cooley's anemia, homozygous, or beta thalassemia major) and thalassemia minor (referred to as thalassemia trait, or beta thalassemia minor). Thalassemia major, if untreated, results in death. Undiagnosed infants become pale and irritable, do not eat, suffer from recurrent fever, and fail to thrive. Eventually the liver, spleen, and heart are damaged as a result of the accumulation of iron contained in the red blood cells. Treatment includes regular blood transfusions, prevention of iron overload with deferoxamine, and bone marrow transplants. Most individuals with thalassemia minor are not aware of it unless they are tested for it. In recent years, prenatal screening programs in Greece, Cyprus, Great Britain, North America, Canada, and Australia, where most of the diaspora resides, have drastically reduced the number of babies being born with thalassemia major. Screen Greek patients with a Mediterranean heritage for thalassemia and advise them of genetic risks.

An additional cultural consideration is the different ways physicians prescribe medications in various countries. For example, in most Asian countries and Great Britain, the preferred practice is to start out with low dosages of medicines and adjust the dosage upward until side effects are seen or therapeutic responses are reached. In the United States, most clinicians start with the maximum dosage and adjust downward as side effects occur.[31] Physical therapists need to investigate the literature for ethnic-specific studies regarding variations in drug metabolism, communicate these findings among colleagues, and educate their patients regarding side effects.

Reflective Exercise

• Which physical therapy interventions influence drug metabolism and pharmacokinetics? • Why is it important for physical therapists to be aware of variations in drug metabolism?

Nutrition

Julio Santos, age 25, was discovered in bed with shaking and chills by his housemates, who took him to the local emergency room. Julio had valvular disease and underwent aortic valve replacement. He had numerous complications after surgery and is now being seen by the physical therapist for conditioning training. He is scheduled for discharge in 2 days, after which a physical therapist will be following him at home. He lives in a group home with six other seasonal farm workers and his sister, who prepares meals for the entire "family." Julio is protein deficient, and this condition is delaying his strength training program.

The cultural domain *nutrition* includes the meaning of food; common foods and food rituals; nutritional deficiencies and food limitations; and the use of food for health promotion and wellness, health restoration, and illness and disease prevention (Fig. 7-10). In most settings, a physical

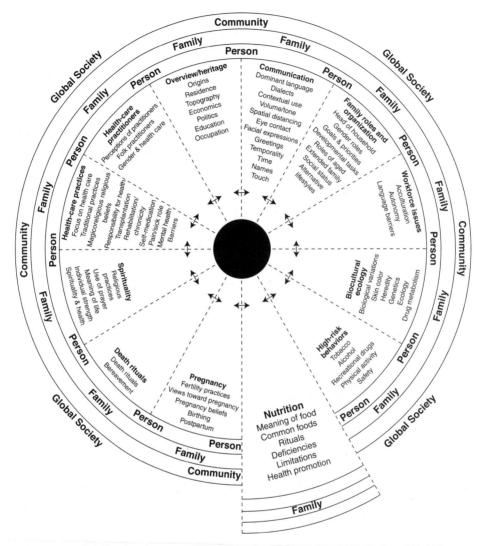

FIGURE 7.10 Nutrition domain. (Adapted from Purnell, L. D., & Paulanka, B. J. (1998). The Purnell Model for Cultural Competence. In L. D. Purnell & B. J. Paulanka (Eds.), *Transcultural health care: A culturally competent approach* (p. 10). Philadelphia: F.A. Davis.)

therapist will be able to refer patients needing nutritional counseling to a dietitian or nutritionist. However, the physical therapist should acquire an understanding of nutritional deficiencies and cultural influences of nutritional practices, as these may impact the physical therapy program. In addition, the more physical therapists understand about the cultural meaning of food, the better

they will be able to appreciate the cultural significance of a food gift or of the diet of patients.

Reflective Exercise

• How might your patient's nutritional status or diet impact the physical therapy program?

Meaning of Food

Food and the absence of food, hunger, have diverse meanings among cultures and individuals. Cultural beliefs, values, and types of foods available influence what people eat, avoid, or alter to make food congruent with cultural lifeways. Food is necessary as a means of survival and relief from hunger, has a significant role in socialization, has symbolic meaning for peaceful coexistence, and is used to prevent disease and illness and to promote healing. Moreover, food is used as an expression of love and caring or as a reward for good behavior, food is withheld as a means of punishment, and special foods are used for special occasions such as birthdays, holidays, funerals, and weddings, to name a few. Some foods are high-status foods, such as lobster in the United States, guinea pig in Ecuador and Peru, and truffles in Great Britain. However, lobster, because it is plentiful, is not a high-status food in the Philippines. Other foods are low-status foods, such as canned sausages in the United States, but not in Panama, where they are high-status foods because they are expensive. Additionally, the appropriate use of food and its consumption vary among and within cultures. For example, eating practices vary from formal dinners to picnics to fast food.

When a guest is invited to dinner for the first time in most European American cultures, the guest frequently, although not required to do so, brings a gift, one of the choices being food. No specific rules exist as to what type of food to bring, but wine, cheese baskets, and special candy are usually appropriate. Some people bring special "ethnic" foods of which they are proud, such as a special bread. Soft drinks, common types of cheese, or candy bars are not usually appropriate in the United States, but are in countries in Central America.

Reflective Exercise

• When you are invited to someone's home for dinner for the first time, do you bring food or beverages?
• What type? • Does your food/beverage selection have a special meaning? • Do you think your food "gift" would be different if you visited the home of an Orthodox Jew versus a Muslim or Vietnamese Buddhist?

Common Foods and Food Rituals

American food and preparation practices reflect the traditional food habits of early settlers who brought their unique cuisines with them. Accordingly, the "typical American diet" has been brought from elsewhere. Americans vary their meal times and food choices according to the region of the country, urban versus rural residence, and weekdays versus weekends. Additionally, food choices vary by marital status, economic status, climate changes, religion, ancestry, availability, and personal preferences.

The diet of most Americans is high in fats and cholesterol and low in fiber, according to the U.S. Department of Agriculture (USDA). The USDA recommends adherence to the food pyramid, originally adapted in 1950 and recently updated in 2005 (Fig. 7-11). The food pyramid is commonly used in elementary and secondary education as a guide for teaching healthy eating to the public. Daily recommendations include 6 ounces of bread, cereal, rice, or pasta; 2.5 cups of vegetables; 2.0 cups of fruit; 3.0 cups of milk, yogurt, or cheese; 5.5 ounces of meat, poultry, fish, dry beans, eggs, or nuts; and limited consumption of fats, oils, and sweets. However, it has been recognized that specific foods in this pyramid must be adapted for non-American food preferences. Additionally, this pyramid has been questioned by prestigious organizations that claim it contributes to obesity and overall poor health. Over half of Americans are overweight, with one-fourth considered obese (30 or more pounds overweight).[39] The American food pyramid may not work with other cultural groups, especially for those who are lactose intolerant or vegetarian. Food choices may be significantly different from the American diet for Hindus, Jews, Muslims, Asians, and Hispanics.[16,21,40–44] In some cases, the person's preferred choices may not be available in the United States, and if they are, they may be very expensive or hard to find, especially in rural areas.

Reflective Exercise

• Do you subscribe to the food pyramid? • Why or why not? • Is it consistent with your cultural background?

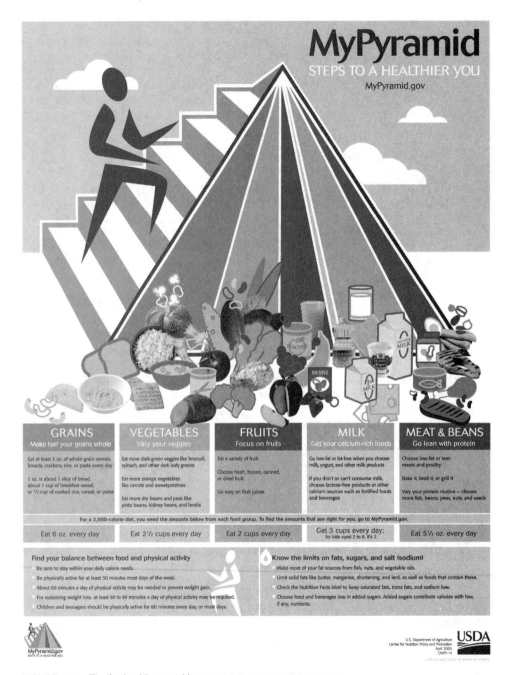

FIGURE 7.11   The food guide pyramid. (From U. S. Department of Agriculture.)

Reflective Exercise

• What foods from your cultural background do you eat? • What foods from your cultural background do you not eat?

Breakfast is usually consumed between 6:00 and 9:00 A.M., depending on the person's work schedule. On weekends, the time may be delayed 1 or 2 hours or extended into "brunch," at 11:00 A.M. to noon. Favorite foods for people in urban areas and for people doing office-type work are hot or cold cereal; pastry; bagels, either plain or with cream cheese; toast with butter or margarine and/or jelly or preserves; fruit; juice; and coffee or tea. For people engaged in physical labor and in farming communities, breakfast more likely includes fried, scrambled, or poached eggs; ham, bacon, sausage, or scrapple (primarily in the southern United States); fried potatoes; toast with butter or margarine and/or jelly or preserves; juice; and coffee or tea. Children traditionally drink milk with breakfast. Most Americans in the work environment enjoy a midmorning "coffee break," although juice, soft drinks, or tea may be consumed instead of coffee.

The noontime meal, typically consumed by 1:00 P.M., is called lunch in urban areas and dinner in rural areas. Urbanites frequently miss lunch completely; otherwise they carry their lunch to work with them, eat salads or sandwiches, and drink iced beverages such as tea or soft drinks, although many also enjoy hot tea and coffee. Americans like choices, and this extends to soft drinks, of which there are wide varieties from which to choose. Unlike people in many other countries, Americans can have their soft drinks with or without caffeine, or in diet (artificially sweetened) or regular (with sugar) form. Most people take an afternoon beverage break, to which they are entitled by law. This short break is not as extensive as the "afternoon tea" that the British and other groups enjoy. In Sweden, a common practice even for professional groups is to routinely gather in a "break room" at a designated time to share coffee or tea and fruit or pastry.

The evening meal, dinner in urban areas or supper in rural areas, is served between 6:00 and

---

Reflection 7.1

I am from Mexico. While studying in the United States, I noticed that many of my friends eat lunch in their car. It seemed their lives are so busy that they did not have time to stop and eat lunch at a table with family or friends. This seemed very unusual to me.

Margarita Gonzalez

9:00 P.M., depending on the family's work pattern. Rural people usually eat earlier than urban people. The evening meal is the largest meal of the day for most people and includes soup and/or a salad; meat, such as beef, pork, or poultry; or fish; a variety of green or yellow vegetables; a starch such as potatoes, pasta, or rice; bread; a dessert such as cake, pie, cookies, ice cream, or pudding; and a choice of beverage. People may begin this meal with an appetizer and enjoy wine before or with the meal. Children and some adults might eat a "bedtime snack." Whereas great variety exists for Americans for any meal, physical therapists immigrating from other countries to the United States may not be accustomed to the dominant American food choices.

Reflective Exercise

• What are your usual mealtime patterns? • How might a patient's pattern of mealtimes impact the physical therapy program?

Many of the elderly and people living alone do not eat balanced meals. They claim that they do not have, or do not want to take, the time to prepare a meal, even though most American homes have labor-saving devices such as stoves, microwave ovens, refrigerators, and dishwashers. For those who are unable to prepare their own meals because of disability or illness, most communities have "Meals on Wheels" programs, where community and church organizations deliver, usually once a day, a hot meal along with a cold meal for later and food for the following morning's breakfast. Other community and church agencies prepare meals for the homeless and/or collect food, which is delivered to those who have none. When people are ill, they generally prefer toast, tea, juice, and other easily digested foods.

Reflective Exercise

• How might you as a physical therapist visiting elderly patients in their homes be involved in their nutritional needs?

Most cities and towns in the United States have an abundance of fast food restaurants that offer chicken, burgers, and pizza; busy people can "eat and drive" or get food to take home to eat. For the most part, these foods are high in fat and cholesterol, although in some places you can buy heart-healthy foods such as salads. Newer immigrants may not be aware of the unhealthy choices offered by many fast food establishments.

Socioeconomic status may dictate food selections—for example, hamburger instead of steak, canned or frozen vegetables and fruit rather than fresh, and fish instead of shrimp or lobster. Given the size of the United States and its varied terrain, food choices differ by region: beef in the Midwest, fish in coastal areas, poultry in the south and along the eastern seaboard, and vegetables, which vary by season, climate, and altitude, although larger grocery stores carry a wide variety of all types of American and international meats, fruits, and vegetables. Television networks advertise food and food products, major newspapers have large sections devoted to foods and preparation practices, and many television stations have entire programs devoted to cooking, testaments to the value that Americans place on food and diversity in food preparation (Fig. 7-12).

Special occasions and holidays among many cultures are frequently associated with ethnic foods. For example, in the United States, hot dogs are consumed at sporting events and turkey is served at Thanksgiving. Many religious groups are required to fast during specific holiday sea-

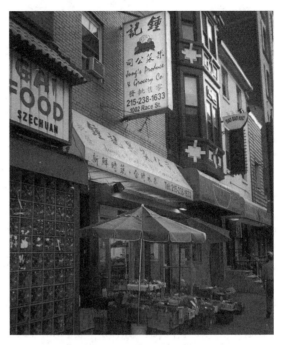

FIGURE 7.12 Ethnic food store.

sons, such as Ramadan for Muslims and Lent for Catholics and various Jewish religious holidays.[40,42,44] However, physical therapists may need to gently remind patients for whom fasting is a concern (those with diabetes, weakened health status, wound healing problems, and febrile states, to name a few) that fasting is not required during times of illness or pregnancy. However, the devout may still wish to fast.

Reflective Exercise

• What are your high-status foods? • What are your low-status foods? • Do you have particular foods for celebrating special occasions such as birthdays, Christmas, Thanksgiving, Ramadan, or other religious/ethnic celebrations?

Dietary Practices for Health Promotion

The nutritional balance of a diet is recognized by most cultures throughout the world. Most cultures have their own distinct theories of nutritional practices for health promotion and wellness and for illness and disease prevention. Common folk practices and selected diets are recommended during periods of illness and for prevention of illness or disease. For example, many societies, such as Iranian, Mexican, Puerto Rican, Greek, Chinese, Asian Indian, Haitian, and Vietnamese, subscribe to the "hot and cold" theory of food selection to prevent illness and maintain health. Although each of these ethnic groups has its own specific name for the "hot and cold" theory of foods—*am* and *dong* for the Vietnamese, *fret* and *cho* for Haitians, and *garm* and *sard* for Iranians—the overall belief is that the body needs a balance of opposing foods. It is important to note that the terms *hot* and *cold* may refer not to the temperature of the food but rather to how the food is used by the body. Thus the recommendation to a patient who needs calcium for bone healing to drink milk may be ignored because of a religious or cultural taboo, or the patient may have a lactose intolerance. Specific cultural food charts are available.[8,21,35,44–47]

In the Western healthcare system, diets that are low in sodium and fats are prescribed for the prevention and treatment of heart conditions. Diets high in fat are recognized as increasing the risk for the development of cardiovascular disease and some types of cancer. Many societies are becoming more health conscious about reducing fat in their diets. Some Asian cultures prepare very spicy foods, which increase the incidence of stomach cancer, ulcers, and gastrointestinal bleeding.[41,43] A thorough history and assessment of dietary practices can be an important diagnostic tool to guide health promotion. Although school lunch programs, Meals on Wheels, and church meal plans, to name a few, are programs through which the physical therapist can encourage and support families in attaining better nutrition, these programs may not provide optimal nutritional selections.

Reflective Exercise

• What foods do you eat to maintain your health?
• What foods do you eat when you are ill? • What foods do you avoid when you are ill? • Do you subscribe to a specific theory of balancing your diet?
• What do you consider a "balanced meal"?

Nutritional Deficiencies and Food Limitations

Because of limited socioeconomic resources or limited availability of their native foods, immigrants may eat foods that were not available in their home country. These dietary changes may result in health problems when they arrive in a new environment. This is more likely to occur when individuals immigrate to a country where native foods are not readily available and they do not know which of the new foods contain the necessary and comparable nutritional ingredients. Consequently, they do not know which foods to select for balancing their diet. Widespread nutritional deficiencies of many types have occurred in recent immigrants from Southeast Asia, in part because of their time spent in refugee camps but also because of changes in food habits with immigration to America. Among Hindus, the consumption of a single grain, such as rice, may result in inadequate intake of lysine and other essential amino acids.[41]

Reflective Exercise

• Do you have difficulty finding your preferred food and beverage choices? • Do you fast for religious or personal reasons?

Reflective Exercise

• When was the last time you referred a patient for nutritional counseling? • How often do you make referrals for nutritional counseling? • How important is nutritional counseling? • How important would it be to refer to a nutritionist who is committed to providing culturally congruent care?

Enzyme deficiencies exist among some ethnic and racial groups. For example, many Vietnamese Americans have lactose intolerance and are unable to drink milk or eat dairy products to maintain their calcium needs.[16] By consuming soups and stews made with pureed bones and cooked to an edible consistency, this deficiency can be overcome. In general, the wide availability of foods in this country reduces the risks of these disorders as long as immigrants have the means to obtain culturally nutritious foods. One must also remember that foods that may be eaten in one culture may not be eaten in another culture; such forbidden foods include pork or pork products for devout Jews[44] and Muslims[40,42] and beef for Hindus,[41] to whom the cow is a sacred animal.

The recent emphasis on cultural foods has resulted in small businesses selling ethnic foods and spices to the general public. The physical therapist's responsibility, when he or she believes that a patient's diet is inadequate, is to refer the patient to a nutritionist for dietary counseling.

CULTURAL SELF-ASSESSMENT EXERCISE 1

Self-Assessment

Answer the following questions to assess the domain *high-risk health behaviors* for yourself.

1. Do you smoke cigarettes, cigars, or a pipe?
2. How many cigarettes/cigars/bowls of tobacco do you smoke each day?
3. For how many years have you smoked?
4. Do you drink alcohol?
5. How frequently do you drink?
6. How much do you drink?
7. Do you use recreational drugs?
8. Which recreational drugs do you use, and how often do you use them?
9. Do you exercise?
10. What type of exercise do you do?
11. How often do you exercise?
12. When you are ill, what over-the-counter medications do you use?
13. How long do you treat yourself before seeing a health practitioner?

CULTURAL SELF-ASSESSMENT EXERCISE 2

Understanding Others / Knowledge and Application

1. Which of the above questions would be important to ask your physical therapy patient?
2. What impact would the answer to each of the questions you identified have on the physical therapy program?
3. Which of the high-risk behaviors noted might you as a physical therapist positively influence?
4. How might you positively influence the high-risk behaviors in a culturally congruent way?

CULTURAL SELF-ASSESSMENT EXERCISE 3

Self-Assessment / Understanding Others

Answer the following questions to assess the cultural domain *biocultural ecology* for yourself.

1. Are you allergic to any medications?
2. Are there any particular allergies that frequently occur in your family?
3. What are the major illnesses and diseases that affect people where you live?
4. What are the most common diseases and illnesses in your family? In other people where you live?
5. Are there any genetic diseases that occur in your family/ancestors?
   a. Which of the above questions would be important to ask your physical therapy patient?
   b. What impact would the answer to each of the questions you identified have on the physical therapy program?

CULTURAL SELF-ASSESSMENT EXERCISE 4

Self-Assessment / Understanding Others

Answer the following questions to assess the cultural domain *nutrition* for yourself.

1. Which foods do you eat to maintain your health?
2. Which foods do you avoid to maintain your health?
3. Why do you avoid these foods?
4. What foods in your culture are taboo, or to be avoided?
5. Which foods do you eat when you are ill?
6. Which foods do you avoid when you are ill?

a. Which of the above questions would be important to ask your physical therapy patient?
b. What impact would the answer to each of the questions you identified have on the physical therapy program?
c. Which of the high-risk behaviors noted might you as a physical therapist positively influence?
d. How might you positively influence the high-risk behaviors in a culturally congruent way?

Vignette Questions

1. What high-risk health behaviors do you see in the Delgado family?
2. How might these high-risk behaviors impact the physical therapy program?
3. Which of these behaviors might you as a physical therapist seek to influence?
4. Which of these behaviors might be linked to culture?
5. How might you influence the high-risk behaviors in a culturally competent manner?
6. Even though Pedro is 45 minutes late for his appointment, would you complete his therapy today or ask him to reschedule?

Vignette Questions

1. What nutritional concerns do you see with Julio?
2. How might these nutritional concerns impact the physical therapy program?
3. What influence might culture have on Julio's nutritional state?
4. What additional culturally related challenges exist?
5. How might you address Julio's nutritional needs in a culturally competent manner?

CASE STUDY SCENARIO I

*M*r. Denny is a 61-year-old male who comes to physical therapy for wound healing and lymphedema management of his bilateral lower extremities. He is grossly overweight and has open wounds on the posterior aspect of his right lower leg and anterior aspect of his left lower leg. Both lower extremities present with moderately pitting edema and changes in the skin. Mr. Denny blames his problem on a burn he sustained on his right leg from a heating pad in the hospital 4 years ago. His wife accompanies him to the appointment. She states that they are having trouble keeping the wounds from oozing and that the dressings for the wounds are expensive.

Mr. Denny smokes a pack of cigarettes a day and states that he cannot exercise because of the pain in his legs. He says that he can walk two blocks before needing to sit down. He can wear only one pair of the shoes that he owns because of the swelling in his feet. The shoes are dirty and smell. Mr. Denny smells of body odor as well. He denies a history of diabetes and states that the vascular tests were negative. He has hypertension, which is controlled by medicine.

1. What high-risk behaviors has Mr. Denny demonstrated?
2. How should the physical therapist address each high-risk behavior?

3. What referrals might the physical therapist make?

4. What is Mr. Denny's understanding of his illness?

5. What approaches or strategies might the physical therapist take to overcome barriers and establish effective interventions?

6. What more should the physical therapist learn in order to better understand Mr. Denny's situation?

CASE STUDY SCENARIO II

*M*r. Lee, age 52, is a Native American who underwent a transfemoral amputation secondary to diabetes. He is now discharged from the rehabilitation hospital and is being seen by a physical therapist in his home. He lives alone on the outskirts of an Indian reservation. The physical therapist makes the visit on the first day and notices that Mr. Lee is very weak and appears to be apathetic. He does not appear to have much food in the house and states that he relies on friends to bring food to him. He states that he has been a diabetic for 20 years and that controlling his blood sugar level has been a challenge. He also indicates that he is not accustomed to formal exercise other than the exercise required for daily work.

1. What cultural norms of communication might factor into this intercultural interaction?

2. What nutritional concerns are present?

3. What should the physical therapist do to resolve the nutritional concerns?

4. What concerns should the physical therapist have regarding Mr. Lee's diabetes and exercise?

5. What referrals might the physical therapist consider?

6. How might the physical therapist advocate for the patient?

REFERENCES

1. Perez-Stable E, Herrera B, Jacob P, Benowitz M. Nicotine metabolism and intake in Black and White smokers. *JAMA.* 1998;280:152–156.

2. World Health Organization. Controlling the global obesity epidemic. Available at: http://www.who.int/nut/obs.htm. Accessed May 30, 2003.

3. Racette SB, Deusinger SS, Deusinger RH. Obesity: Overview of prevalence, etiology, and treatment. *Phys Ther.* 2003;83:276–288.

4. Fuchs J, Levinson R, Stoddard R, Mullet A, Jones D. Update on the search for DNA markers linked to manic-depressive illness in Old Order Amish. *J Psychiatr Res.* 1990;26:305–308.

5. Wenger AFZ. The culture care theory and the Old Order Amish. In: Leininger MM, ed. *Culture Care Diversity and Universality: A Theory of Nursing.* New York, NY: National League for Nursing; 1991.

6. Wenger AF, Wenger M. The Amish. In: Purnell L, Paulanka B, eds. *Transcultural Health Care: A Culturally Competent Approach.* 2nd ed. Philadelphia, Pa: FA Davis; 2003:54–72.

7. Flegal KM, Carroll MD, Ogden CL, Johnson CL. The prevalence and trends in obesity among US adults, 1999–2000. *JAMA.* 2002;228:1723–1727.

8. Colin J, Paperwalla G. People of Haitian ancestry [chapter on CD-ROM]. In: Purnell L, Paulanka B, eds. *Transcultural Health Care: A Culturally Competent Approach.* 2nd ed. Philadelphia, Pa: FA Davis; 2003.

9. U.S. Department of Energy, Office of Science. Human Genome Project information. Available at: http://www.ornl.gov/sci/techresources/Human_Genome/home.shtml. Accessed January 12, 2002.

10. Glanville C. People of African American heritage. In: Purnell L, Paulanka B, eds. *Transcultural Health Care: A Culturally Competent Approach.* 2nd ed. Philadelphia, Pa: FA Davis; 2003:40–53.

11. Purnell L. People of Appalachian heritage. In: Purnell L, Paulanka B, eds. *Transcultural Health Care: A Culturally Competent Approach.* 2nd ed. Philadelphia, Pa: FA Davis; 2003:73–89.

12. Steckler J. People of German heritage [chapter on CD-ROM]. In: Purnell L, Paulanka B, eds. *Transcultural Health Care: A Culturally Competent Approach.* 2nd ed. Philadelphia, Pa: FA Davis; 2003.

13. From M. People of Polish heritage. In: Purnell L, Paulanka B, eds. *Transcultural Health Care: A Culturally Competent Approach.* 2nd ed. Philadelphia, Pa: FA Davis; 2003:284–306.

14. Wilson S. People of Irish heritage. In: Purnell L, Paulanka B, eds. *Transcultural Health Care: A Culturally Competent Approach.* 2nd ed. Philadelphia, Pa: FA Davis; 2003:194–203.

15. Giger JN, Davidhizar RE. *Transcultural Nursing: Assessment and Intervention.* 3rd ed. St. Louis, Mo: Mosby; 2003.

16. Nowak T. People of Vietnamese heritage. In: Purnell L, Paulanka B, eds. *Transcultural Health Care: A Culturally Competent Approach.* 2nd ed. Philadelphia, Pa: FA Davis; 2003:327–344.

17. Centers for Disease Control and Prevention. Cardiovascular disease. Available at: http://www.cdc.gov/nccdphp/cvk/cvdaag. Accessed January 12, 2004.

18. Still O, Hodgins D. Navajo Indians. In: Purnell L, Paulanka B, eds. *Transcultural Health Care: A Culturally Competent Approach.* 2nd ed. Philadelphia, Pa: FA Davis; 2003:279–283.

19. Pacquiao D. People of Filipino heritage. In: Purnell L, Paulanka B, eds. *Transcultural Health Care: A Culturally Competent Approach.* 2nd ed. Philadelphia, Pa: FA Davis; 2003:138–159.

20. Sharts-Hopko N. People of Japanese heritage [chapter on CD-ROM]. In: Purnell L, Paulanka B, eds. *Transcultural Health Care: A Culturally Competent Approach.* 2nd ed. Philadelphia, Pa: FA Davis; 2003.

21. Zoucha R, Purnell L. People of Mexican heritage. In: Purnell L, Paulanka B, eds. *Transcultural Health Care:*

A Culturally Competent Approach. 2nd ed. Philadelphia, Pa: FA Davis; 2003:264–278.

22. National Cancer Institute. Current and accurate cancer information. Available at: http://cancernet.nci.nih.gov/dictionary.html. Accessed January 12, 2004.

23. CDC National Center for HIV, STD, and TB Prevention. Divisions of HIV/AIDS Prevention. "Basic Statistics" June 20, 2005. Available at: http://www.cdc.gov/hiv/stats.html. Accessed July 27, 2005.

24. Purnell L, Paulanka B. Appendix: Cultural and racial illnesses and diseases. In: Purnell L, Paulanka B, eds. *Transcultural Health Care: A Culturally Competent Approach.* 2nd ed. Philadelphia, Pa: FA Davis; 2003:345–351.

25. Centers for Disease Control and Prevention. National diabetes fact sheet. Available at: http://www.cdc.gov/health/diabetes.htm. Accessed January 12, 2004.

26. AIDS challenges religious leaders. *Washington Post.* August 8, 2001: A10.

27. International HIV/AIDS Alliance. Supporting community action on AIDS in developing countries. Available at: http://www.aidsalliance.org/. Accessed January 12, 2004.

28. Joint United Nations Programme on HIV/AIDS. UNAIDS. Available at: www.UNAIDS.org. Accessed January 12, 2004.

29. Purnell L. People of Brazilian heritage [chapter on CD-ROM]. In: Purnell L, Paulanka B, eds. *Transcultural Health Care: A Culturally Competent Approach.* 2nd ed. Philadelphia, Pa: FA Davis; 2003.

30. Johnson JA. Influence of race and ethnicity on pharmacokinetics of drugs. *J Pharmacol Sci.* 1997;86:1328–1333.

31. Levy R. Ethnic and racial differences in response to medications: Preserving individualized therapy in managed pharmaceutical programs. *Pharm Med.* 1993;7:139–165.

32. Lin K, Anderson S, Poland R. Ethnicity and psychopharmacology: Bridging the gap. *Psychiatr Clin North Am.* 1995;18:635–647.

33. Matthews HW. Racial, ethnic and gender differences in response to medicines. *Drug Metab Drug Interact.* 1995;12:77–91.

34. Salerno E. Race, culture, and medications. *J Emerg Nurs.* 1995;21:560–562.

35. Wang Y. People of Chinese heritage. In: Purnell L, Paulanka B, eds. *Transcultural Health Care: A Culturally Competent Approach.* 2nd ed. Philadelphia, Pa: FA Davis; 2003:106–121.

36. Hillman S. People of Italian heritage. In: Purnell L, Paulanka B, eds. *Transcultural Health Care: A Culturally Competent Approach.* 2nd ed. Philadelphia, Pa: FA Davis; 2003:205–217.

37. Purnell L. People of Egyptian heritage [chapter on CD-ROM]. In: Purnell L, Paulanka B, eds. *Transcultural*

Health Care: A Culturally Competent Approach. 2nd ed. Philadelphia, Pa: FA Davis; 2003.

38. Purnell L, Papadopoulos R. People of Greek heritage [chapter on CD-ROM]. In: Purnell L, Paulanka B, eds. *Transcultural Health Care: A Culturally Competent Approach.* 2nd ed. Philadelphia, Pa: FA Davis; 2003.

39. Food Guide Pyramid. U.S. Department of Agriculture. Available at: http://www.nal.usda.gov:8001/py/pmap.htm. Accessed January 12, 2004.

40. Hafizi H, Lipson J. People of Iranian heritage. In: Purnell L, Paulanka B, eds. *Transcultural Health Care: A Culturally Competent Approach.* 2nd ed. Philadelphia, Pa: FA Davis; 2003:177–193.

41. Jambanathan J. People of Hindu heritage [chapter on CD-ROM]. In: Purnell L, Paulanka B, eds. *Transcultural Health Care: A Culturally Competent Approach.* 2nd ed. Philadelphia, Pa: FA Davis; 2003.

42. Kulwicki A. People of Arab heritage. In: Purnell L, Paulanka B, eds. *Transcultural Health Care: A Culturally Competent Approach.* 2nd ed. Philadelphia, Pa: FA Davis; 2003:90–105.

43. Purnell L, Kim S. People of Korean heritage. In: Purnell L, Paulanka B, eds. *Transcultural Health Care: A Culturally Competent Approach.* 2nd ed. Philadelphia, Pa: FA Davis; 2003:249–263.

44. Selekman J. People of Jewish heritage. In: Purnell L, Paulanka B, eds. *Transcultural Health Care: A Culturally Competent Approach.* 2nd ed. Philadelphia, Pa: FA Davis; 2003:234–248.

45. Juarbe T. People of Puerto Rican heritage. In: Purnell L, Paulanka B, eds. *Transcultural Health Care: A Culturally Competent Approach.* 2nd ed. Philadelphia, Pa: FA Davis; 2003:307–326.

46. Kittler P, Sucher K, eds. *Food and Culture.* 3rd ed. Albany, NY: Wadsworth; 2003.

47. Purnell L. Panamanians' practices for health promotion and the meaning of respect afforded them by healthcare providers. *J Transcult Nurs.* 1999;10:333–340.

Chapter 8

Exploring Spirituality and Cultural Death Rituals

- Jill Black Lattanzi, PT, EdD
- Larry D. Purnell, PhD, RN

Cultural Death Rituals

George Carrington, age 34, has been a patient for 3 weeks—first in the intensive care unit and then on the rehabilitation unit. Mr. Carrington had multiple injuries from an automobile accident. He had been progressing with his injuries and was expected to be discharged to home within the week. As the therapist enters his room, Mr. Carrington's wife, Bernice, is leaning over the bed and wailing. Her husband had died 5 minutes before. The nurse is quietly working to remove the crash cart. As the physical therapist approaches the bed, Mrs. Carrington grabs the physical therapist tightly and screams, "He's dead, he's dead! What are I and the children going to do without him? Why did God let this happen?"

At times physical therapists are faced with the death of a patient, particularly those working in the ICU and in home care with oncology patients and other severely ill patients. While physical therapists are not social workers or clergy, it is important that they know how to respond appropriately and sensitively and in as culturally congruent a manner as possible. The cultural domain *death rituals* includes how the individual and the society view death and end-of-life issues, rituals to prepare for death, burial practices, and bereavement. Death practices, beliefs, and rituals vary significantly among cultural and religious groups and change slowly over time[1-4] (Fig. 8-1).

Concerns among physical therapists in regard to patient care may ensue because some staff may not understand the value of customs with which they are not familiar, such as ritual washing of the body in Islamic and Jewish religions. To avoid cultural taboos, physical therapists must become knowledgeable about unique practices related to death, dying, and bereavement if they are to help their patients and families cope with these processes.

Death Rituals and Expectations

For many American physical therapists, educated in a culture of mastery over the environment,

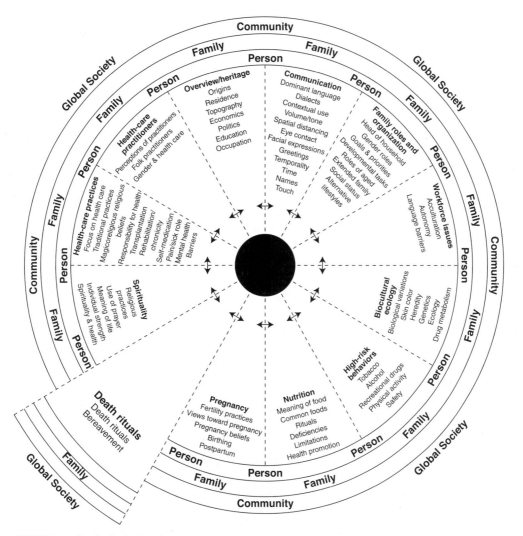

FIGURE 8.1 Death rituals domain. (Adapted from Purnell, L. D., & Paulanka, B. J. (1998). The Purnell Model for Cultural Competence. In L. D. Purnell & B. J. Paulanka (Eds.), *Transcultural health care: A culturally competent approach* (p. 10). Philadelphia: F.A. Davis.)

death is seen as one more disease to conquer, one more impairment to overcome, one more functional limitation to rehabilitate; and when this does not happen, death becomes a personal failure. Thus, for many, death does not take a natural course because it is "managed" or "prolonged," making it difficult to die with dignity. Accordingly, death and responses to death are not easy topics for many Americans to verbalize. Rather than

verbalize that a person died, many euphemisms are used, such as "he/she passed on/away," "he/she is no longer with us," and "he/she went to visit the 'Grim Reaper' (or in China, "he/she went to visit Mao").

In the culture of the United States, death is often institutionalized and hidden. Eighty percent of deaths take place in the hospital as opposed to the home, in the presence of family and friends.[5] The body is embalmed to look lifelike and the rituals of the viewing and funeral are typically very orderly and proper, characterizations of the American values of cleanliness, sterility, and emotional control. The dominant American culture's belief in self-determination and autonomy extends to people making their own decisions about end-of-life care.[4,6–8] Mentally competent adults have the right to decide what medical treatment and interventions they wish to use to extend life, such as artificial life support, artificial feeding, and therapeutic interventions.

Reflective Exercise

• What words/euphemisms are used in your culture to talk about death?

Reflective Exercise

• Do you feel that the patient should be allowed to refuse therapeutic interventions that might prolong life?

Most Americans believe that a dying person should not be left alone, and accommodations are usually made for a family member to be with the dying person at all times. Healthcare personnel are expected to care for the family as much as for the patient during this time. Most people are buried or cremated within 3 days of death, but extenuating circumstances may lengthen this period to accommodate family and friends who must travel a long distance to attend a funeral or memorial service.[9] The family can decide if the deceased will have an open casket for viewing by family and friends, or if the casket will remain closed.

Significant variations in burial and bereavement practices occur among other ethnocultural groups in the United States. The tradition among Orthodox Jews is to bury their deceased before sundown the next day and perform post-death rituals that last for several days.[10] Other groups stage elaborate ceremonies in commemoration of the dead, such as the *velorio* among Mexican Americans, which may last for days.[11] To some

people, such a ritual looks like a celebration; in reality, it is a celebration of the person's life. In the Greek Orthodox society, there are successive stages of mourning that include memorial services 40 days after burial and again at 3 months and 6 months, with yearly rituals thereafter.[12] When Muslims approach death, they may wish to face Mecca and recite passages from the Holy Qur'an; the physical therapist may need to help determine the direction of Mecca and help position the bed accordingly.[13] Whether in the hospital, in the extended-care facility, or at home in the community, the furniture may need to be rearranged to accomplish this important ritual.

Reflective Exercise

• What are the customary burial practices in your culture? • Are you in agreement with these practices? • How would you be treated in the community if you decided to go against the cultural burial practices?

Responses to Death and Grief

American society, medical and otherwise, has launched a major initiative to assist patients to die as comfortably as possibly without pain. As a result, more people are choosing to remain at home or to enter a hospice for end-of-life care, where their comfort needs are better met. The modern hospice movement began in Great Britain in the 1960s. The first hospice in the United States was in New Haven, Connecticut, in 1974. Hospice is a concept of committed care to patients and their families facing the end stages of life. Hospice neither prolongs life nor hastens death, but rather emphasizes the quality of one's last days by caring for one's comfort and dignity.[14] Hospice care is not, however, accepted equally by all ethnocultural groups and individuals. African Americans are less receptive to hospice care than are white Americans;[15] they are also less likely than white Americans to choose assisted death, wanting every treatment available to them.[9,16]

When death does occur, most Americans conservatively control their grief, although women are usually more expressive than men. Men, in particular, are expected to be stoic in their reactions to death, at least in public.[3,17] Generally, tears are shed, but loud wailing and uncontrollable sobbing rarely occur. The belief is that the person has progressed to a better existence and no longer has to undergo the pressures of life on earth. However, this is not the expectation among all Puerto Ricans and Italians, who may tend to express their grief openly.[18,19]

Reflective Exercise

• What are your personal beliefs about hospice care? • What is the role of the physical therapist in hospice care?

The expression of grief in response to death varies among cultural groups. For example, in the East Indian Hindu culture, loved ones are expected to suffer the grief of death in silence, with little display of emotion.[20,21] The bereavement time for Chinese people may be a week or longer, depending on the relationship of the family member to the deceased and the degree of acculturation. The family of a deceased Chinese or Korean American may need extra leave time from work to fulfill their cultural obligations.[1,22,23] Such variations in the grieving process may cause confusion for physical therapists, who may perceive some patients as overreacting and others as not caring. The behaviors associated with the grieving process must be placed in the context of the specific ethnocultural belief system in order to provide culturally competent care. Physical therapists should encourage ethnically specific bereavement practices when providing support to family and friends. Bereavement support strategies are listed in Box 8-1.

Reflective Exercise

• What would your response be to Mrs. Carrington in the introductory vignette in this chapter?

Reflective Exercise

• What are the traditional bereavement practices in your culture? • Are they different for men than they are for women?

BOX 8.1

Bereavement Support Strategies

(a) Being physically present
(b) Encouraging a reality orientation
(c) Openly acknowledging the family's right to grieve
(d) Permitting varied behavioral responses to grief
(e) Acknowledging the patient's pain
(f) Giving the patient and family permission to grieve
(g) Assisting the patient and family to express their feelings
(h) Encouraging interpersonal relationships
(i) Promoting interest in a new life
(j) Making referrals to other resources, such as a priest, minister, rabbi, or pastoral care person with the patient's and/or family's permission[1-4]

Spirituality

H iram Kravitz, age 62, is an Orthodox Jew with multiple sclerosis. Ms. Miller is the physical therapist assigned to him. She is supposed to help evaluate his abilities for self-care. When she speaks with Mr. Kravitz, he acknowledges her but will not maintain eye contact with her. After a 15-minute conversation, Ms. Miller begins to examine him. He immediately thanks her for coming and states that he is now okay and that she can leave.

The domain *spirituality* involves more than formal religious beliefs related to faith and affiliation and the use of prayer. For some people, religion shapes nutrition practices, healthcare practices, and other cultural domains. Spirituality includes all behaviors that give meaning to life and provide strength to the individual. Furthermore, it is difficult to distinguish religious beliefs from cultural beliefs because for some, especially the very devout, religion guides their dominant beliefs, values, and practices even more than culture (Fig. 8-2).

Spirituality, a component of health related to the essence of life, is a vital experience that is shared by all humans. Spirituality helps provide balance among the mind, body, and spirit. Trained and folk religious leaders provide comfort to both the patient and family. Spirituality does not have to be scientifically proven and is patterned unconsciously from a person's worldview. Accordingly, people may deviate somewhat from the majority view or position with regard to their formally recognized religion.

Spirituality and religious beliefs relate powerfully to health and wellness, and the physical therapist should consider a patient's beliefs for the following reasons (adapted from Koenig,[24] p. 5):

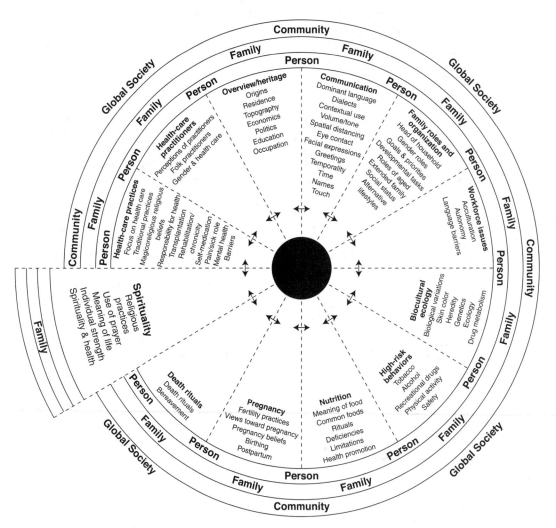

FIGURE 8.2 Spirituality domain. (Adapted from Purnell, L. D., & Paulanka, B. J. (1998). The Purnell Model for Cultural Competence. In L. D. Purnell & B. J. Paulanka (Eds.), *Transcultural health care: A culturally competent approach* (p. 10). Philadelphia: F.A. Davis.)

1. Religious beliefs help many patients to cope with stress and illness.
2. Religious beliefs influence medical decisions, especially in cases of serious illness.
3. Religious beliefs and activities such as prayer are related to better health and quality of life.
4. Studies and polls demonstrate that patients would like to have clinicians address their spiritual needs.
5. The practice of medicine is rooted in a long historical relationship between religion, medicine, and healthcare.

Reflective Exercise

• With what religion do you identify? • Do you accept/ practice all of the church's tenets? • Which ones do you modify to fit your personal beliefs? • How influential are your spiritual and/or religious beliefs on your worldview? • How do your spiritual and/or religious beliefs affect your views on health, illness, and death?

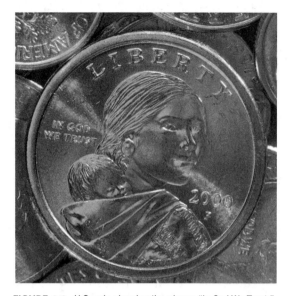

FIGURE 8.3 U.S. coin showing the phrase "In God We Trust."

Dominant Religion and Use of Prayer

Many groups settled in the United States to escape religious persecution in Europe and other continents. These early settlers sought to establish a government allowing religious freedom and separation of church and state so that their descendants would not undergo similar religious persecution. The new government was rooted largely in Judeo-Christian principles, as evidenced by the founding documents and the national anthem. For example, the Declaration of Independence states that "all men are created equal, that they are endowed by their Creator with certain unalienable rights."[25] The repetitious use of the phrase "one nation under God" depicts both a political and a spiritual legacy where the United States is under God rather than under a sovereign king. Even the currency of the United States bears the phrase "In God we trust." The phrase first appeared on U.S. coins in 1864, and on July 30, 1956, Congress recognized "In God We Trust" as the national motto[25] (Fig. 8-3).

The chronological history of the national Thanksgiving holiday and the National Day of Prayer also speak to the Judeo-Christian heritage of the United States. In 1795, George Washington gave a national Thanksgiving proclamation when he asked God to "impart all the blessing we possess, or ask for ourselves, to the whole family of mankind." In 1863, President Lincoln reestablished the national Thanksgiving proclamation when he stated, "We have been recipients of the choicest bounties of Heaven … we have grown in numbers, wealth and power as no other nation has ever grown. But we have forgotten God…. Intoxicated with unbroken success, we have become too self-sufficient to feel the necessity of redeeming and preserving grace, too proud to pray to the God that made us." Lincoln went on to proclaim the third Thursday in November to be a national holiday designed to allow all Americans to stop and thank the God that has made us and has blessed us. In 1981 President Ronald Reagan reestablished the first Thursday in May as the National Day of Prayer, reviving the early spring prayer and fall Thanksgiving practiced by the Continental Congress. Congress in 1988 unanimously confirmed this date as the National Day of Prayer.[26]

Today, 85% of Americans claim to be Christian, 2% Jewish, 1.5% Muslim, and 1% Buddhist; 9.4%

claim no religion and the remaining percentage hold to traditional ethnic, Hindu, Baha'i, Sikh, and Chinese beliefs and practices.[27] Moreover, specific religious groups are concentrated regionally in the United States, with Baptists in the South, Lutherans in the North and Midwest, and Catholics in the Northeast, East, and Southwest.[28] Within this context, there is a separation of church and state, and the U.S. government cannot support any particular religion or prevent people from practicing their chosen religion. However, this does not include cults or extremist groups, who usually devote themselves to esoteric ideals and fads.[29]

In contrast to many countries that support a specific church or religion and where people discuss their religion frequently and openly, religion is not an everyday topic of conversation for most Americans, and yet the heritage of the democratic nation of the United States of America is rich with Judeo-Christian principles and ethics (Figs. 8-4 and 8-5).

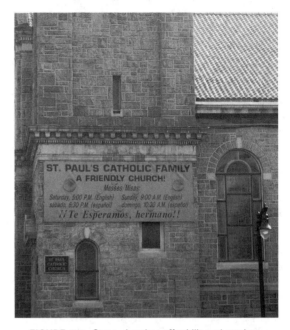

FIGURE 8.4 Some churches offer bilingual services.

Reflective Exercise

• How would you modify a prayer service or the opening ceremony of a conference to be inclusive of all religious denominations?

Use of Prayer

Prayer takes different forms and has different meanings. Some people pray daily and may have altars in their homes. Others may consider themselves devoutly religious and say prayers only on special occasions or in times of crisis or illness. Recent research involving a double-blind, randomized, controlled clinical trial demonstrates the effectiveness of intercessory prayer in health outcomes for those admitted to a coronary care unit. Patients receiving the intercessory prayer had less need for antibiotics, diuretics, and ventilator support and overall had improved health outcomes compared with the control group.[30] Positive therapeutic effects resulted from intercessory prayer in a coronary care unit population. Townsend and colleagues[31] conducted a systematic review of the research relating to religion and health and concluded that religious beliefs and activities (including prayer) appear to improve

blood pressure, immune function, depression, and length of life.

Among the Amish, faith-related behavior includes corporate (group) worship, prayer, and

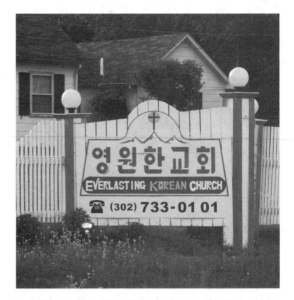

FIGURE 8.5 Some churches exist for specific ethnic groups.

singing, which help build conformity and maintain harmony within the group.[32] Prayer is a significant source of individual strength for Muslims, who pray five times a day.[13] According to a Century Foundation poll, 82% of Americans believe that prayer can cure a serious illness. As for intercessory prayer, 73% believe in its effectiveness for curing others, and 64% of Americans reported that they would like their physicians to pray with them.[33] Physical therapists may need to make special arrangements for individuals to say prayers in accordance with their belief systems and may want to consider praying with their patients if the patient and physical therapist so desire. Additionally, scheduling appointments around scheduled prayer times may improve attention to therapy and improve attendance.

Reflective Exercise

• What does prayer mean to you? • Do you pray for good health? • How often do you pray?

Reflection 8.1

I recall an awkward moment when I was working a bedside rotation at a hospital. I entered the room of my patient early in the morning to find her two daughters and son huddled around her. I knew it was a bad time but didn't understand why. One of the daughters stepped out of the room with me and explained that her family was Hindu, and it was customary to have a time of prayer both at the start and the end of the day. She requested that her mother be allowed this time every day, as she felt it would greatly help her recovery. We agreed to a later time for her therapy session that would not interfere with her time of prayer.

Camilla Carter, PT

Meaning of Life and Individual Sources of Strength

What gives meaning to life varies among and within cultural groups. To some people, their formal religion may be the most important facet of fulfilling their spirituality needs, whereas for others, religion may be replaced as a driving force by other life forces and worldviews. Among some groups, family is the most important social entity and is extremely important in helping meet their spiritual needs. For others, what gives meaning to life is good health and well-being. For a few, spirituality may include work or money.

A person's inner strength comes from different sources. Among the Navajo, the inner self is dependent on being in harmony with one's surroundings.[34] For Christians, a belief in God and His mercy through His son, Jesus Christ, gives personal hope and strength. For some people, spirituality includes a combination of these factors. Knowing these beliefs allows healthcare providers to assist individuals and families in their quest for strength and self-fulfillment.

Reflective Exercise

• What gives meaning to your life? • Is religion the primary source of strength for you? • From where do you get your inner strength to cope with life's difficulties?

Spiritual Beliefs and Healthcare Practices

Spiritual wellness brings fulfillment from a lifestyle of purposeful and pleasurable living that embraces free choices, satisfaction in life, and self-esteem. For example, when Navajo Indians are not in harmony with their surroundings and experience insomnia from anxieties, the Blessingway ceremony, ritual dancing, and herbal treatments, combined with prayers and songs, are performed for total body healing and the return of spirits to the body.[34,35] Practices that interfere with a person's spiritual life can hinder physical recovery and promote physical illness.

Taking a spiritual history serves many purposes and sends a powerful message. First, it communicates that the physical therapist is concerned about the entire person, and not just the disability. Second, it provides important information regarding the person's motivations and behaviors related to health. Third, the physical therapist may glean information about support systems and resources within the home and community by taking a spiritual history; and finally, it communicates to the patient that this is an area open to discussion should the need arise in the future.[24]

The physical therapist who is aware of the patient's religious practices and spiritual needs and who acknowledges the relationship between religion, spirituality, and health is in a better position to promote culturally competent health care (Fig. 8-6). The physical therapist must demonstrate an appreciation of and respect for the dignity and spiritual beliefs of patients by avoiding negative comments about religious beliefs and practices. Patients may find considerable comfort in speaking with religious leaders in times of crisis and serious illness, and physical therapists should be ready to offer a referral to a religious leader/counselor of the patient's choice.

Physical therapists should inquire if the person wants to see a member of the clergy, even if he or she has not been active in church. Sometimes a crisis such as an illness leads one to ponder spiritual issues not pondered previously, and spiritual counseling may be something the patient is newly considering. Religious emblems should not be removed, as they provide solace to the person and removing them may increase or cause anxiety. A thorough assessment of spiritual life is essential for the identification of solutions and resources that can support health and well-being.

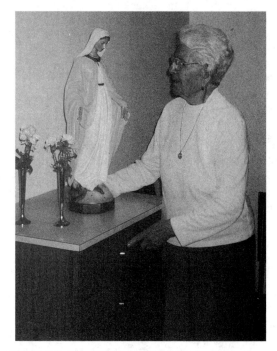

FIGURE 8.6 This patient appreciates that her therapy includes ambulating to the Catholic chapel in the rehabilitation hospital.

Reflective Exercise

• How are spirituality and health connected in your life?

CULTURAL SELF-ASSESSMENT EXERCISE 1

Self-Assessment

Answer the following questions related to the domain of death rituals for yourself.
1. If something unexpected happens and your heart or lungs stop functioning, do you want cardiopulmonary resuscitation?

2. If you were declared brain-dead, would you want life support equipment discontinued?
3. If you were unaware of your surroundings, would you want to be fed artificially?

4. Do you have a "living will"?
5. Do you have a durable power of attorney?
6. Who do you want to make life decisions for you if you are unable to do so?
7. Where do you prefer to die? In a healthcare facility? Your home? Someplace else?
8. Do you want your body returned to your home country (if appropriate)?
9. Where do you want to be buried?
10. Do you want interment or cremation?
11. Who do you want at your bedside when you are ill?
12. Would you want to be told if you have a terminal illness?
13. What do you expect family/friends to do when you die?
14. Do you believe people have the right to take their own lives?
15. Are there any circumstances in which it is okay to withhold life support?
16. Are there any circumstances in which it is okay to withdraw artificial feeding?
17. Would you want to see a clergyperson if you were dying?
18. Do you say special prayers for health?
21. What do you normally do to express your grief?
22. What do you normally do when you receive bad news?

CULTURAL SELF-ASSESSMENT EXERCISE 2

Understanding Others

1. Which of the above questions would be important to ask your physical therapy patient?

2. Why would it be important for you as a physical therapist to understand the answers to the questions you noted?

CULTURAL SELF-ASSESSMENT EXERCISE 3

Self-Assessment

Answer the following questions related to the domain of spirituality for yourself.
1. With what religion(s) do you identify?
2. Does everyone in your household identify with the same religion as you?
3. Is there a specific holy day that you observe?
4. How often do you pray?
5. Do you pray alone or in a group?
6. Would you like someone to pray with you?

(continued)

CULTURAL SELF-ASSESSMENT EXERCISE 3 *(Continued)*

7. Do you need any special items or arrangements to pray?
8. Which religious holidays do you celebrate?
9. What does your religion mean to you personally?
10. What diet does your religion require?
11. What medications does your religion restrict you from taking? Vaccinations? Immunizations?
12. What things do you believe in or have faith in?
13. How has this illness influenced your faith?
14. What role does faith play in regaining your health?
15. Do you have someone to talk with about religious or spiritual things?
16. Would you like to talk about religious or spiritual things with someone?
17. What does spirituality mean to you personally?
18. What is the most important thing in your life?
19. What other things in life are important to you?

CULTURAL SELF-ASSESSMENT EXERCISE 4

*U*nderstanding Others

1. Which of the above questions about spirituality would be important to ask your physical therapy patient?
2. Why would it be important for you as a physical therapist to understand the answers to the questions you noted?

Following are observations that might be helpful in understanding a patient's spirituality.

1. Does the patient have religious books or objects in his or her possession or at the bedside?
2. Does the patient wear any religious articles, clothing, or headdress?
3. Does the patient receive greeting or get-well cards of a religious nature?
4. Does a religious person visit the patient?

*V*ignette *Q*uestions

1. How would you respond to Mrs. Carrington?
2. What comfort might you be able to provide for her?
3. How comfortable are you in dealing with death and dying?
4. Where might you go to learn about cultural death ritual patterns?

Vignette Questions

1. Mr. Kravitz did not maintain eye contact with Ms. Miller and dismissed her when she began her physical evaluation of him. What might these behaviors mean?
2. What should Ms. Miller do now?
3. Was Ms. Miller wrong or did she act inappropriately?
3. How might Ms. Miller better understand Mr. Kravitz's culture?
4. How might the situation have been avoided?
5. What accommodations might Ms. Miller and the clinic make to better serve Mr. Kravitz's needs in a culturally competent manner?
6. What might both parties learn from the encounter?

CASE STUDY SCENARIO I

You are a physical therapist working in the home care setting. You have an appointment with your patient, an 80-year-old, second-generation German male who recently underwent a transfemoral amputation secondary to diabetes. His name is Hal Schmidt and he has a cardiac history. You arrive at the door and no one answers your knock. You can hear noise inside, and you become concerned. You find that the door is unlocked, and you cautiously open the door and call into the room. Your patient's wife, who moved to the United States from Korea after marrying her husband, emerges from the patient's bedroom and is wailing, "Hal is dead! He is dead! He is dead!" You rush to the bedside and you can see by his coloring that he is lifeless. You check for a pulse and cannot find one. His wife hysterically insists that you do something. She repeatedly wails, "He can't die here, he must get to the hospital!"

1. What would you do first?
2. How would you help Mrs. Schmidt?
3. What do you know about the death rituals of Korean culture?
4. What do you know about the death rituals of German culture?
5. Where might you get this information?

CASE STUDY SCENARIO II

Refer to the case scenario for Sandra Yoder, the young Amish woman, in Chapter 5. Mrs. Yoder is now in the rehabilitation hospital. Challenges exist with the occupational therapist (OT) assisting her with dressing. Mrs. Yoder is extremely modest and prefers that the OT not be present

(continued)

for dressing; she would rather one of her sisters or sisters-in-law help her. Her dress is also a challenge in the physical therapy gym. The long skirts and petticoats are cumbersome in her transfer to the mat, performing exercises, and gait training. Mrs. Yoder's dress and head covering are an important part of the Ordnung, the understood order of Amish life.

Last week, Mr. Yoder told the rehabilitation team that it was very important that Mrs. Yoder be home for a biannual council meeting and communion service the following week. The council meeting is a day-long event involving every member of the Amish community. It serves to unify and affirm membership in the community. On the following week is the day-long communion service, another important biannual event. The ministers of the church conduct the service, which includes prayers, songs, sermons, and confession. Mr. Yoder emphasizes the importance for Mrs. Yoder to attend these events. He also notes that it would be important to her if she could kneel for the prayers with the rest of the community.

1. What challenges does the rehab team face in the accomplishment of rehabilitation goals within Mrs. Yoder's culture?

2. How might the therapist handle activities of daily living (ADL) training for Mrs. Yoder?

3. How might the physical therapist manage Mrs. Yoder's dress in the clinic?

4. Why is it that Mr. Yoder speaks for Mrs. Yoder? How do you feel about this?

5. Should the rehabilitation team make an effort to allow Mrs. Yoder to attend the council meeting and/or communion service?

6. How might the rehabilitation team meet these challenges?

REFERENCES

1. Braun L, Pietsch J, Blanchette P. *Cultural Issues in End-of-Life Decision Making.* Thousand Oaks, Calif: Sage; 2000.
2. Leash RM. *Death Notification.* Hinesburg, Vt: Upper Access; 1994.
3. Leming M, Dickinson G. *Understanding Death, Dying, and Bereavement.* Ft Worth, Tex: Harcourt Brace; 2002.
4. Purnell L. The Purnell Model for Cultural Competence. In: Purnell L, Paulanka B, eds. *Transcultural Health Care: A Culturally Competent Approach.* 2nd ed. Philadelphia, Pa: FA Davis; 2003:8–40.
5. Turner B. *Medical Power and Social Knowledge.* 2nd ed. London: Sage; 1995.
6. Althen G. *American Ways: A Guide for Foreigners in the United States.* Yarmouth, Me: Intercultural Press; 1988.
7. Datesman M, Crandall J, Kearney E. *The American Ways.* White Plains, NY: Prentice-Hall; 1997.
8. Kim EY. *The Yin and Yang of American Culture.* Yarmouth, Me: Intercultural Press; 2001.
9. Glanville C. People of African American heritage. In: Purnell L, Paulanka B, eds. *Transcultural Health Care: A Culturally Competent Approach.* 2nd ed. Philadelphia, Pa: FA Davis; 2003:40–53.
10. Selekman J. People of Jewish heritage. In: Purnell L, Paulanka B, eds. *Transcultural Health Care: A Culturally Competent Approach.* 2nd ed. Philadelphia, Pa: FA Davis; 2003:234–248.
11. Zoucha R, Purnell L. People of Mexican heritage. In: Purnell L, Paulanka B, eds. *Transcultural Health Care: A Culturally Competent Approach.* 2nd ed. Philadelphia, Pa: FA Davis; 2003:264–278.
12. Purnell L, Papadopoulos I. People of Greek heritage [chapter on CD-ROM]. In: Purnell L, Paulanka B, eds. *Transcultural Health Care: A Culturally Competent Approach.* 2nd ed. Philadelphia, Pa: FA Davis; 2003.

13. Kulwicki A. People of Arab heritage. In: Purnell L, Paulanka B, eds. *Transcultural Health Care: A Culturally Competent Approach.* 2nd ed. Philadelphia, Pa: FA Davis; 2003:90–105

14. Hospice Foundation of America. Hospice care. Available at: http://www.hospicefoundation.org/what_is/. Accessed June 4, 2004.

15. Neubauer B, Hamilton C. Racial differences in attitudes toward hospice care. *Hospice J.* 1990;16:37–48.

16. O'Brien L, Siegert E, Grisso J. Tube feeding among nursing home residents. *J Gen Intern Med.* 1997;12: 354–371.

17. Purnell L. People of Appalachian heritage. In: Purnell L, Paulanka B, eds. *Transcultural Health Care: A Culturally Competent Approach.* 2nd ed. Philadelphia, Pa: FA Davis; 2003:73–89.

18. Hillman S. People of Italian heritage. In: Purnell L, Paulanka B, eds. *Transcultural Health Care: A Culturally Competent Approach.* 2nd ed. Philadelphia, Pa: FA Davis; 2003:205–217.

19. Juarbe T. People of Puerto Rican heritage. In: Purnell L, Paulanka B, eds. *Transcultural Health Care: A Culturally Competent Approach.* 2nd ed. Philadelphia, Pa: FA Davis; 2003:307–326.

20. Jambanathan J. People of Hindu heritage [chapter on CD-ROM]. In: Purnell L, Paulanka B, eds. *Transcultural Health Care: A Culturally Competent Approach.* 2nd ed. Philadelphia, Pa: FA Davis; 2003.

21. Miller WS, Goodin JN. East Hindu Americans. In: Giger JN, Davidhizar RE, eds. *Transcultural Nursing: Assessment and Intervention.* 3rd ed. St Louis, Mo: Mosby; 1999:459–481.

22. Purnell L, Kim S. People of Korean heritage. In: Purnell L, Paulanka B, eds. *Transcultural Health Care: A Culturally Competent Approach.* 2nd ed. Philadelphia, Pa: FA Davis; 2003:249–263.

23. Wang Y. People of Chinese ancestry. In: Purnell L, Paulanka B, eds. *Transcultural Health Care: A Culturally Competent Approach.* 2nd ed. Philadelphia, Pa: FA Davis; 2003:106–121.

24. Koenig HG. *Spirituality in Patient Care: Why, How, When, and What.* Philadelphia, Pa: Templeton Foundation Press; 2002.

25. Infoplease. Declaration of Independence. Available at: http://www.infoplease.com/ipa/A0101022.html. Accessed July 3, 2003.

26. Thanks-Giving Square. The history of Thanksgiving in the United States. Available at: http://www.thanksgiving.org/2chron.html. Accessed June 14, 2003.

27. Operation World. Dawn Ministries. Available at: http://www.24-7prayer.com/ow/country2.php?country_id=51. Accessed June 14, 2003.

28. Largest Religious Groups in the United States of America. http://www.adherents.com/rel_USA.html. Accessed July 26, 2005. ©2005 by Adherents.com.

29. What Types of Cults Exist. http://www.csj.org/studyindex/studycult/cultqa2.htm (no publication date). Accessed July 26, 2005.

30. Byrd R. Positive therapeutic effects of intercessory prayer in a coronary care unit population. *South Med J.* 1988;81: 826–829.

31. Townsend M, Kladder V, Ayele H, Mulligan T. Systematic review of clinical trials examining the effects of religion on health. *South Med J.* 2002;95:1429–1434.

32. Wenger AF, Wenger M. The Amish. In: Purnell L, Paulanka B, eds. *Transcultural Health Care: A Culturally Competent Approach.* 2nd ed. Philadelphia, Pa: FA Davis; 2003:54–72.

33. Century Foundation. Public Opinion Watch. *Time* [serial online]. June 24, 2003. Available at: http://www.tcf.org/Opinions/Public_Opinion_Watch/June24–28.html. Accessed July 3, 2003.

34. Still O, Hodgins D. Navajo Indians. In: Purnell L, Paulanka B, eds. *Transcultural Health Care: A Culturally Competent Approach.* 2nd ed. Philadelphia, Pa: FA Davis; 2003:279–283.

35. Wilson U. Nursing care of the American Indian patient. In: Orque MS, Block B, Monrroy LSA, eds. *Ethnic Nursing Care: A Multicultural Approach.* St Louis, Mo: Mosby; 1993.

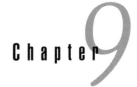

Chapter 9

Exploring Cultural Healthcare Practices and Roles of Healthcare Practitioners

- Jill Black Lattanzi, PT, EdD
- Larry D. Purnell, PhD, RN

Healthcare Practices

Kim Chung Nam, age 42 years, has lived in the United States for 5 years. She lived in Canada for 4 years before coming to the United States. She is originally from Korea. She has undergone a total hip replacement and is recuperating at home, where she uses acupuncture and herbal therapies for pain control and to manage her diabetes mellitus. She lives with her mother, her father-in-law, her husband, and her son. Her mother answers the door when the physical therapist arrives and indicates (she does not speak English) that the physical therapist should remove his shoes.

Healthcare practices and beliefs are linked intimately to culture. One learns healthcare practices and beliefs from family and community and from lived experiences. The physical therapist interfaces directly with the client's healthcare practices and beliefs whether the physical therapist realizes it or not. The goal of this chapter is to help the physical therapist understand his or her healthcare beliefs and to better recognize, respect, and understand the physical therapy implications of the client's healthcare beliefs and practices.

The domain *healthcare practices* is interconnected with all other domains of culture and includes the focus of healthcare (acute vs. preventive); traditional, magicoreligious, and biomedical beliefs; individual responsibility for health; self-medicating practices; and views toward mental illness, chronicity, rehabilitation, and organ donation and transplantation. In addition, responses to pain and the sick role are shaped by specific ethnocultural beliefs. Significant barriers to healthcare may be shared among cultural and ethnic groups (Fig. 9-1). The concepts of chronicity, rehabilitation, pain, and sick role hold particular relevance for the physical therapist.

Health-Seeking Beliefs and Behaviors

Health-seeking beliefs and behaviors determine the acceptance of proposed health practices. Therefore, it is important that the physical therapist attain an understanding of a client's underlying health beliefs and behaviors, also termed the "explanatory model of health and illness."[1] The physical therapist working with clients from the dominant U.S. culture will most likely encounter clients who believe in a biomedical explanation of illness. The biomedical model attributes health and illness to physiological, biological, and scientifically explainable changes in one's body. Thus, the most acceptable interventions would be those that are scientifically proven. In congruence with the individualistic nature of U.S. culture, the bio-

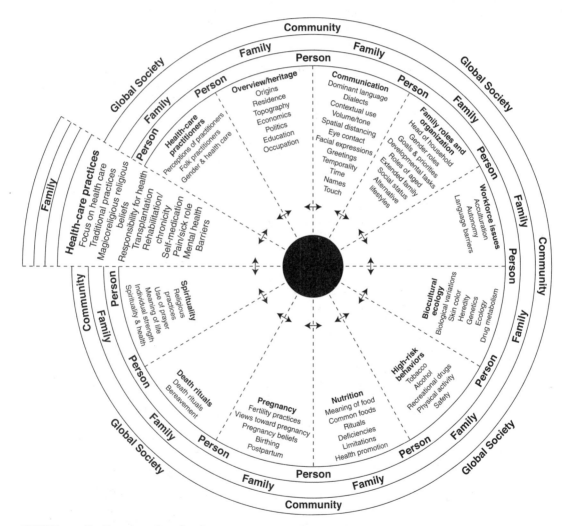

FIGURE 9.1 Healthcare practices domain. (Adapted from Purnell, L. D., & Paulanka, B. J. (1998). The Purnell Model for Cultural Competence. In L. D. Purnell & B. J. Paulanka (Eds.), *Transcultural health care: A culturally competent approach* (p. 10). Philadelphia: F.A. Davis.)

medical model emphasizes the treatment of the individual's body and minimizes the links to households, communities, or the supernatural. Murdock[2] published a survey of 189 different cultures' beliefs regarding health and wellness; interestingly, the biomedical model was a minority view among these cultures.

The biomedical model has led to great advances in combating disease, illness, and disability with an emphasis on scientific research and the discovery of new interventions. The physical therapy profession has grown in respectability and effectiveness as the profession has emphasized and encouraged evidence-based practice and clinical research. The fact remains, however, that science is not able to explain everything about health and illness, and a level of faith is required. A point exists within physical health and wellness where science fails to yield precise answers and the unexplainable occurs.

Reflective Exercise

• How strongly do you hold to biomedical explanations of health and illness? • How has physical therapy altered or reinforced your explanatory model of health and illness?

Traditional and folk healing practices have maintained people's health for centuries, and in many cultures they are the dominant healthcare practices. Currently, the United States is undergoing a paradigm shift from a high value placed on curative and restorative medical practices with sophisticated technological care, to one of health promotion and wellness, illness and disease prevention, and health maintenance and restoration.[3] Most ethnocultural groups believe that the individual, family, and community have the ability to influence their health. However, among other populations, good health may be seen as divine providence, with individuals having little control over their health and illness.[4-9] This fatalistic view toward health might make it difficult for a client and/or the client's family to embrace a program of physical rehabilitation. Why pursue rehabilitation of an impairment, functional limitation, or disability if one has no control over it? The Garifuna, a people of African descent in

BOX 9.1

Kleinman's Explanatory Model

1. How and/or why has the problem occurred?
2. What is the cause of the problem?
3. What else might cause it?
4. How might other people in your family explain the cause of a problem such as this?
5. How might other people in your country explain the cause?

Belize, hold to a fatalistic belief system and may not embrace the concept of physical rehabilitation (Black and Purnell, personal experiences, January 2000). Regardless of the client's map of health understandings, it is essential that the physical therapist seek to understand that map if interventions are to be effective. Kleinman[1] suggests that the physical therapist use the questions listed in Box 9-1 to understand the client's explanatory model.

Reflective Exercise

• How much control do you feel you have over your health and wellness? • What do your family members believe about this?

Cultures may be more past, present, or future oriented.[10,11] Physical therapy inherently requires a present orientation, and the nature of goal setting and program planning necessitates a degree of future orientation. The hard work that goes into a physical rehabilitation program is an investment in potential future gain. Cultures with a past orientation may practice ancestor worship or simply focus on the past and do not plan for the future as readily.[8,12-14] Thus, clients from these cultures may be less amenable to a physical therapy program that focuses on setting short- and long-term, future-oriented goals.

Other cultures, particularly when the secondary cultural characteristic of low socioeconomic status is present, are more attuned to a present-oriented temporality. A present orientation arises where individuals must focus the majority of their energies on the needs of today. Sometimes the present needs are so encompassing that their urgency disallows a future focus. In this case, the future-oriented physical therapy program may not be a priority in meeting the immediate needs of the present.

Reflective Exercise

• Do you consider yourself more past oriented, present oriented, or future oriented? • Give reasons for your answer.

Reflective Exercise

• Is your profession more past oriented, present oriented, or future oriented? • Give reasons for your answer.

The primacy of patient autonomy has been accepted as an enlightened perspective in European American cultures. To this end, advance directives are an important part of medical care. Patients can specify their wishes concerning life-and-death decisions before entering an inpatient facility. Advance directives, a living will, and a durable power of attorney allow patients to name a family member or significant other to speak for them and make decisions if they are unable to do so. Each inpatient facility has forms on which to document the patient's wishes. Patients may use these forms or bring their own forms. The practice and acceptance of using advance directives and living wills are not uniform across ethnocultural groups. Only 12% of African Americans, 13% of Korean Americans, 47% of Mexican Americans, and 69% of white Americans favor advance directives[15,16] (Fig. 9-2). Collectivist cultures, where the family decision making is deemed more important then the individual's decision making, are less likely to have advance directives.[4,9,17,18]

Undergoing surgery is always a major concern and decision for most people. Beliefs about surgery vary among ethnocultural groups. For example, many Hispanics believe that undergoing surgery for cancer will cause the cancer to spread and thus are less likely to believe that surgery for breast cancer will cure the disease.[9,19] Other

> ## Reflection 9.1
>
> I am from India and received my PTA training in the United States. I find that the interaction between the therapist and the patient is given more importance in the United States compared with India. In the United States, therapists explain the procedures in simple language to make clients better understand the effectiveness of the therapy, and patient consent for treatment is not taken for granted and is never to be forced. In India, not as much importance is given to these matters. Patients are expected to do whatever the doctor tells them. The doctor knows best.
>
> *Deepali Hazariwala, PTA*

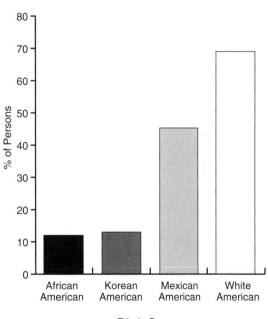

FIGURE 9.2 Bar graph indicating acceptance of advanced directives across ethnic groups.

cultural beliefs suggest that the more invasive the procedure, the better it is; thus, people in these cultures opt for immediate surgical interventions over a trial period of physical therapy.[20,21]

Reflective Exercise

• Do you have a living will or other document that guides your healthcare decision making? • How do you feel about living wills and advance directives?

The concept and practice of exercise and physical fitness vary among cultures. The culture of the United States has increasingly embraced exercise and physical fitness programs over the past 40 years. Physical therapists should not be surprised if their elder clients are not accustomed to formal exercise programs. Much of their exercise may come in the physical activities of daily routines as opposed to more formal fitness regimens (Fig. 9-3). Exercise and the emphasis on physical fitness do not cross all cultures. Physical therapists prescribing exercise programs to their clients are wise to remember that this may be a foreign concept to some. In some cultures, such as the Egyptian culture, exercise is not typically a part of the lifestyle.[22] Iranian women are supposed to refrain from exercise during their menstrual period so as not to encourage additional hemorrhage.[20]

Reflective Exercise

• What value do you place on exercise and physical fitness? • From where does that value come? • What values do your physical therapy clients place on physical fitness? • Why might that be important to understand in establishing a physical therapy plan of care?

Responsibility for Healthcare

Most Western nations and many Eastern cultures are moving to a paradigm where people take increased responsibility for their health. In a society where individualism is valued, one is expected to be self-reliant.[13] In fact, the individual is expected to exercise some control over disease, including controlling the amount of stress in one's life. If the person does not maintain a healthy lifestyle,

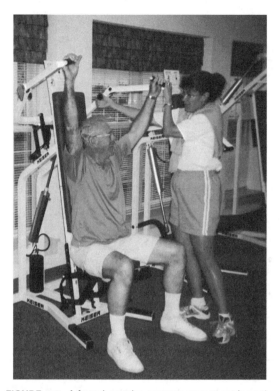

FIGURE 9.3 A formal exercise program on gym equipment may be unfamiliar to some elder patients.

some believe it is the person's own fault if he or she gets a disease or illness. Unless one is very ill, he or she should not neglect social and work obligations.[23]

On the other hand, collectivist cultures emphasize group responsibility in the face of illness and disability. Often, the individual is not the decision maker with regard to his or her health.[21,24] Simpson, Mohr, and Redman[25] suggest asking the following questions:

1. Who makes the healthcare decisions in the family?
2. Whom would you like the physical therapist to address?
3. How much information should the client be given?

The United States government recently enacted the Health Insurance Portability and Accountability Act (HIPAA). It is interesting to note that the regulations aimed at protecting the individual's privacy reflect a purely U.S., individualistic cultural value. Many of the collectivist cultures, such as the Chinese,[24] Korean,[8] Japanese,[26] Vietnamese,[18] and Arab[21] cultures, would not appreciate the exclusion of the group.

Reflective Exercise

• How has HIPAA influenced your physical therapy practice? • Why might HIPAA be offensive to some cultures?

Many beliefs exist across cultures as to what causes illness and disease. To prevent the onset of illness, one is told, for example, not to go out in the cold with wet hair,[27] not to place one's warm feet on a cold floor, and not to shower immediately after exercising.[9] For some, illness or disease is due to fate or is God's will. For others, it may be due to lack of faith in a higher being or to sinful behavior.[28]

The healthcare delivery system of the country of origin may shape the client's and employee's beliefs regarding personal responsibility for healthcare. In the United States, any person, regardless of socioeconomic or immigration status, can receive acute care services. However, the person will be charged a fee for the service, and nonacute follow-up care may not be available unless the person proves that he or she is able to pay for the service. Even if the person is covered by health insurance, an insurance company representative may need to approve the visit and then supply a list of the procedures and interventions for which they will reimburse or limit the number of sessions they will approve. However, Great Britain, Australia, Germany, Japan, Korea, and Canada, to name only a few countries, provide free healthcare at the point of entry to the healthcare system, with reimbursement coming from the government. Individuals who did not need health insurance in their native country may not realize the importance of having health insurance in the United States.

Many of the working poor cannot afford to purchase economic essentials for the family, and thus cannot even consider the purchase of health insurance when the government or the employer does not provide it. Physical therapists should not assume that clients who do not have health insurance or practice health prevention do not care about their health. The physical therapist must assess clients individually and provide culturally congruent education regarding health promotion and wellness, illness and disease prevention, and health maintenance activities.

Reflective Exercise

• How do you feel about the U.S. government's and the insurance industry's view of healthcare reimbursement? • Do you think that all people should have equal access to healthcare? • What is your opinion about socialized medicine, where all people receive healthcare free at the point of entry into the healthcare system?

Reflective Exercise

• Do you have health insurance? • What would you recommend for someone who does not have the financial means to afford health insurance?

The use of herbal medicine has increased in the United States over the last decade. Most herbs that people can purchase are harmless, but many can have serious negative health effects if taken in large quantities or in combination with prescription medicine. Some of the more popular herbal medicines are listed in Box 9-2.

Reflective Exercise

• Why might it be important for a physical therapist to know of the client's herbal remedy practices? • How might the client's herbal remedy practices impact the physical therapy program?

A potential high-risk behavior in the self-care context involves self-medicating practices. Self-medicating behavior in itself may not be harmful, but when combined with prescription medications or used to the exclusion of prescription medications, it may be detrimental to a person's

BOX 9.2

Common Herbal Medicines

(a) Echinacea, an immune stimulant and anti-infective, is contraindicated in patients with immune system disorders and can be hepatotoxic with persistent use.

(b) Feverfew, which is used for migraines, arthritis, and menstrual irregularities. may cause increased clotting time and hypersensitivity with ragweed allergies.

(c) Garlic, which is used as an antihypertensive and antibiotic, and for lowering cholesterol, may increase clotting time and decrease blood glucose levels when taken in large amounts.

(d) St. John's wort, which is used as an antidepressant, can cause insomnia, falsely elevate digoxin levels, and potentiate MAO inhibitors.

(e) Ginkgo, which is used to increase peripheral vascular circulation and increase cerebral blood flow, may interact with anti-thrombotic therapy and affect platelet agglutination.

health. A common practice with prescription medications is to take the medicine until the symptoms disappear, and then discontinue the medicine prematurely. This practice commonly occurs with antihypertensive medications and antibiotics, resulting in poor control of hypertension and antibiotic resistance or superinfection.

Reflective Exercise

• For what conditions do you self-medicate? • When prescribed medication, do you *always* take it as ordered and for the required duration, or do you discontinue it prematurely? • Look in your medicine cabinet. How many medicines are there? • How many are outdated?

Each country has some type of control over the purchase and use of medications. The United States is more restrictive than many countries and provides warning labels and directions for the use of over-the-counter medications. In many countries, pharmacists may be consulted before physicians for fever-reducing and pain-reducing medicines. In parts of Central America[6,7] and Turkey,[29] a person can purchase antibiotics, intravenous fluids, and a variety of medications over the counter; most grocery stores sell medications, and vendors sell drugs in corner shops and on public transportation systems. People who are accustomed to purchasing medications over the counter in their native country may see no problem in sharing their medications with family and friends. To help prevent conflicting or exacerbated effects of prescription medication and treatment regimens, physical therapists should ask about clients' self-medicating practices. One cannot ignore the ample supply of over-the-counter medications in American pharmacies, in addition to the numerous television and Internet advertisements for self-medication and media campaigns for new medications, all encouraging viewers to ask their doctor or healthcare provider about a particular pharmaceutical product.

Reflective Exercise

• Do you routinely ask clients if they are taking over-the-counter medications? • Why might this information be important for the physical therapist to know?

Folk Practices

Some societies favor traditional, folk, or magicoreligious healthcare practices over biomedical practices, or use them simultaneously. What are considered alternative or complementary healthcare practices in one country may constitute mainstream medicine in another culture. In the United States, interest has increased in alternative and complementary health practices. The U.S. government's Office of Alternative Medicine at the National Institutes of Health has grants to bridge the gap between traditional and nontraditional therapies.[30]

As an adjunct to biomedical treatments, many people use acupuncture, acupressure, acumassage, herbal therapies, and other traditional treatments (Fig. 9-4). These terms can cause

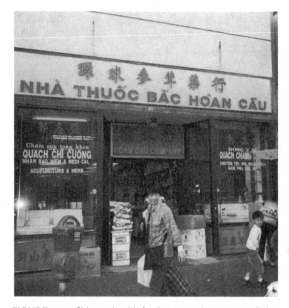

FIGURE 9.4 Chinese health food store and acupuncturist's office.

others, is essential. Many times these traditional, folklore, and magicoreligious practices are rightfully incorporated into the plans of care for clients. However, physical therapists must ask clients about these practices so that conflicting treatment modalities are not used. An example specifically related to physical therapy is a client choosing to apply hot herbal compresses to an acute inflammatory condition. This would be in direct conflict with the physical therapist's recommendation to apply cold. If clients perceive that physical therapists do not accept or are unwilling to consider their beliefs, they may be less compliant with prescriptive treatment and less likely to reveal their use of these practices.

Reflective Exercise

• Do you observe any complementary/alternative practices (acupressure, acupuncture, herbal medicines, megavitamins, massage therapy, etc.)?

confusion. "Traditional" may or may not be "alternative." Many people, such as Hispanics, commonly visit traditional healers because modern medicine is viewed as inadequate.[4,6,7,9,31] Examples of folk medicine include covering a boil with axle grease, wearing copper bracelets for arthritis pain, mixing wild turnip root and honey for sore throats, and drinking herbal teas.[13] Native American traditions include ceremonial dances and songs.[32] The Chinese subscribe to the "yin and yang" theory of treating illnesses,[24] and Hispanic groups believe in the "hot and cold" theory of foods for treating illnesses and disease.[4,9,31] Moreover, the "hot and cold" theory extends to Haitians,[12] Vietnamese,[18] Arabs,[21] and many other cultures, although the words used to describe the opposing forces vary. Traditional schools of pharmacy in Brazil grow, sell, and teach courses on folk remedies.[33] Most Americans practice folk medicine in some form, including the use of family remedies passed down from previous generations.

Inquiring about the full range of therapies being used, such as food items, teas, herbal remedies, nonfood substances, over-the-counter medications, and medications prescribed or loaned by

An awareness of the possibility of combined practices when treating or providing health education to individuals and families helps ensure that therapies do not conflict with each other, intensify the treatment regimen, or cause an overdose. Such practices may also be harmful, conflict with, or potentiate the effects of prescription medications. Traditional and folk medicines are the only choice for some, because allopathic medicine cannot cure such illnesses as the evil eye, a common folk illness in many cultural groups. To help protect against the evil eye, one may wear beads, tie a string around the wrist, or wear a red (Ashkenazi Jews) or a blue (Sephardic Jews) ribbon.[34] One notable culture-bound syndrome in Westernized cultures that does not exist in non-Western cultures is anorexia, which affects women more than men.

Reflective Exercise

• Do you routinely ask clients about complementary and alternative therapies? • In your experience, do patients generally volunteer this information? • How might these practices affect the physical therapy intervention?

Barriers to Healthcare

In order for people to receive adequate healthcare, a number of considerations need to be addressed.

1. *Availability:* Is the service available and at a time when needed? Is the clinic open and with appointments available when the client can get there? For example, clinic hours may coincide with clients' work hours, making it difficult for them to schedule appointments for fear of workplace reprisals.
2. *Accessibility:* Are transportation services available? Do features of the geographical terrain, such as rivers and mountains, make it difficult for people to obtain needed healthcare services when no physical therapist is available in their immediate region? For example, it can be difficult for a single parent with four children to make several bus transfers to get one child to therapy.
3. *Affordability:* The service may be available, but does the client have the financial resources to afford the physical therapy?
4. *Appropriateness:* Are the appropriate physical therapy services available? For example, a physical therapy clinic in a rural setting might provide general physical therapy services, but a pediatric or hand specialist might be the specific therapy that is needed.
5. *Accountability:* Do physical therapists take accountability for their own education and learn about the cultures of the people they serve?
6. *Adaptability:* A mother brings her child to the clinic for physical therapy. Can she undergo her physical therapy for her back pain at the same time, or must she make another appointment on another day?
7. *Acceptability:* Are services and client education offered in a language preferred by the client? Are the interventions proposed congruent with the client's understanding of his or her illness?
8. *Awareness:* Is the client aware that needed services exist in the community? The service may be available, but if clients are not aware of it, the service will not be used.
9. *Attitudes:* Adverse subjective beliefs and attitudes from healthcare providers mean that the client will not return for needed services until the condition is more compromised. Do physical therapists have negative attitudes about patients' home-based traditional practices?
10. *Approachability:* Do clients feel welcomed? Do physical therapists and receptionists greet patients in the manner in which they prefer? This includes greeting patients with their preferred names.
11. *Alternative practices and practitioners:* Do biomedical providers incorporate clients' alternative/complementary practices into treatment plans? An overreliance on traditional and folk medicine may also be a barrier to adequate healthcare.
12. *Additional services:* Are child and adult care services available if a parent must bring children or an aging parent to the session?[3]

Physical therapists can help reduce some of these barriers by calling an area ethnic agency or church for assistance, establishing an advocacy role, involving professionals and lay people from the same ethnic group as the client, and using cultural brokers. If all of these elements are in place and used appropriately, they have the potential of generating culturally responsive care.

Cultural Responses to Health and Illness

In the United States, significant research has been conducted on patients' responses to pain, which has been called the "fifth vital sign." Most Americans believe that patients should be made comfortable and not have to tolerate high levels of pain. Accrediting bodies, such as the Joint Commission on Accreditation of Healthcare Organizations, survey healthcare organizations to ensure that the patient's pain level is assessed and that appropriate interventions are instituted. Beliefs regarding pain are one of the oldest culturally related research areas in healthcare. A 1969 study revealed that Irish Americans are stoic in their responses to pain, while Jewish Americans and Italian Americans are more vocal.[34] The Navajo regard pain and discomfort as a way of life,[32] and many Filipinos[5] view pain as part of life and an opportunity to atone for past transgressions; thus, they may be tolerant and stoic while experiencing pain. Astute observations and careful assessments must be completed

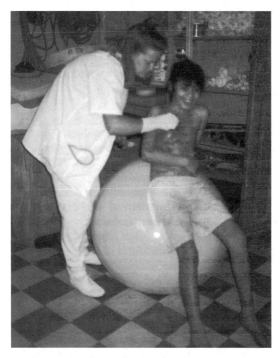

FIGURE 9.5 Physical therapists work with patients with burns, likely one of the most painful conditions treated.

Visual Graph

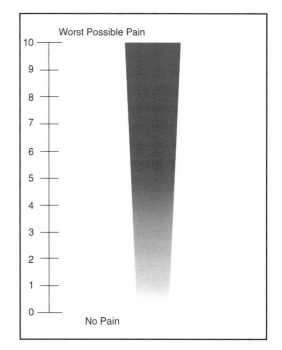

FIGURE 9.7 A visual analogue graph pain scale.

to determine the level of pain a person can and is willing to tolerate (Fig. 9-5).

At a minimum, physical therapists should have pain scales in the language of their clients, both with words and with pictures of the cultural group. Because facial expressions differ among racial groups, it may be difficult for a Chinese person to distinguish pain in the facial expressions of white people.[24] The reverse is true as well. Figures 9-6, 9-7, and 9-8 depict three different styles of

pain scales that may be helpful. Two of these pain scales have been translated into a number of different languages and are available on the Web.

Physical therapists must investigate the meaning of pain to each person within a cultural explanatory framework to interpret diverse behavioral responses and provide culturally competent care. The physical therapist may need to encourage the client to take the pain medication and explain that it will help the healing process.

FIGURE 9.6 A numeric pain scale, which can be translated into many languages.

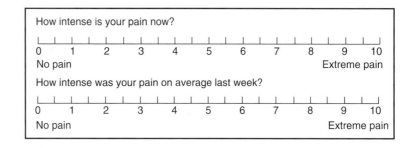

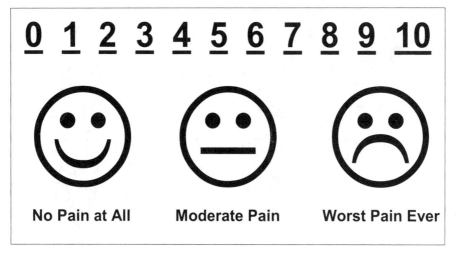

FIGURE 9.8 Wong Baker visual analogue scale, based on smiles and frowns with corresponding rank by number.

Research needs to be conducted in the areas of ethnic pain experiences and management of pain.

Reflective Exercise

• Do you feel that you have a high or low pain tolerance? As a child growing up, what were you taught to do when you had pain? • Based on your cultural background, how do men and how do women generally respond to pain?

Mental illness is perceived and expressed differently among ethnocultural groups, and this has a direct effect on how individuals present themselves and, consequently, on how healthcare providers interact with them. In some societies, such as American and Asian, mental illness may be seen by many as not as important as physical illness.[8,18,24] Mental illness is culture bound; what may be perceived as a mental illness in one society may not be considered a mental illness in another. Among most Asian American groups, mental illness or emotional difficulty is considered a disgrace and taboo. As a result, the family is likely to keep the mentally ill person at home as long as they can. This practice may be reinforced by the belief that all individuals are expected to contribute to the household for the common good of the family, and when a person is unable to contribute, further disgrace occurs.[8,18,24]

Filipinos may not readily accept professional mental health care but may be open to support and advice from family and friends.[5] In Korea, mentally disturbed children are stigmatized, and the lack of supportive services may cause families to abandon their loved ones because of the cost of long-term care and the family's desire and desperate need for support. Such children are kept from the public eye in hopes of saving the family from stigmatization. Koreans in the United States may hold these same values.[8,35]

Reflective Exercise

• Do you place a greater value on physical or mental illness? • In your culture, how is mental illness viewed?

Culturally congruent mental health services for these clients specific to physical therapy are listed in Box 9-3.

Physical Disabilities
Persons with physical disabilities may be treated differently in diverse cultures; sometimes nothing

BOX 9.3

Mental Health Considerations

1. Avoid emphasizing the independence of children and adolescents on the first encounter.[36]
2. Maintain formality and conversational distance.[37]
3. Do not expect an open public discussion of emotional problems.[38]
4. Expect somatization of emotional problems.[39,40]
5. Avoid discussion of hospitalization and seek alternative care services if possible.[37]

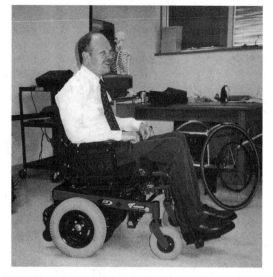

FIGURE 9.10 In the United States, it is not uncommon to see people with disabilities in the business world.

at all is done to provide accessibility for them (Fig. 9-9). In previous decades in the United States, individuals with physical disabilities were seen as less desirable than those who did not have a physical disability. If the handicap was severe, the person was sometimes hidden from the public's view.

In 1992, the Americans with Disabilities Act took effect, protecting individuals with a disability or handicap from discrimination. The Americans with Disabilities Act shifted the focus from changing the person with the disability to changing the social and political environment by removing the barriers restricting the person with the disability. Public places must be accessible, and it is not uncommon in the United States to see persons with physical disabilities in the workplace and elsewhere in society[41] (Figs. 9-9 and 9-10). In other countries, especially those with

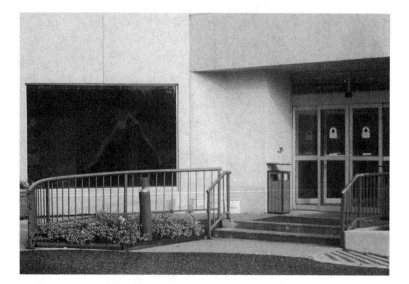

FIGURE 9.9 An entrance that meets ADA regulations in the United States.

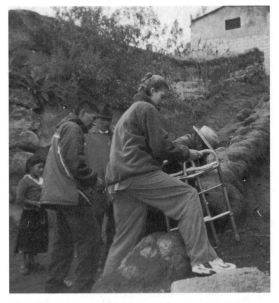

FIGURE 9.11 Accessibility is sometimes a critical issue.

challenging geographical terrain, accessibility can be a critical issue (Fig. 9-11).

Reflective Exercise

• What is your understanding of disability?
• How has that understanding changed since you became a physical therapist? • Do you attempt to change the person with disability, the environment, or both?

Despite the strides toward acceptance of and respect for people with disabilities, negative stereotypes, discrimination, and misunderstandings continue to exist and be perpetuated. The individualistic U.S. cultural values of autonomy, youth, and productivity are not totally incongruent with rehabilitation. People with disabilities can be productive members of society. While a collectivist culture might be more likely to keep the person with a disability hidden and protected from society, the cultural norms of group and family importance lead the family to value and care for the individual with a disability within their group. The collectivist culture does not hold

the same expectations of autonomy and productivity for the individual with a physical disability. Likewise, a person with a disability within the collectivist culture may not need or desire to reach his or her full potential to the extent that the physical therapist from the dominant U.S. culture might envision.

Rehabilitation

In the United States, rehabilitation and occupational health services focus on returning individuals with disabilities to productive lifestyles in society as soon as possible. The goal of the American healthcare system is to rehabilitate everyone: criminals, people with alcohol and drug problems, as well as those with physical conditions. Among Greek Americans[42] and Egyptian Americans,[22] rehabilitation programs that include drastic changes in lifestyle are more appealing when clients and their families are convinced that the programs are scientifically supported. To establish rapport, healthcare practitioners working with clients suffering from chronic disease must avoid assumptions regarding health beliefs and provide rehabilitative health interventions within the scope of the client's cultural customs and beliefs. Failure to respect and accept clients' values and beliefs can lead to misdiagnosis, lack of cooperation, and alienation of clients from the healthcare system (Figs. 9-12 and 9-13).

Reflective Exercise

• How would you handle working with a client who does not share your value of independence and autonomy?

Sick role behaviors are culturally prescribed and vary among ethnic societies. Unlike the American practice of fully disclosing the health condition to the client, the Filipino family prefer to be informed of the bad news, and then they, in turn, slowly break the news to the sick family member.[5] The sick role may not be readily accepted by Italian Americans[43] and Polish Americans,[44] resulting in some individuals keeping an illness hidden from the family until it

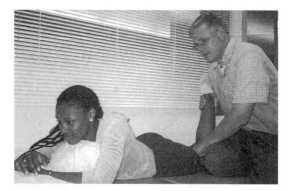

FIGURE 9.12 Diversity in physical rehabilitation encounters in the United States.

reaches a more advanced stage. Given the ethno-cultural acceptance of the sick role, physical therapists must assess each client and family individually and incorporate culturally congruent therapeutic interventions to return the client to the optimal level of functioning.

Reflective Exercise

• How is illness treated in your culture? • Are people expected to go to work or complete everyday activities if they are not seriously ill?

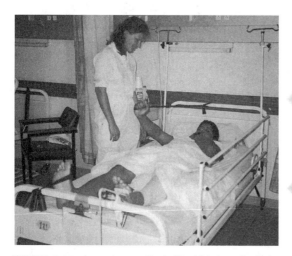

FIGURE 9.13 Assessing a patient at bedside in a physical rehabilitation facility in Belize.

Healthcare Practitioners

M ina Said, age 39, is seeing the physical therapist for hydrotherapy on a leg wound. She was accompanied to the clinic by her husband, Mustafa. When a young male physical therapist greeted her and began to escort her to the treatment area, her husband immediately intervened and stopped her from proceeding to the treatment area. He stated that his wife could not be treated by a male physical therapist and that he wanted an older, female therapist who "knew what they were doing."

The domain *healthcare practitioners* includes the status, use, and perceptions of traditional, magicoreligious, and biomedical healthcare providers. In addition, the gender of the physical therapist is significant for some people (Fig. 9-14).

Traditional versus Biomedical Care Providers

Most people use biomedical healthcare practitioners in conjunction with traditional practices, folk healers, and magicoreligious healers. The healthcare system abounds with individual and family folk practices for curing or treating specific illnesses. A significant portion of all care is delivered outside the perimeter of the formal healthcare arena. Many times herbalist-prescribed therapies are handed down from family members and may have their roots in religious beliefs.

Reflective Exercise

• What types of traditional and folk practitioners do you use?

Reflective Exercise

• In your experience, do clients readily disclose their use of traditional and folk practitioners? • What are the most common folk practitioners you see in your practice?

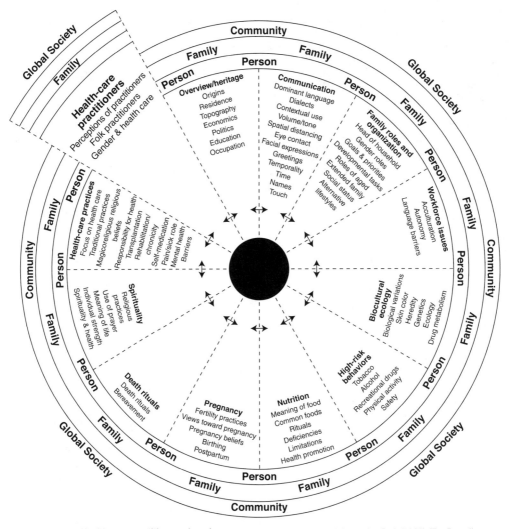

FIGURE 9.14 Healthcare practitioners domain. (Adapted from Purnell, L. D., & Paulanka, B. J. (1998). The Purnell Model for Cultural Competence. In L. D. Purnell & B. J. Paulanka (Eds.), *Transcultural health care: A culturally competent approach* (p. 10). Philadelphia: F.A. Davis.)

The American healthcare practice is to assign staff to patients regardless of gender differences, although often an attempt is made to provide a same-gender provider when intimate care is involved, especially when the patient and caregiver are of the same age. However, physical therapists should recognize and respect differences in gender relationships when providing culturally competent care, because not all ethnocultural groups accept care from someone of the opposite gender. For example, many Hispanics are traditionally seen as being modest, even with physical therapists, and may feel uncomfortable and refuse care provided by someone of the opposite gender.[3,4,6,9] Because any open display of affection is taboo, Hindu and Korean women may be especially modest and generally seek out female healthcare providers for gynecological examinations.[8,17] Physical therapists need to respect clients' modesty by providing adequate privacy and assigning a same-gender caregiver whenever possible. In providing care to a Hasidic male client, a female caregiver should touch him only when providing care, and then preferably with gloves. Therapeutic touch is inappropriate with these clients.[34]

Reflective Exercise

• For what conditions do you prefer same-gender healthcare providers? • Under what conditions do you assign same-gender healthcare providers to your clients?

Status of Healthcare Providers

Western healthcare practitioners are perceived differently among diverse ethnocultural groups. Individual perceptions of selected practitioners may be closely associated with previous contacts and experiences with healthcare providers. Unfortunately, some groups have not always been treated fairly or respectfully by the traditional healthcare system.[28] The revelation of previous mistreatment of African American subjects in studies led to the passage of the National Research Act of 1974, requiring that all studies involving human subjects undergo rigorous ethical scrutiny.[45] Even so, recent studies reveal discrepancies in the treatment of minority cultures within the traditional healthcare system.[46,47]

Reflective Exercise

• In what ways might clients be unfairly treated in physical therapy practice? • How might you as a physical therapist guard against inequities?

Julia[48] notes that distrust of healthcare providers and unfamiliarity with the Western medical system poses major barriers to healthcare for some. Collectivist cultures in particular may struggle with strict hospital visiting hours. Within Latin America, family members often stay in a patient's room overnight and assist with the patient's self-care. The U.S. system of limited

visiting hours conflicts with their cultural norms.[9] Physical therapists should make use of the visiting family members and structure ways in which they might contribute positively to the program for their loved one. The physical therapist should also be cognizant of the stress that the patient might be feeling within the foreign hospital environment.[49]

Reflective Exercise

• How might the family hinder the physical therapy care? • How might the physical therapist demonstrate respect for the family's strong commitment to the client and yet avoid family hindrance of care? • How might the physical therapist work to incorporate the family in the physical therapy care?

In many Western societies, healthcare providers, especially physicians, are viewed with great respect, although recent studies show that this is declining among some groups. Within the Iranian culture, the physician may rely more on physiological cues than on technology for a diagnosis. When physicians order many tests or ask clients what they think the problem is, clients may view them as incompetent.[20,21] Likewise, the physical therapist may risk losing the respect or the confidence of the client if he or she appears

---

Reflection 9.2

I am from Nepal. When I first came to the United States, I received physical therapy for a torn ligament in my knee. At first, I wondered about the competence of the doctor and the physical therapist because both of them asked me many questions and sent me for tests. In my country, the doctors don't ask so many questions. They simply tell you what to do and you follow

Anonymous patient

indecisive or asks a lot of questions of the client. Some cultures expect the educated physical therapist to be the authority and they respect an authoritative tone from the physical therapist (Fig. 9-15). This is in contrast to U.S. culture, where people are expected to question authority and take an active and participatory role in their personal health.

Based on status and power differences among various healthcare providers, Iranian immigrant physicians may misunderstand the assertive behaviors of American physical therapists. On the other hand, Iranian physical therapists may be considered less assertive than they should be in the American culture. Furthermore, many Middle

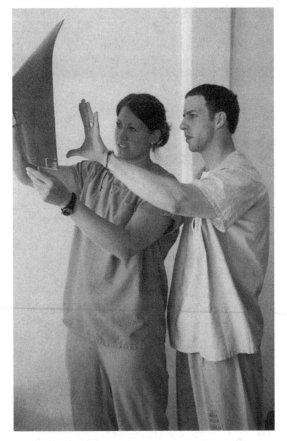

FIGURE 9.15 Attitudes and expectations toward healthcare practitioners vary in different cultures and may be influenced by age, gender, and dress.

Easterners perceive older male physicians as being of higher rank and more trustworthy than younger health professionals.[13,20,21] Chinese[24] and Korean[8] Americans are taught from a very early age to respect elders, and to show deference to healthcare providers, regardless of gender or age.

Reflective Exercise

• Does the age of the healthcare provider make a difference to you in receiving care? • Do you believe that one type of biomedical healthcare provider has higher status than another?

In some cultures, folk and magicoreligious healthcare providers may be deemed superior to biomedically educated physicians, physical therapists, and nurses. It may be that folk, traditional, and magicoreligious healthcare providers are well known to the family and provide more individualized care.[3] In such cultures, physical therapists need to take time to get to know clients as individuals and engage in small talk totally unrelated to the healthcare problem to accomplish their objectives. Establishing satisfactory interpersonal

Reflection 9.3

I am from Germany, where I received my PT training. A big difference I see in the United States practice of physical therapy is the volume of patients you have to see in a short period of time and the use of the physical therapist assistants to help with treatment. In my country, we don't have the physical therapist assistant and we see one patient at a time. Communication between therapists and doctors is poor in my country because we don't have the acknowledgment as a profession that you do in the United States.

Christina Parsons, PT

relationships is essential for improving healthcare and education in these ethnic groups.

Reflective Exercise

• Do you believe that biomedical healthcare providers have higher status than folk or traditional practitioners? • Why or why not?

Reflective Exercise

• What steps do you take to establish trust with clients? • How might you establish trust with a client in a very busy clinic?

Conclusion

Healthcare practices and regard for healthcare practitioners vary across and within cultures. Patients' healthcare beliefs and practices, as well as their attitudes, expectations, and comfort level with the healthcare provider, will impact the success of the physical therapy program. The culturally competent physical therapist should first understand his or her own healthcare beliefs, attitudes, and expectations and then seek to understand those of the patient or the patient's family in order to establish the most culturally congruent and, thus, most effective physical therapy plan of care.

CULTURAL SELF-ASSESSMENT EXERCISE 1

Cultural Self-Assessment

Answer the following questions related to the domain of healthcare practices for yourself.

1. Do you have a physician or nurse whom you see regularly for health checkups?
2. When was the last time you saw a physician or nurse for a health checkup?
3. When was the last time you saw a physician or nurse for a health problem?
4. Do you consider yourself to be in good health?
5. What do you think is responsible for good health?
6. What do you think is responsible for bad health?
7. How do you feel about your weight?
8. How do you maintain/reduce your weight?

9. Do you routinely get exercise? How often?
10. What prescription medicines do you take on a regular basis?
11. What over-the-counter medications do you take on a regular basis?
12. Besides a physician or nurse, what other practitioners do you see when you have health-related problems? (If the provider knows the titles of commonly used folk practitioners, it is best to name them specifically, such as *curandero, espiritista, sobador,* etc.)
13. What other health providers do you see besides physicians or nurses, such as a chiropractor, acupuncturist, herbalist, massage therapist, homeopathic practitioner, naturopathic practitioner, etc.? (Try to be specific according to the availability of complementary/alternative practitioners in your community.)

(continued)

CULTURAL SELF-ASSESSMENT EXERCISE 1 *(Continued)*

14. What do you usually do when you have a minor illness such as a cold or the flu?
15. What do you usually do when you experience pain?
16. What herbs do you take on a regular basis?
17. What herbs do you take when you are ill?
18. What vitamins do you take on a regular basis?
19. What do you do to maintain your health?
20. What things do you avoid to maintain your health?
21. What home remedies do you take when you are ill?
22. What traditional healthcare practices do you use? (Try to be specific according to what is seen in the community, such as coining, moxibustion therapy, acupressure, acumassage, meditation, etc.)
23. How are people with physical disabilities in your culture viewed?
24. How are people with mental disabilities in your culture viewed?
25. What do you usually do to control stress in your life?
26. What prevents you from seeing a physician or nurse when you are ill?
27. What do you do when you have a minor illness such as a sore throat, cold, or headache?

CULTURAL SELF-ASSESSMENT EXERCISE 2

Recognizing, Respecting, and Understanding Others

1. Which of the above questions would you want to ask your physical therapy client?
2. Why would understanding these things be important?
3. Identify three ways in which the answers to the questions might impact the physical therapy program.
4. How would you manage each of the potential impacts in a culturally respectful manner?

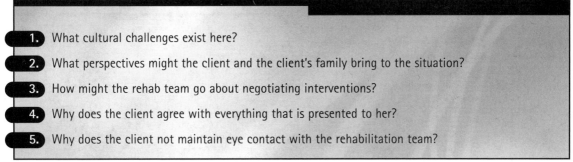

Case Study Scenario II Continued

1. What cultural challenges exist here?

2. What perspectives might the client and the client's family bring to the situation?

3. How might the rehab team go about negotiating interventions?

4. Why does the client agree with everything that is presented to her?

5. Why does the client not maintain eye contact with the rehabilitation team?

REFERENCES

1. Kleinman A. *Patients and Healers in the Context of Culture.* Berkeley, Calif: University of California Press; 1978.
2. Murdock GP. *Theories of Illness: A World Survey.* Pittsburgh, Pa: University of Pittsburgh Press; 1980.
3. Purnell L. The Purnell Model for Cultural Competence. In: Purnell L, Paulanka B, eds. *Transcultural Health Care: A Culturally Competent Approach.* 2nd ed. Philadelphia, Pa: FA Davis; 2003:8–40.
4. Juarbe T. People of Puerto Rican heritage. In: Purnell L, Paulanka B, eds. *Transcultural Health Care: A Culturally Competent Approach.* 2nd ed. Philadelphia, Pa: FA Davis; 2003:307–326.
5. Pacquiao D. People of Filipino heritage. In: Purnell L, Paulanka B, eds. *Transcultural Health Care: A Culturally Competent Approach.* 2nd ed. Philadelphia, Pa: FA Davis; 2003:138–159.
6. Purnell L. Panamanians' practices for health promotion and the meaning of respect afforded them by healthcare providers. *J Transcult Nurs.* 1999;10:333–340.
7. Purnell L. Guatemalans' practices for health promotion and wellness and the meaning of respect afforded them by healthcare providers. *J Transcult Nurs.* 2000;11:40–46.
8. Purnell L, Kim S. People of Korean heritage. In: Purnell L, Paulanka B, eds. *Transcultural Health Care: A Culturally Competent Approach.* 2nd ed. Philadelphia, Pa: FA Davis; 2003:249–263.
9. Zoucha R, Purnell L. People of Mexican heritage. In: Purnell L, Paulanka B, eds. *Transcultural Health Care: A Culturally Competent Approach.* 2nd ed. Philadelphia, Pa: FA Davis; 2003:264–278.
10. Hall E. *The Hidden Dimension.* New York, NY: Doubleday; 1990.
11. Hall E. *The Silent Language.* New York, NY: Doubleday; 1990.
12. Colin J, Paperwalla G. People of Haitian heritage [chapter on CD-ROM]. In: Purnell L, Paulanka B, eds. *Transcultural Health Care: A Culturally Competent Approach.* 2nd ed. Philadelphia, Pa: FA Davis; 2003.
13. Purnell L. People of Appalachian heritage. In: Purnell L, Paulanka B, eds. *Transcultural Health Care: A Culturally Competent Approach.* 2nd ed. Philadelphia, Pa: FA Davis; 2003:73–89.
14. Wenger AF, Wenger M. The Amish. In: Purnell L, Paulanka B, eds. *Transcultural Health Care: A Culturally Competent Approach.* 2nd ed. Philadelphia, Pa: FA Davis; 2003:54–72.
15. Hanson L, Rodgman E. The use of living wills at the end of life: A national study. *Arch Intern Med.* 1996;156:1018–1022.
16. McKinley E, Garrett J, Evans A, Danis M. Differences in end-of-life decision making among black and white ambulatory cancer patients. *J Gen Intern Med.* 1996;11:651–656.
17. Jambanathan J. People of Hindu heritage [chapter on CD-ROM]. In: Purnell L, Paulanka B, eds. *Transcultural Health Care: A Culturally Competent Approach.* 2nd ed. Philadelphia, Pa: FA Davis; 2003.
18. Nowak T. People of Vietnamese heritage. In: Purnell L, Paulanka B, eds. *Transcultural Health Care: A Culturally Competent Approach.* 2nd ed. Philadelphia, Pa: FA Davis; 2003:327–344.
19. Fulton J, Rakowski W, Jones A. Determinants of breast cancer screening among inner-city Hispanic women in comparison with other inner-city women. *Public Health Rep.* 1995;110:476–482.
20. Hafizi H, Lipson J. People of Iranian heritage. In: Purnell L, Paulanka B, eds. *Transcultural Health Care: A Culturally Competent Approach.* 2nd ed. Philadelphia, Pa: FA Davis; 2003:177–194.
21. Kulwicki A. People of Arab heritage. In: Purnell L, Paulanka B, eds. *Transcultural Health Care: A Culturally*

Competent Approach. 2nd ed. Philadelphia, Pa: FA Davis; 2003:90–105.

22. Purnell L. People of Egyptian heritage [chapter on CD-ROM]. In: Purnell L, Paulanka B, eds. *Transcultural Health Care: A Culturally Competent Approach.* 2nd ed. Philadelphia, Pa: FA Davis; 2003.

23. Steckler J. People of German heritage [chapter on CD-ROM]. In: Purnell L, Paulanka B, eds. *Transcultural Health Care: A Culturally Competent Approach.* 2nd ed. Philadelphia, Pa: FA Davis; 2003.

24. Wang Y. People of Chinese heritage. In: Purnell L, Paulanka B, eds. *Transcultural Health Care: A Culturally Competent Approach.* 2nd ed. Philadelphia, Pa: FA Davis; 2003:106–121.

25. Simpson G, Mohr R, Redman A. Cultural variations in the understanding of traumatic brain injury and brain injury rehabilitation. *Brain Inj.* 2000;14:125–140.

26. Sharts-Hopko N. People of Japanese heritage. In: Purnell L, Paulanka B, eds. *Transcultural Health Care: A Culturally Competent Approach.* 2nd ed. Philadelphia, Pa: FA Davis; 2003:218–233.

27. Wilson S. People of Irish heritage. In: Purnell L, Paulanka B, eds. *Transcultural Health Care: A Culturally Competent Approach.* 2nd ed. Philadelphia, Pa: FA Davis; 2003:194–204.

28. Glanville C. People of African American heritage. In: Purnell L, Paulanka B, eds. *Transcultural Health Care: A Culturally Competent Approach.* 2nd ed. Philadelphia, Pa: FA Davis; 2003:40–53.

29. Towle C, Arslanoglu T. People of Turkish heritage [chapter on CD-ROM]. In: Purnell L, Paulanka B, eds. *Transcultural Health Care: A Culturally Competent Approach.* 2nd ed. Philadelphia, Pa: FA Davis; 2003.

30. University of Pittsburgh. Alternative medicine resources. Available at: http://www.pitt.edu/~cbw/internet.htm. Accessed January 16, 2004.

31. Purnell L. People of Cuban heritage. In: Purnell L, Paulanka B, eds. *Transcultural Health Care: A Culturally Competent Approach.* 2nd ed. Philadelphia, Pa: FA Davis; 2003:122–137.

32. Still O, Hodgins D. Navajo Indians. In: Purnell L, Paulanka B, eds. *Transcultural Health Care: A Culturally Competent Approach.* 2nd ed. Philadelphia, Pa: FA Davis; 2003:279–283.

33. Purnell L. People of Brazilian heritage [chapter on CD-ROM]. In: Purnell L, Paulanka B, eds. *Transcultural Health Care: A Culturally Competent Approach.* 2nd ed. Philadelphia, Pa: FA Davis; 2003.

34. Zborowski M. *People in Pain.* San Francisco, Calif: Jossey-Bass; 1969.

35. Kim L. Psychiatric care of Korean Americans. In: Gaw A, ed. *Culture, Ethnicity, and Mental Illness.* Washington, DC: American Psychiatric Press; 1993:347–357.

36. Gaw C. Psychiatric care of Chinese Americans. In: Gaw A, ed. *Culture, Ethnicity, and Mental Illness.* Washington, DC: American Psychiatric Press; 1993:245–280.

37. Yamamoto J. Therapy for Asian Americans and Pacific Islanders. In: Wilkinson C, ed. *Ethnic Psychiatry.* New York, NY: Plenum; 1986:89–141.

38. Sue DW, Sue D. *Counseling the Culturally Different: Theory and Practice.* 2nd ed. New York, NY: Wiley; 1990.

39. Ho M. *Minority Children and Adolescents in Therapy.* Newbury Park, Calif: Sage; 1992.

40. Hughes C. Culture in clinical psychiatry. In Gaw A, ed. *Culture, Ethnicity, and Mental Illness.* Washington, DC: American Psychiatric Press; 1993:347–357.

41. U.S. Equal Employment Opportunity Commission. Facts about Americans with Disabilities Act. Available at: http://www.eeoc.gov/facts/fs-ada.html. Accessed January 16, 2004.

42. Purnell L, Papadopoulos I. People of Greek heritage [chapter on CD-ROM]. In: Purnell L, Paulanka B, eds. *Transcultural Health Care: A Culturally Competent Approach.* 2nd ed. Philadelphia, Pa: FA Davis; 2003.

43. Hillman S. People of Italian heritage. In: Purnell L, Paulanka B, eds. *Transcultural Health Care: A Culturally Competent Approach.* 2nd ed. Philadelphia, Pa: FA Davis; 2003:205–217.

44. From M. People of Polish heritage. In: Purnell L, Paulanka B, eds. *Transcultural Health Care: A Culturally Competent Approach.* 2nd ed. Philadelphia, Pa: FA Davis; 2003:284–306.

45. Gamble V. Under the shadow of Tuskegee: African Americans and health care. *Am J Public Health.* 1997;87:1773–1778.

46. Bach PB, Cramer LD, Warren JL, Begg CB. Racial differences in the treatment of early-stage lung cancer. *N Engl J Med.* 1999;34:1198–1205.

47. Institute of Medicine. Unequal treatment: Confronting racial and ethnic disparities in health care. Available at: http://www.iom.edu/report.asp?id=4475. Accessed January 19, 2004.

48. Julia M. *Multicultural Awareness in the Health Care Professions.* Boston, Mass: Allyn & Bacon; 1996.

49. Black JD, Purnell LD. Cultural competence for the physical therapy professional. *J Phys Ther Educ.* 2002;16:3–10.

50. Selekman J. People of Jewish heritage. In: Purnell L, Paulanka B, eds. *Transcultural Health Care: A Culturally Competent Approach.* 2nd ed. Philadelphia, Pa: FA Davis; 2003:234–248.

PART

2

Resources for Integration:
A Closer Look at
Selected Cultures

SECTION 1

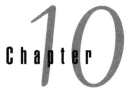

Chapter 10

Cultural Considerations for the African American/ Black Cultures

● Kim Nixon-Cave, PT, PhD, PCS

*M*rs. Saunders, a 76-year-old African American born in Mississippi, is now living in a northeast urban environment in a two-story house with her daughter and 3 of her 15 grandchildren. She is the matriarch and the primary caregiver in her immediate and extended family, all of whom live in the same neighborhood. Mrs. Saunders is an active member of the Baptist church and assists church members when they are ill. Mrs. Saunders has a history of hypertension and diabetes type II. She is admitted to a rehabilitation center following a stroke and is referred to you for physical therapy. During your initial examination, she appears apprehensive and is very brief and guarded when answering your questions. At the end of the session, Mrs. Saunders tells you that she is skeptical and suspicious of the medical care she is receiving and that she must return home immediately to care for her family.

This chapter describes cultural characteristics of African Americans in the United States in order to assist the physical therapist in providing culturally competent care to this population. A lack of knowledge about the African American culture can lead to inaccurate assessments and less-than-optimal clinical outcomes. The Purnell Model for Cultural Competence is used as a guide in the development of this chapter.

Overview/Heritage

The African American population in the United States is a diverse group, many of whom are descendants of slaves who came primarily from the west coast of Africa beginning in the mid-seventeenth century (Fig. 10-1). There is no general agreement among this ethnocultural group as to their preferred name. Some prefer *African*

American, some prefer *black,* some prefer *person of color,* and a few prefer *colored* or *Negro.* When it is necessary to use one of these terms, ask the person how he or she prefers to be identified. For the purposes of this chapter, the terms *black* and *black American* are used to denote race, and *African American* is used to denote culture. Although most people in this group have varying degrees of light brown to darker black skin coloring, some people with white skin may also identify with the African American culture. Dark-skinned people from the Caribbean may also self-identify with the African American culture, but most prefer to be recognized by more specific terms, such as *Haitian, Jamaican,* or *Dominican Republican.* Newer immigrants with dark skin coming from Africa prefer such terms as *Nigerian, Tanzanian,* or *Eritrean* and may have little in common with the African American community in the United States (Box 10-1).

Contemporary life for most African Americans continues to be deeply rooted in customs and traditions, which are influenced by the history of slavery and the experiences that they have endured in this country. The African American community comprises over 13% of the population in the United States. The majority live in the South or in urban settings in the northern states.

Reflective Exercise

• Given the heritage and diversity of the African American population in the United States, what social and cultural issues do you consider important in working with patients from this culture?

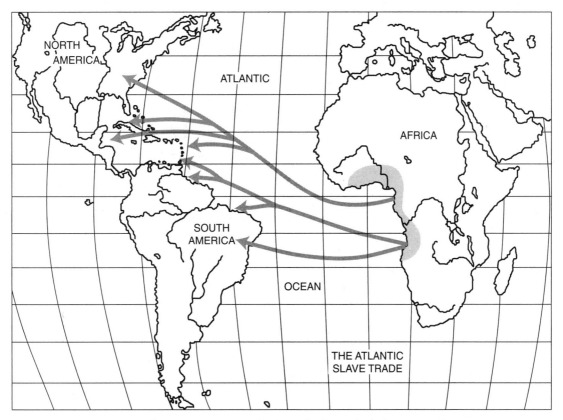

FIGURE 10.1 Map depicting African slave migration to North and South America in the seventeenth century.

B O X   1 0 . 1

A Cultural Journey[6]

ORIGINS

1. When you think about your roots, what country(ies) other than the United States do you identify as a place of origin for you or your family?
2. Are there any foods that you or someone else prepares that are traditional for your country(ies) of origin? What are they?
3. Are there any celebrations, ceremonies, rituals, or holidays that your family continues to celebrate that reflect your country(ies) of origin? What are they? How are they celebrated?

BELIEFS, BIASES, AND BEHAVIORS

1. Have you ever heard anyone make a negative comment about people from your country(ies) of origin? If so, what was it?
2. Have you ever been with someone in a work situation who did something because of his or her culture, religion, or ethnicity that seemed unusual to you? What was it?

Reflection 10.1

Test Your Knowledge of Black/African American History
Question: Was slavery the first time that African Americans/blacks arrived in America?
Answer: The first African American arrived in this country as a free man before slavery in 1619. Some reports indicate that blacks arrived in the fifteenth century.

Reflective Exercise

• What is your knowledge of the social and historical issues that have affected black Americans? • How might that experience affect your interaction and intervention with this population?

Communication

Dominant Language and Dialects

The dominant language spoken in the African American community is English; however, other dialects are common, such as Black English and Gullah. Black English, an informal form of English, also referred to as Ebonics, has recently gained recognition.[2] Black English is an everyday variation spoken by African Americans, especially those in urban neighborhoods and rural communities. Examples of Black English are "Mama and 'em were sayin' it is hot" and "Cause you always be da man, G." Gullah, a Creole language that is a combination of several languages, developed during slavery when slaves, who did not have a common language, were forced to find a way to communicate with each other. Today, Gullah is spoken primary in Georgia, South Carolina, and some areas of New Orleans.[2]

Cultural Communication Practices

African American communication uses phraseology and rhythmic cadence of expression; it involves reaching out, keeping the lines open, and showing interest in what the other person is

Educational Status and Occupations

Thirty-seven to 40% of African Americans have completed high school, and 12–15% have completed 4 or more years of college.[1] African Americans are represented in every socioeconomic group, with increasing numbers represented in the middle- and upper-middle-class income levels. However, a disproportionate number work in low-paying jobs in polluted inner-city environments, which increases their risk of violence and respiratory illnesses. Although many have not attained the overall status of the dominant white cultures in the United States, there is a continuing increase in the number of African Americans entering professional jobs and attending graduate programs to seek professional careers. Physical therapists must recognize and be sympathetic to the social and historical issues that some African Americans have experienced with healthcare and the long-standing mistrust of the white mainstream healthcare system.

saying.[3] As stated by Genovese,[4] "in black urban ghettos verbal ability contributes at least as much as physical strength to individual prestige. Language for African Americans is a manner of identification because those who speak the same language or dialect have something in common with one another" (p. 432). In general, the communication style of African Americans is loud and highly contexted, relying less on verbal communication and more on an understanding through shared experiences and history that are deeply rooted in the past. Among intimates, no words are necessary; one look and they know what each other means. Communication within the African American family is open and characterized by trust; however, for individuals outside of the family, communication is limited, and family matters are viewed as private.[2]

Reflective Exercise

• Ms. Smith is a 70-year-old African American patient with whom you have been working for several weeks. You sense a lack of rapport with her. As a physical therapist you need to build a rapport with Mrs. Smith. What are some ways to communicate effectively with her and build rapport?

Reflective Exercise

• In your next treatment session with Ms. Smith, you attempt to build a rapport with her. When she seems uncomfortable, you move very close to her to give a sense of warmth and friendliness. Her reaction is to withdraw. What cultural considerations should you have addressed? • What can you do to improve your rapport with Ms. Smith? • What specific verbal and nonverbal strategies would be most effective?

Nonverbal communication is expressive and animated; facial expressions and gesturing are common. Most are comfortable with physical closeness, standing within 18 to 24 inches with strangers but closer with family and intimates. Direct eye contact without staring is maintained by most, but more sustained eye contact can be viewed as aggressive behavior. A few more traditional, usually older, people do not maintain direct eye contact with people in hierarchical positions.

Humor and music are important forms of communication among African Americans. Humor is used to deal with stress and anger, and to address and ease issues related to racial tension.[2] Music is an integral part of African American cultural life, ranging from rhythm and blues to contemporary forms of hip-hop and rap music. Many writers have described the nature of music and black culture, examining the relationship between racial and social issues, black cultural priorities, and popular resistance to black music such as rap.[5] These writers have increased the understanding of the role of music in the black community. Physical therapists need to consider the importance of music in the black community and find ways to incorporate it into the rehabilitation plans of patients, especially children and young adults.

Reflective Exercise

• Jamal is 16-year-old African American who injured his knee playing basketball. He has been receiving physical therapy for 2 weeks but seems disinterested and removed from the sessions. Jamal always comes to therapy with a Walkman. How can you incorporate his interest in music into his rehabilitation program?

Time and Temporality

Many African Americans with temporality based in the present may fail to be on time for healthcare appointments. The healthcare provider should recognize that African Americans believe it is more important to make the appointment than to be on time. Whenever possible, be flexible in scheduling appointments. If punctuality is important, carefully explain the reason and the possible consequences of lateness.

Most young and middle-aged adults are oriented to the present whereas older African Americans are more oriented to the past, focusing on events of their childhood or ancestors. The more educated and those of higher socioeconomic status are usually more future-oriented.

Greeting

Clearly, formal and informal manners are important in addressing this group. Most African Americans are taught to address adults formally to show respect for them as persons and for their position in the community. Adults are addressed as Mr., Ms., Mrs., Miss, or some other title unless they are family members; then they are usually addressed as Aunt or Uncle. Adults who are not blood relatives but are considered to be a part of the family are also referred as Aunt or Uncle. The physical therapist should always address African American clients formally until told to do otherwise.

Family Roles and Organization

Head of Household and Gender Roles

Many African American families are matriarchal with a large, strong extended family network that the grandmother or mother may be responsible for directing and guiding. Other households are patriarchal, and still others are egalitarian in their decision making. In most families, men and women share in child rearing, household chores, and financial resources. A long-standing myth is that African American families are disorganized as a result of slavery and the practice of splitting up families to work on various plantations. This is not an established historical fact.[3] On the contrary, the family has strong bonds and kinship with a clear organization. Family includes blood relatives and special friends and individuals not related by blood.[6] The physical therapist should recognize the importance of the nuclear and extended family in the African American community, which is also an important network for providing care, support, and a sense of belonging.[3]

Prescriptive, Restrictive, and Taboo Practices

Families value self-reliance, independence, unity, education, and shared economics. Self-reliance and independence are important because they prepare one to stand on one's own feet and to have one's own things. These values empower individuals to make it on their own in the world, to provide for their basic needs, and to raise a family and achieve their goals in life.

Children are valued because they are the future.[3] Children are taught from an early age that they must be respectful to adults and older people in the community. They are expected to be obedient and conform to the practices of the family and community, which will lead to good behavior. As a result, discipline is a very important aspect of child rearing and socialization of the child in the African American community. The old African proverb "It takes a village to raise a child" rings true in the African American culture and has been passed down through the generations. Adults in the African American community are expected be involved in the training and in some cases the discipline of the children. Children are given protection and guidance and the opportunity to develop their knowledge, because education is seen as crucial to succeeding in the world.[3] Finally, play for a child is viewed as important, and there is an attempt to allow the child to be a child as long as possible and not to push him or her into adulthood too early.[3] Play is viewed as important for both physical and social development. Marian Wright Edelman,[7] in her book *The Measure of Our Success*, discusses the importance of passing on the legacy and lessons that are important for children to know about the African American culture. She describes 25 lessons of life that clearly outline the philosophy, values, and beliefs that African Americans consider important in raising children. Some of the lessons are listed below.

Reflection 10.2

1. Never work just for money or for power. They won't save your soul or help you sleep at night.
2. Try to live in the present.
3. Forming families is serious business.

Reflective Exercise

• How would you address discipline with a family that you feel is being too physically aggressive with their 2-year-old son? How do you respect the cultural values and beliefs about child rearing and discipline?

Older people are important and respected in the African American community. They often guide and direct younger members and are responsible for passing on cultural traditions and beliefs. Most older people are affiliated with the black church, which is central in their lives. Respected grandmothers are often referred to as "Big Mama," "Nana," or "Mama" because they provide insight into life. Grandmothers frequently provide child care for their grandchildren and in some cases provide financial support to the family.

The physical therapist may want to capitalize on the kinship bonds and focus on family strengths, recognizing the extended family's role in caregiving and including them in the care of the patient. The use of informal support networks such as the church, neighbors, and friends is a way to increase the effectiveness of intervention. Acknowledge and recognize the strong kinship/family relationships that exist in the black family.

Alternative Lifestyles

Alternative lifestyles are as common in the African American community as they are in other cultures. However, a high social stigma is attached to being lesbian or gay. African American gay and bisexual men are less likely to disclose their sexuality or to associate with gay groups than are white men and women.[8] Perceived homophobia and racism in the African American community combine to make it difficult for individuals who are homosexual. Acceptance of homosexuality within families is variable; some individuals are not willing to jeopardize their family relationships by admitting their homosexuality. As a result, gay men are less likely to participate in preventive programs for HIV/AIDS or other sexually transmitted diseases.

Single parenting is common in the African American community, with many households headed by single females (Fig. 10-2). A high percentage of single parents live in poverty. However, there is a strong family network of grandmothers and extended family who assist with child rearing. This practice is seen throughout the African American community, especially among teenage mothers; grandmothers direct and guide the household and are the primary caregivers. Additionally, the number of single fathers in the African American com-

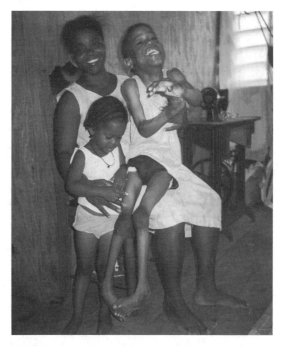

FIGURE 10.2 A single mother bears the responsibility of rearing her two children.

munity is growing because of the increasing divorce rate.

Reflective Exercise

• Ms. Bailey, a single mother, has been followed in physical therapy two times a week for the past month for low back pain. When Ms. Bailey arrives for therapy, she appears rushed and always has two of her three children with her. She is having difficulty focusing on the intervention, needing to attend to the children. What strategies can you employ to increase the benefit of your therapeutic intervention for Ms. Bailey? • What cultural factors would help Ms. Bailey address the issue of needing therapy and having to care for her children?

Workforce Issues

Culture in the Workforce

Although increasing numbers of African Americans are completing higher educational degrees and entering professional careers, many still lag behind the dominant white population in the United States, especially in healthcare. Himmelstein, Lewontin, and Woolhandler[9] looked at medical employment rates of African American women in the United States in 1993. They reported that one-fifth of all employed African American women work in the healthcare sector. Most are employed as paraprofessional caregivers in nursing homes and home care. A small percentage are employed in practitioners' offices. Unfortunately, paraprofessional workers in nursing homes typically have lower wages than other healthcare positions and often lack medical insurance benefits. This pattern of employment, unskilled positions with low wages and no health insurance, is not uncommon in work environments where large numbers of African Americans are employed. As stated by Lowenstein and Glanville,[10] "culture and politics affect the employment of blacks in the healthcare industry, often relegating African Americans to nonskilled roles." Thus, African Americans continue to deal with inequities in employment.

Issues Related to Autonomy

Autonomy is an issue in the workplace and an area of frustration for African Americans, especially men. According to Glanville,[2] this problem has historical roots in slavery, resulting in some African Americans having difficulty taking direction from European Americans. The issue is exacerbated by the fact that few African Americans are in leadership roles. Although this is changing, there continues to be a lack of leaders and role models in the black community.

Racial and ethnic stress, discrimination, and unfair treatment are central issues in the work environment for some African Americans. The research literature suggests that these stressors can lead to physical illness and depression. Krieger and Sidney[11] examined the association between blood pressure and self-reported experiences of racial discrimination and workers' responses to unfair treatment. The results indicate that for black adults who typically accepted unfair treatment but had not experienced racial discrimination, systolic blood pressure was about 7 mm Hg higher compared with those who challenged the unfair treatment and experienced racial discrimination. For black professionals, systolic blood pressure was 9 to 10 mm Hg lower than that of professionals who challenged unfair treatment without reports of racial discrimination. From this study and others, similar studies, there appears to be an association between racial and ethnic discrimination in the workplace that may lead to health conditions such as high blood pressure for African Americans. In spite of these obstacles, African Americans have a strong work ethic with a focus on materialism.

Biocultural Ecology

Skin Color and other Biological Variations

Over one hundred racial strains have been identified among the African American population, resulting in variations in skin color and hair texture.[2] The complexions of African Americans can range from very light to very dark because of genetic influences and mixing with other racial and ethnic groups. The therapist must become familiar with skin color to make correct assessments of oxygenation status. The skin coloration resulting from injury or inflammation may be darker or a color other than red, which is seen in white-skinned people. To assess for cyanosis and jaundice in dark-skinned people, it is necessary to examine the sclera, oral mucosa, and the palms of the hands and soles of the feet rather than relying on skin color. To assess for rashes, palpate the area and feel for increased heat.

Diseases and Health Conditions

African Americans have an increased tendency for keloids, vitiligo, melasma, and pseudofolliculitis. Keloids are due to overgrowth of connective tissue associated with protection against infection and repair after injury. African American also have a greater prevalence of birthmarks, about 20% as opposed to other groups at 1–3%. A notable type of skin discoloration or birthmark is referred to as a mongolian spot, which is common in newborns for the first several months of life. There is a clear discoloration of the baby's skin, which to the unfamiliar person may be seen as bruising; however, these spots disappear over time. The physical therapist should be careful not to misjudge the natural skin color changes that occur for the African American infant and not assume that mongolian spots are indicative of bruising or abuse.

Melasma, or mask of pregnancy, is more commonly seen in darker-skinned females. For males, pseudofolliculitis, or razor bumps, is more common in black people than among other racial groups. African Americans also have a higher incidence of vitiligo, which is pigment discoloration due to an autoimmune disease. This disease essentially strips the individual of skin pigmentation, changing the skin from brown to white with no pigmentation.

African Americans have a high prevalence of hypertension, diabetes mellitus, obesity, asthma, end-stage organ disease, kidney and liver failure, and coronary heart disease, resulting in a lower life expectancy compared with whites. Research suggests that environmental factors such as stress and racism, perceived or real, may contribute to these diseases[12,13] (Box 10-2).

BOX 10.2

Chronic Illness Among African Americans and the Incidence of the Disease

- Stroke
  - Black men are twice as likely to die from a stroke as white men
- Coronary heart disease
  - Black women are more likely to die from coronary heart disease than white women.
- Cancer
  - Higher incidence in black men
- Diabetes
  - Higher incidence in black men and women
- Low birth weight babies/infant mortality
  - Twice as likely to occur for black females
- AIDS/HIV
  - Fastest growing group of infected individuals with a widening gap seen in females and children. Leading cause of death between 25 and 44 years.
- Homicide
  - Higher incidence in black men and women

Reflective Exercise

- Based on the information you now have about skin color and other biological variations for African Americans, what changes would you make in your examination techniques?

The incidence of cardiovascular disease (CVD) has declined in the general population; however, in the African American population, this decline has not equaled that for other ethnocultural groups. As a result, African Americans in the United States have a disproportionate share of CVD.[14] Gorelick[15] found that African Americans are almost twice as likely to die from a stroke compared with their white counterparts. This disparity is even more pronounced among black men age 45 to 49.

The mortality rate for blacks is higher in comparison with whites, with the leading causes of death including violence, accidents, cancer, CVD, hypertension, diabetes, and sexually transmitted diseases. Additionally, a project conducted by the Institute of Medicine[22] found that for some racial and ethnic groups, a lower quality of care may contribute to the disparities in healthcare, resulting in a greater prevalence of acute and chronic diseases, with an accompanying increase in mortality.

Asthma also has a higher prevalence in minority groups and low-income populations. Persky et al.[16] examined the relationship between race and socioeconomic status and the prevalence, severity, and symptoms of asthma among school-age children in Chicago. They found a higher incidence of childhood asthma in schools more heavily populated by African American students from low income neighborhoods. The majority of African Americans live in the inner city, with increased exposure to pollutants, which are factors contributing to asthma and other respiratory diseases and illnesses. The researchers found that decreased access to healthcare might be related to the high rates of asthma-related deaths in inner-city environments such as Chicago.[16]

Sexually transmitted disease is a significant problem in the African American community, especially for women and young adults. Black women, especially teenagers, are the fastest-growing population diagnosed with HIV/AIDS. African Americans' mortality rate for HIV/AIDS is about 1.6 times higher than for whites.[17]

Violence is another health concern in the African American population, resulting in an epidemic of black-on-black crime, with black males having a higher incidence of being victims of crime. Homicide is the leading cause of death for black males.[2,18]

Reflective Exercise

• What preventive measures and environmental adaptations will decrease the incidence of illness and disease for African Americans? • Identify cultural issues that may affect interventions among African Americans.

The most common genetic disorder among African Americans is sickle cell anemia, a disorder that causes an abnormality of the globin genes in hemoglobin. Symptoms include fever with pain in the joints and abdomen. Significant research in this area is increasing life expectancy as well as quality of life for individuals diagnosed with sickle cell anemia.

Variations in Drug Metabolism

Most medical research has focused on white populations; more recent research is focusing on minority groups because of a clear statement from funding agencies that research must include minority groups. African Americans have been found to respond differently to some drugs compared with the groups on whom the drug research was conducted. Flaws and Bush[19] looked at the drug tamoxifen, which is one of the most common drugs used in the treatment of breast cancer. Their preliminary evidence suggests that tamoxifen is less effective in nonwhites than in whites.

In the treatment of hypertension, studies have found that calcium channel blockers are more effective among blacks than beta-blockers, which are more effective among whites.[20] Other drugs that appear to act differently in African Americans include alcohol, psychotropics, and caffeine. Clearly, further racial/ethnic-specific research studies need to be conducted to address drug interventions and metabolism in minority groups.

Reflective Exercise

• What resources might you seek for drug metabolism differences among ethnic/racial groups? • How does the variation in drug metabolism affect your intervention?

High-Risk Behaviors

High-risk behaviors among African Americans are the same as for the rest of the population, varying only in the degree, including nonuse of helmets while riding bicycles and motorcycles, unprotected sexual activity and substance abuse, and HIV/AIDS and sexually transmitted diseases. National statistics on HIV/AIDS report a decline in the incidence of the disease in the overall population; however, within the African American population, HIV/AIDS has continued to increase, especially among females. Researchers hypothesize that this increase may be related to cultural beliefs about HIV and continued high-risk sexual behaviors and substance abuse.[21] Current research and intervention efforts are focusing on changing high-risk behaviors, improving the decision making of individuals, and providing more culturally congruent and sensitive educational programs.

Reflective Exercise

• You have received a referral for physical therapy for a young, single mother recently diagnosed with HIV. She has two children, ages 3 and 5. How would you go about developing a relationship with her? • What salient issues would you address for her and her two children?

Nutrition

Meaning of Food

African Americans have a sociohistorical memory of deprivation, resulting in foods taking a particular meaning, especially ones high in calories. Eating food is an important part of many celebrations and symbolizes good health and wealth. One common ritual is to offer guests food. Even in low-income homes, it is still important to offer whatever is available, and the rule is to offer good food.

Dietary Staples and Practices for Health Promotion

The diet for many African Americans stems from the time of slavery and making do with what you have. Ancestors were very skilled at making use of whatever was given to them and whatever they could grow in small slave gardens on the plantation. The slaves were typically given the leftovers or, in many cases, the garbage that the owners did not desire.

Today's African American diet varies widely but continues to include dark, leafy vegetables, red meat, and cheese. Potatoes, rice, bread, and fruits are typical staples. The African American diet can be high in fat and sodium and low in fiber. Foods are frequently fried. In the African American community this diet is termed "soul food," with fat, pork, and red meat as primary components. However some religious tenets, such as Islam, indicate that red meat should not be consumed.[2] One important dietary note for African Americans is the high incidence of lactose intolerance, which includes about 75% of the African American population.

Reflective Exercise

• Mr. Smith, age 49, has a long history of hypertension and has recently had a stroke and is currently undergoing rehabilitation. You are in his room when the family arrives with fried chicken, cornbread, collard greens with bacon bits, and deep-fried pork rinds. How do you address your concerns about the appropriateness of this meal given Mr. Smith's hypertension and stroke? • How do you include the family in addressing food choices and preparation practices?

Meals in the African American home are served at set times. Not all family members necessarily sit down at the same time, and food is "left on the stove" for family members to eat whenever they are ready.[3] Babies are often introduced to table food well before the recommended time, with solid food, primarily cereal, introduced at about 2 months of age. The general belief is that formula is not enough to keep the baby full and satisfied.[3] At about 1 year of age, children are usually switched completely to table food, the same food that everyone else in the family is eating.

Pregnancy and Childbearing Practices

Fertility Practices and Views toward Pregnancy

African Americans have a high fertility rate and a high incidence of multiple births. However, blacks are twice as likely to have a preterm, low-birth-weight infant compared with white ethnocultural populations. Research supports that this higher incidence may not be linked to African Americans being an underserved minority group, but may be related to racial factors.[23]

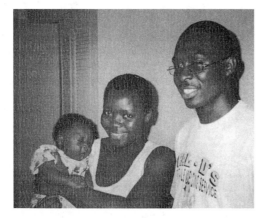

FIGURE 10.3 This couple recently emigrated from Togo in Africa and gave birth to their son here in the United States.

Current research is looking at stress, racism, and low self-esteem to address the incidence of low-birth-weight infants.[24] African Americans use a variety of fertility control methods, including tubal ligation, birth control pills, intrauterine devices, and foams and creams (Fig. 10-3).

Prescriptive, Restrictive, and Taboo Practices in the Childbearing Family

In the African American family, older people guide and direct the expectant mother during her pregnancy, including sharing taboos and traditions about pregnancy. Taboos include not taking the pregnant mother's picture, because this may lead to a stillbirth and/or capture the soul of the mother.[2] Another taboo is not purchasing clothes for the infant until after birth because of the possibility of bringing bad luck to the child.

Reflective Exercise

• In a postpartum exercise program a young mother informs you that she does not need to do the exercises because her great-grandmother provides her with herbs and home remedies to help her return to full health. How do you encourage this young mother to consider your exercises while using her home remedies?

Fathers, mothers, or other female relatives are welcomed in the delivery room and assist as coaches. After delivery, the mother receives support and care from her mother or other relatives to ensure that she returns to health, which requires rest. At this time, there is concern that the mother is at a high risk for illness.

Death Rituals

Death Rituals and Expectations

Most African Americans believe that life does not end with death, but that there is a place for the redeemed to go after life or a place where the individual will be in the presence of God. Depending on the denomination, this belief may have variations; however, most African Americans believe that they can continue their relationship with their loved ones after death.

Responses to Death and Grief

In the acute-care setting, the provider can expect many nuclear and extended family members, as well as non–blood relatives, to visit the dying person and express their concerns openly. Most burials or funerals are held 5 to 7 days after the death of the family member. This tradition dates back to the days when family members had begun to move north from the South, allowing for travel time so that everyone can have the opportunity to attend the funeral services. Funeral services are usually spiritual and very emotional. In this environment, African Americans who usually do not express their feelings openly can freely express their feelings in public. Cremation is not common in the African American community; however a few are choosing this option.

Spirituality

Religious Practices and Use of Prayer

African Americans belong to a wide variety of religious denominations, including African Methodist Episcopal, Jehovah's Witnesses, Seventh-Day Adventists, Pentecostal, Presbyterian, Lutheran, Roman Catholic, Nation of Islam, and Church of God in Christ; however, most are affiliated with Baptist and Methodist denominations. Spirituality/religion is a cultural value that is taught early in a child's life. Children are taught that in order for one's life to be meaningful, religion must be a part of it.[3]

Prayer is an important aspect of religion and spirituality along with "laying on of hands" and "speaking in tongues."[2] Healthcare professionals should acknowledge and respect the role of the church, spirituality, and religion in the African American community. The church and the clergy can be allies in addressing illness issues and should be sought out for assistance, especially for the elderly.[3,25] Stolley and Koenig[25] report that African Americans, especially females, rely heavily on religion. Religion is an important social support and a mechanism for coping with stressful life events, serving more than a spiritually oriented purpose.[25–29]

Reflective Exercise

• Mrs. Wilson, a 64-year-old patient, is in the middle of completing a difficult functional task that has taken her weeks to accomplish. She always responds best to immediate, detailed feedback. The family asks you to stop the session because the minister from the local church has arrived and must pray for the patient. This is the first session where the patient has made progress in her therapy. Would you stop the treatment and allow the minister to say a prayer with Mrs. Wilson? • What cultural factors must you consider in this situation?

Spirituality Beliefs and Healthcare Practices

African Americans view life as a process rather than a state. According to Spector,[18] a person's nature is viewed in terms of energy rather than in terms of matter. All things, whether living or dead, influence one another. African Americans view religion as a "source of spiritual sustenance."[3] The influence of religion and a strong sense of spirituality provide a support system in everyday life, comfort in times of distress, and a mechanism for coping with and counteracting detrimental effects.[30] Religion and spirituality have allowed people to deal with the stress and psychological concerns associated with long-standing, deep-seated issues associated with racism and discrimination that most minorities experience in the United States.[25] According to

Ferraro and Koch,[31] African Americans are more likely to turn to religion in times of stress and illness than are European Americans.

Reflective Exercise

• You notice that your elderly male African American patient appears distracted and ill at ease with his lack of progress in strength conditioning, indicating that he cannot continue the exercises by himself at home. What are some sociocultural supports that you can explore with him?

Meaning of Life and Individual Sources of Strength

The black church is a central institution in the African American community.[25] In the history of African Americans as slaves and free individuals, the black church and spirituality have been sources of survival and strength.[2] Research reports that up to 75% of older African Americans are church members, 50% attend church every day, and 93% pray daily.[25,32,33] The black church shapes the community, provides organization, and offers guidance for the young. It is a place where everyone can come together for a sense of community. The church is not as influential as it has been in the past, but it does impact the lives of most members of the community. African Americans take their religion very seriously, believing that life events such as marriages, births, and deaths must be validated by a religious spiritual event.

It is important that physical therapists recognize the formal and informal community networks such as the black church and assist patients in accessing them.

Reflective Exercise

• Recognizing the importance of religion in the African American culture, what strategies can you use to support and enhance patient care? • How can you incorporate the role of the church into the patient's care?

Healthcare Practices

Responsibility for Healthcare

Culture has a strong influence in the healthcare practices for all patients. Ethnocultural beliefs concerning health and illness guide the patients' and providers' healthcare values and ultimately influence the therapeutic relationship. Culture is like a second skin; we carry our cultural values and beliefs with us in every experience and relationship in which we participate.[34]

Reflective Exercise

• Both you and the patient bring your cultural values and beliefs into the therapeutic relationship. How can you ensure that you respect the patient's culture and not let your personal cultural values have an undue influence on your clients?

Data on African Americans report a low usage of healthcare services. Some refrain from seeking mainstream allopathic services due to mistrust of the healthcare system, lack of access to health services, and overuse of home or folk remedies. Many wait until they are very ill to seek healthcare, by which time their symptoms have become more severe, requiring greater use of medical resources. The use of emergency rooms for minor healthcare problems is common for some African Americans.

Some African Americans believe that healthcare providers, especially physicians, are out to make a profit and want to use them to experiment with drugs and treatments. It is not uncommon in a black family to hear an elder discourage someone from going to the doctor or seeking traditional healthcare with the statement "They're just going to experiment on you at that hospital."

The use of medical care and preventive care can vary widely within the African American community depending on the socioeconomic level of the family. The majority of middle/upper-income families use the healthcare system and healthcare facilities as needed (Fig. 10-4). African Americans who are present oriented are less likely to worry about future problems that can result from conditions such as hypertension. They may not be concerned about taking medication for hypertension to prevent a possible future stroke.

Reflective Exercise

• What education tools could you use that are culturally sensitive to address the prevention and wellness of the African American patient? • What part of the APTA patient care disablement management model could you use to increase the patient's understanding of his/her disease?

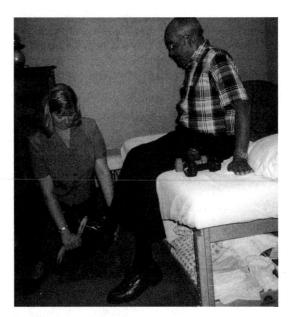

FIGURE 10.4 Physical therapy is an acceptable healthcare practice.

African Americans' faith and spirituality are influential in making end-of-life decisions. Most believe that everything is in God's hands, and God will determine whether they live or die, and when. Thomas's[35] study reported that African Americans believe in praying for a miracle as opposed to accepting terminality.

Traditional and Folk Practices

Traditional and folk medicine have been used for many generations in the black community. Many of these traditions started in Africa and have been continued with some variations into today's African American communities. Some believe that home/folk remedies are more effective than mainstream healthcare. Usage of these remedies has little association with educational level, socioeconomic status, or the availability of medical facilities. These folk remedies have been tried and tested for generations and are believed to cure illness and diseases as well as or better than mainstream medicine. Physical therapists must respect and incorporate nonharmful folk practices into allopathic prescriptions.

Reflective Exercise

• Mrs. Robinson developed herpes zoster after a brief fever while in the hospital for pneumonia, which resulting in deconditioning. During your treatment session she informs you that there is nothing that anyone at the hospital can do for her; she must be discharged so she can go south to visit a lady in the community who can get this root off of her. How do you assess the medical and cultural implications of the patient's belief?

Many African Americans believe that there can be two causes of illness, one a result of natural causes and the other a result of unnatural causes. Voodoo is the belief that unnatural and evil spirits cause illness or mental problems stemming from an interpersonal conflict and supernatural activity. An example is a young man who suddenly behaves differently and wants nothing more than to be with a woman who treats him badly. He also develops an unexplained rash that appears once a month. These unexplained events lead the elders to assume that the young man has been "rooted" because he may have done an injustice to the young woman.

Barriers to Healthcare

Significant barriers to healthcare exist in the African American community. The barriers include lack of access to healthcare facilities and providers, financial limitations, and cultural bias toward healthcare. Many disenfranchised groups, including African Americans, feel that the healthcare system has far too often treated them with disrespect. Some have had experiences that were degrading and in some cases humiliating. The Tuskegee experiment is a landmark event in the African American community, creating distrust in healthcare providers and hospitals. This experiment used black men diagnosed with syphilis as research subjects, to test the outcome of syphilis if left untreated. They misled the men into believing that they were receiving treatment. Events such as the Tuskegee experience fostered mistrust along with more contemporary events, such as abuses from sickle cell screening and minority-focused sterilization initiatives in the 1970s.[34]

Reflective Exercise

• You have been working with Mr. Johnson, a 78-year-old African American who is in rehabilitation following a stroke. He is now scheduled for prostate cancer surgery while in rehab for the stroke. He appears very nervous the day before the surgery and talks about canceling, believing that the doctors are not telling him the truth. What strategies can you use to reassure the patient that his fears are unfounded?
• What cultural history must you consider and recognize during your discussion?

Lack of access to healthcare can be related to several factors, from distance to a facility as well as the availability of specific services in a given community. Healthcare cost is steadily rising, and for African Americans in the lower socioeconomic groups, health insurance is not always affordable.

Blood Transfusions and Organ Donation

Unless the client is a Jehovah's Witness, there is no taboo to receiving blood or blood products for African Americans. However, some are reluctant to receive blood out of fear of contracting HIV.

African Americans are less likely than white ethnic groups to have addressed the use of end-of-life directives. This means that they may be less informed or even unaware of such directives, as they are not typically discussed.[36]

African Americans are less likely to donate their organs or a family member's organs than are white ethnic groups.[36] With increasing education, more African Americans are becoming a part of donor programs, but the cultural belief is that you leave this world with "what you arrived with." African Americans' long-standing mistrust of mainstream white medicine influences organ donation. Some fear that organs may be taken prematurely; others believe that lifesaving methods may not be fully employed in an eagerness to procure the organs. If African Americans do donate their organs, they prefer to donate them to other African Americans.[37]

Healthcare Practitioners

Status of Healthcare Providers

In the African American community, healthcare providers are viewed as important, with physicians receiving the highest regard, followed by nurses and other healthcare providers (Fig. 10-5). Folk and traditional healers are also well respected, mostly because they are known in the community. Along with allopathic healthcare providers, folk healers, mostly older women in the community, are commonly used. Other healers include spiritual leaders such as ministers, voodoo practitioners, and priests.[2] Each individual serves a different purpose within the community. The spiritual leaders focus on religion and foster the spiritual growth of the members of the community. Voodoo practitioners focus on removing curses or hexes that some individuals feel have been placed on them.

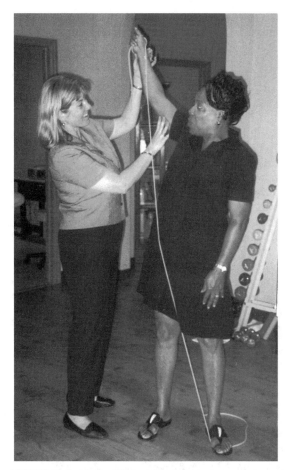

FIGURE 10.5 Physical therapists are among respected healthcare practitioners.

Reflective Exercise

• Recognizing that your African American patient may not have seen an allopathic health professional or may have no healthcare insurance, from what other healthcare professionals might a patient benefit? • What strategies can you use to reduce the barriers to obtaining healthcare for this patient?

The gender of the healthcare provider usually is not an issue among African Americans. Some may prefer a same-gender provider for intimate care and examinations.

CASE STUDY SCENARIO

*M*s. Keya Jackson, a 62-year-old widowed African American, has a history of hypertension, coronary artery disease, hypercholesterolemia, diabetes mellitus type I, and arthritis. She lives in a second-floor walk-up apartment with a railing on the right side of the stairs. Her teenage daughter and two grandchildren live with her. She has three children, all of whom live nearby. Ms. Jackson is the primary caregiver for her grandchildren. Her family is very supportive, and she also has the support of close friends and extended family in the area. Her 65-year-old sister lives down the block, and her brother lives about 10 minutes away.

Ms. Jackson completed high school and has worked for over 30 years as a nurse's aide in a local nursing home. She retired last year but still has some "side jobs" as a home health aide. She receives social security and a small pension from her nursing home position. Her hobbies include taking her grandchildren to the playground, doing crossword puzzles, and watching old movies on television. She is an active member of the Solid Rock Baptist Church, is on the mother's board, and assists church members when they are ill. She is also a member of the church choir and works with the children's ministry. Ms. Jackson enjoys going to bible study weekly. Her daughter is also very active in the church and is head of the usher board.

Ms. Jackson has been referred to physical therapy for examination and treatment for her arthritis, which is causing her pain and discomfort in both hips and her back. Her minister and church sister, May, bring Ms. Jackson to physical therapy.

The therapist assigned to Ms. Jackson is a young female of European American ancestry. The therapist addresses Ms. Jackson by her first name, Keya. The therapist experiences difficulty obtaining the health history and information about Ms. Jackson's home and family environment. As the questions become more specific, Ms. Jackson gives the therapist only one-word answers. When the therapist begins to ask Ms. Jackson about her activity level, her diet, and responsibilities at home, Ms. Jackson gives little to no response to the inquiries.

The therapist does ascertain that Ms. Jackson is the primary caregiver and matriarch in her family. She is also very involved with her extended family and church. Ms. Jackson also says that she doesn't understand why her doctor sent her to physical therapy because she has her own oils and remedies that she has used for years, and that they work well. Moreover, she cannot attend therapy on a regular basis because she has to take care of her grandchildren and a sick church member

1. What cultural issues of the patient should be considered in this case?

2. What cultural issues of the therapist should be considered in this case?

3. What challenges exist for the patient and the therapist?

4. What strategies can be used to build rapport with Ms. Jackson?

5. What resources would you consider important for Ms. Jackson?

6. What issues are important to address with Ms. Jackson and her family about her diagnosis and care?

7. How can the patient's strong connections with the church be used in planning care?

R E F E R E N C E S

1. Educational attainment in the United States: 2003. Issued June 2004. Available at http://www.census.gov/prod/2004pubs/p20-550.pdf. Accessed August 2, 2005.
2. Glanville CL. People of African American heritage. In: Purnell L, Paulanka B, eds. *Transcultural Health Care: A Culturally Competent Approach.* 2nd ed. Philadelphia, Pa: FA Davis; 2003:40–54.
3. Willis W. Families with African-American roots. In: Lynch EW, Hanson MJ. *Developing Cross-Cultural Competence.* Baltimore, Md: Paul H. Brookes; 1992.
4. Genovese ED. *Roll, Jordan, Roll: The World Slaves Made.* New York: Pantheon; 1974.
5. Rose T. *Black Noise: Rap Music and Black Culture in Contemporary America.* Hanover, NH: University Press of New England; 1994.
6. Lynch EW, Hanson MJ. *Developing Cross-Cultural Competence.* Baltimore, Md: Paul H. Brookes; 1992.
7. Edelman MW. *The Measure of Our Success: A Letter to My Children and Yours.* Boston, Mass: Beacon Press; 1992.
8. Kennamer JD, Honnold J, Bradfield J, Hendricks M. Differences in disclosure of sexuality among African American and White gay/bisexual men: Implications for HIV/AIDS prevention. *AIDS Educ Prev.* 2000;12:519–531.
9. Himmelstein DU, Lewontin JP, Woolhandler S. Medical care employment in the US, 1968 to 1993: The importance of health sector jobs for African-Americans and women. *Am J Public Health.* 1996;86:525–528.
10. Lowenstein A, Glanville CL. Cultural diversity and conflict in the health care workplace. *Nurs Econ.* 1995; 13:203–209.
11. Krieger N, Sidney S. Racial discrimination and blood pressure: The CARDIA study of young black and white adults. *Am J Public Health.* 1996;86:1370–1378.
12. Broman CL. The health consequences of racial discrimination: A study of African Americans. *Ethn Dis.* 1996;6:148–153.
13. Polednak AP. Segregation, discrimination and mortality in US Blacks. *Ethn Dis.* 1996;6:99–108.
14. Crook ED, Clark BL, Bradford ST, et al. From 1960s Evans County Georgia to present-day Jackson, Mississippi: An exploration of the evolution of cardiovascular disease in African Americans. *Am J Med Sci.* 2003;325:307–314.
15. Gorelick P. Cerebrovascular disease in African Americans. *Stroke.* 1998;29:2656–2664.
16. Persky VW, Slezak J, Contreras A, et al. Relationships of race and socioeconomic status with prevalence, severity, and symptoms of asthma in Chicago school children. *Ann Allergy Asthma Immunol.* 1998;8:266–271.
17. Buka SL. Disparities in health status and substance use: Ethnicity and socioeconomic factors. *Public Health Rep.* 2002;117(suppl):S118–S125.
18. Spector RE. *Cultural Diversity in Health & Illness.* 5th ed. Upper Saddle River, NJ: Prentice-Hall; 2000.
19. Flaws JA, Bush TL. Racial differences in drug metabo-lism: An explanation for higher breast cancer mortality in blacks? *Med Hypotheses.* 1998;50:327–329.
20. Brownley KA, Hurwitz BE, Schneiderman N. Ethnic variations in the pharmacological treatment of hypertension: Biopsychosocial perspective. *Hum Biol.* 1999;71: 607–639.
21. Plowden K, Miller JL, James T. HIV health crisis and African-Americans: A cultural perspective. *ABNF J.* 2000; 11:88–93.
22. Institutional and policy-level strategies for increasing the racial-ethnic diversity of the US healthcare workforce. Available at: http://www.iom.edu/ project.asp?id=4888. Accessed January 14, 2004.
23. Collins JW, Hammond NA. Relation of maternal race to the risk of preterm, non–low birth weight infants: A population study. *Am J Epidemiol.* 1996;143:333–337.
24. Murrell NL. Stress, self-esteem, and racism: Relationships with low birth weight and preterm delivery in African American women. *J Natl Black Nurs Assoc.* 1996;8:45–53.
25. Stolley JM, Koenig H. Religion/spirituality and health among elderly African Americans and Hispanics. *J Psychosoc Nurs Ment Health Serv.* 1997;35:32–38.
26. Courtenay BC, Poon KW, Martin P, Clayton GM, Johnson MA. Religiosity and adaptation in the oldest-old. *Int J Aging Hum Devel.* 1992;34:47–56.
27. Idler EL, Kasl SV. Religion, disability, depression, and the timing of death. *Am J Sociol.* 1992;97:1052–1079.
28. Koenig HG, Cohen HJ, Blazer DG. Religious coping and depression among elderly, hospitalized medically ill men. *Am J Psychiatr.* 1992;149:1693–1700.
29. Williams DR. Measurements of religion. In: Levin JS, ed. *Religion, Aging, and Health.* Thousand Oaks, Calif: Sage; 1994.
30. Tripp-Reimer T, Johnson R, Rios H. Cultural dimensions in gerontological nursing. In: Stanley M, Beare PG, eds. *Gerontological Nursing.* Philadelphia, Pa: JB Lippincott; 1995.
31. Ferraro K, Koch J. Religion and health among black and white adults: Examining social support and consolation. *J Sci Stud Relig.* 1994;4:362–375.
32. Levin JS, Chatters LM, Taylor RJ. Religious effects on health status and life satisfaction among black Americans. *J Gerontol.* 1994;50:154–163.
33. Levin JS, Taylor RJ. Gender and age differences in religiosity among Black Americans. *Gerontologist.* 1993; 33:16–23.
34. Berger JT. Culture and ethnicity in clinical care. *Arch Intern Med.* 1998;158:2085–2090.
35. Thomas N. The importance of culture throughout all of life and beyond. *Holist Nurs Pract.* 2001;15:40–46.
36. Plawecki H, Plawecki J. Improving organ donation rates in the black community. *J Holist Nurs.* 1992;10:34–36.
37. American Medical Association, Council on Scientific Affairs. Unequal treatment: Confronting racial and ethnic disparities in health care. Available at: http://www.ama-assn.org/ama/ pub/article/2036-7223.html.

Chapter 11

Cultural Considerations for the Chinese Culture

● Theresa Kraemer, PT, PhD, ATC

Madame Sue Li is a 64-year-old female who suffered a left cerebral vascular accident. She recently emigrated from China to the United States to live with her son after the death of her husband. She has limited English skills, does not maintain eye contact, and assumes a passive role in treatment. Her son and daughter-in-law are very involved in her care and assist her with activities of daily living. She does not complain of pain or discomfort and appears very cooperative.

Introduction

Chinese, the cultural group this chapter describes, includes ethnic people from China, Taiwan, and Hong Kong. Great diversity exists among this group in terms of its economics, extent of globalization and modernization, and healthcare practices. Chinese Americans are an even more diverse group according to the primary and secondary characteristics of culture as described in Chapter 1. Table 11-1 compares the dominant Asian and Western values but should be used only as a guide to assessing and understanding the differences and similarities of people from these cultures. Due to the complexity of these values, it is impossible to develop specific cultural interventions appropriate for all Chinese clients. This chapter uses the Purnell Model for Cultural Competence as an organizing framework to describe Chinese cultural characteristics. The information in this chapter serves as a guide for beginning to enhance one's cultural awareness, sensitivity, and competence in working with people of Chinese heritage.

Overview/Heritage

The People's Republic of China (PRC) boasts the world's oldest continuous civilization, with more than 4,000 years of recorded history. Historically, China has been ruled by strong dynasties, the first being the Hsia, which was founded around 2200 B.C., and the last being the Ch'ing dynasty, which ended in 1911. Beijing, or Peking, has been the capital of China for over 800 years and is the country's political, economical, and cultural hub. Foreigners often refer to the People's Republic of China as Mainland China, Communist China, or Red China.[1]

When Taiwan became a Chinese province in the mid-1680s, migration increased to the point

TABLE 11.1

A Comparison of Traditional Asian versus Mainstream U.S. Cultural Values

ASIAN VALUE	U.S. (AMERICAN) VALUE
Group orientation	Individual orientation
Submission to authority	Resistance to authority
Humility, self-effacement, humbleness	Superiority, brashness, imperialism
Extended family	Nuclear/blended family
Stable	Mobile
Tradition	Innovation
Implicit trust in one another	Self-reliance
Friendship	Personal achievement
Public service is a moral responsibility	Public service is a personal choice
Encourages strong network of social ties	De-emphasizes strong social ties
Relationships based on social ties	Relationships are fluid
Hierarchical	Lateral; decline in hierarchy
Formal	Informal
Rank, protocol, status	Competence
Communist government	Democratic republic
Strong societal network	Fluid society
Equity	Wealth
Conservation and saving resources	Consumption
Education is an investment; prestige reflects economic well-being of entire family	Education is a means of personal development and success
Strong collectivist work ethic	Decline in Protestant "work ethic"
Conformity	Competition
Conflict to be avoided at all costs	Conflict is an energy to be managed
Respect for the past	Future oriented
Long-term orientation	Short-term/immediate orientation
Group/familial motivation	Individual motivation
Respect for elders	Emphasis on youth
Traditional Chinese (considered complementary/alternative to U.S.)	Biomedical/biotechnological
Initial meeting: social	Initial meeting: business
Prefer side-by-side interactions	Prefer face-to-face interactions
Indirect eye contact	Direct eye contact
Non-touch orientation	Touch orientation
Low context	High context
Prefer quiet environments	Prefer noisy/active environments
Value silence	Value directness
Subtle, calming behaviors	Loud, boisterous behavior

where the Chinese dominated the aboriginal population. In 1895, following the first Sino-Japanese war, Taiwan was annexed to Japan. At the end of World War II, Taiwan again came under Chinese control in the form of a non-Communist provisional government, which is still in effect today. In 1997, control of Hong Kong was returned to the PRC after 150 years of British control, subject to certain treaty provisions allowing democratic government and some independence from the central government.[2]

The PRC is the most populous nation in the world, with over 1.3 billion inhabitants; 94% are Han, with the remainder divided among 54 ethnic groups and 56 nationalities and religious groups. Only 13% of China's people live in urban areas. Taiwan adds 20.5 million residents and Hong Kong another 6.5 million[1] (Fig. 11-1).

Residence and Reasons for Migration
The largest Chinese communities in the United States are in New York City, San Francisco, and

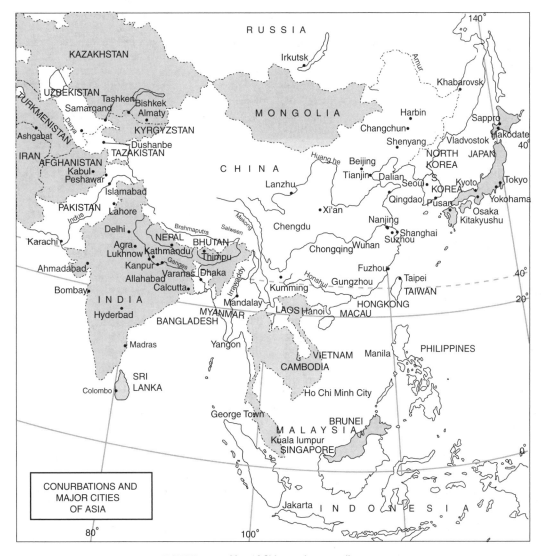

FIGURE 11.1 Map of China and surrounding area.

the state of Washington, although other U.S. cities have formed their own "Chinatowns."[3] Every year the quota for the immigration of Chinese to the United States has been filled, with more than 40,600 arriving from the PRC, Taiwan, and Hong Kong. Most of the Chinese have immigrated to the United States at three points in history: the 1800s, the 1950s, and more recently.[4] Reasons for immigration include education and increased economic opportunities.[3] The earliest immigrants were male peasants from the Guangdong and Fujian provinces who came without their families to make their fortunes on the transcontinental railroad and in the California Gold Rush of 1849.[3] Many believed they could make money in the United States to help their families and later return to China. Unfortunately, most found that opportunities were limited to hard labor and other vocations that were not desired by European Americans. Because of their cultural diversity and their unusual physical features, it was difficult for the Chinese to assimilate into American society. They looked different, and unlike European cultures, they could not simply change their names to try to blend with others. Racial violence and prejudice against them were common.

The Chinese Exclusion Act in 1882 drastically decreased immigration. In 1943, the Chinese Exclusion Act of 1882 was repealed, resulting in more women immigrating and reducing the male-to-female ratio imbalance. In 1952 the McCarran-Walters Bill relaxed immigration laws and permitted more Chinese to enter. In 1965, Public Law 89–232 removed ethnic-based immigration barriers and made it possible for all Asians to immigrate more easily.[5]

Education Status and Occupations
Six years of education is compulsory in China, and most children receive the equivalent of a ninth-grade education.[6] Only a small percentage of people graduate from high school and attend one of the approximately 450 universities and colleges. A university education is valued above all; however, few have the opportunity to achieve this goal because openings in better educational institutions are limited. Competition for top universities is keen, and many families select less-valued universities to ensure that their child is

accepted into a university rather than being slated for a technical school education. Many young adults come to Western countries to attend universities, which is considered prestigious in China.

In the United States, the educational levels of Chinese are divided between the highly educated and the poorly educated.[7] This dichotomy results in healthcare providers categorizing their clients in a similar manner. Many people falsely believe that Chinese occupations are limited to restaurants, service employment, and the garment industry. Student immigrants are expected to return to China when their education is completed. However, many do not return and elect to remain in Western countries, leading to "brain drain" in one of China's most important resources, its young scholars. As a result, it has become increasingly difficult for Chinese students to come to the West to study. Another group of Chinese immigrants are professionals from Hong Kong who moved to Canada, the United States, and other Western countries to avoid the repatriation in 1997. These immigrants usually have family connections or close friends in Western countries who are characterized by high levels of education and skills.

Reflective Exercise

• Do you know any people of Chinese descent?
• When and why did they (or their ancestors) come to the United States?

Reflective Exercise

• What prejudices and stereotypes do you have about the people from various Asian countries?
• How might these influence your interactions with clients of diverse Asian backgrounds?

Communications

Dominant Language and Dialects
Due to the linguistic diversity and variety of tones and dialects within the Chinese culture,

communication problems occur among the Chinese in China and in the United States. In China and Taiwan, the official language is Mandarin, based on the Northern Beijing dialect (Pu tong hua), which is spoken by more than 70% of the population. Nearly all Chinese are bilingual, speaking the national language and a native dialect. Other major dialects are Cantonese and Shanghaiese. Because the dialects are so different, many groups cannot understand one another verbally. However, the written language is the same. Written Chinese consists of characters, better known as ideographs, that represent an object or idea (Fig. 11-2). Each Chinese character consists of only one syllable. Each character has its own meaning. Tones within the language change the meaning of a syllable or a word. The Chinese language has a limited number of verbs, does not have tenses, and does not use plurals. Most Chinese business representatives and students can speak, understand, and correspond in English to some degree. Hong Kong has two official languages, Cantonese and English.

Contextual Use of the Language
China is a collectivist culture with a highly contextualized language wherein nonverbal communication is as important as the spoken word. Few words are used to express a thought. For example, facial expressions, movements, tensions, and speed of speech are perceived during interactions and have some meaning.[8] Chinese people have a tendency to view what is immediately perceptible, especially visually, and seek intuitive understanding through direct perception. Hence, intuitive understanding is valued more than logical reasoning.[9] Therefore, it is essential that the physical therapist understand both a Chinese individual's nonverbal cues and their contextual meaning in order to communicate effectively.

Reflective Exercise

• What considerations should you as a physical therapist familiar with low-contextual communication have when communicating with someone familiar with high-contextual language?

Cultural Communication Patterns
The Chinese value silence. Individuals are expected to conduct themselves with restraint and to refrain from loud, boisterous speech and actions. Although many times Chinese sound loud when talking with other Chinese, they generally speak in a moderate to low voice. To raise one's voice in order to make a point is interpreted by the Chinese as anger and is a sign of loss of control. Americans are considered loud to most Chinese. Hence, the physical therapist must be aware of and sensitive to voice volume and tone and avoid a loud voice volume when interacting with Chinese clients so that his or her intentions are not misinterpreted.

Negative inquiries or questions stated in a negative format are difficult for Chinese to understand. For example, a Chinese individual may have a difficult time understanding a phrase such as "You know how to do that, don't you?" A better way to present a query is to say, "Do you know how to do that?" Do not use compound or complex sentences (i.e., with "ands" and "buts"), as a Chinese individual may have difficulty deciding what to respond to first.

When Chinese Americans encounter difficulty in communicating, they often experience feelings of shame and embarrassment. Moreover,

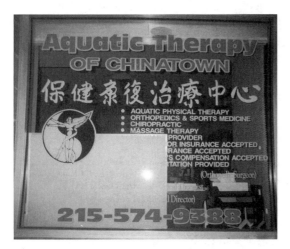

FIGURE 11.2 Chinese characters advertising a physical therapy aquatic practice.

many Chinese, especially those with language difficulties, apologize frequently for inconveniencing the other person with their lack of linguistic inabilities.

It is often easier for Chinese individuals to understand instructions when they are placed in a specific order. For example, when instructing a client in an exercise program, the physical therapist should say/write, "One, at nine o'clock every morning lie on the floor on your back; two, bend one knee; three, bring the bent knee to your chest; four, hold your knee to your chest for a slow count of 5; five, put the foot back on the floor; six, stretch out the leg until it is straight; seven, relax."

Chinese avoid disagreeing or criticizing one another to maintain harmonious relationships, at least on the surface. To avoid confrontation, the word *no* is rarely used because it can cause the person to lose face. The word "yes" can mean "no" or "perhaps." When asked whether they understand what was just said, Chinese individuals will invariably answer "yes," even when they do not understand what you have said. Such an admission of "failure" (in this case, to understand) causes loss of face. Hence, it is better to have the person repeat instructions or give a demonstration to assess the level of comprehension, especially in relation to directions for medically related matters such as medication usage, treatments, and home exercise programs.

Some Chinese Americans feel that they are disturbing or inconveniencing the physical therapist when they ask questions. Many suppress feelings (e.g., anxiety, fear, depression, pain) and are quiet, polite, and unassertive. Therefore, it is important that the physical therapist observe the client's nonverbal behaviors, accurately interpret their cultural meanings, and encourage the client to verbalize concerns and ask questions. If an interpreter is needed, identify which dialect the client speaks.

Reflective Exercise

• What communication considerations should the physical therapist have when communicating with someone of Chinese culture?

Nonverbal Communication

Even though most Chinese do not express their emotions, some may narrow their eyes to express anger and disgust.[10] Chinese Americans typically demonstrate less eye contact than Americans because direct eye contact may indicate rudeness. Direct eye contact is rarely used with the elderly, regardless of social status. Gazing around and looking to one side when listening to another is considered polite.

Chinese rarely show facial expressions and emotions in public. In formal business situations or when greeting persons of high rank, the Chinese typically limit their use of body movements and facial expressions. As a result, the Chinese are often viewed as cold and unfeeling. However, among family and friends, facial expressions are used extensively. The physical therapist must observe for changes in facial expression or other nonverbal cues in order to note changes in the client's physical or psychological status (e.g., the onset of pain). Finally, the Chinese love to laugh and joke, but Western humor does not translate well.

When standing or sitting, Chinese prefer a side-by-side or right-angle arrangement, feeling uncomfortable with a face-to-face position. The person of higher status has the prerogative of sitting as desired; thus, the burden of correct behavior falls to the person of lesser status.[11] The Chinese may communicate in closer physical proximity than is common among European Americans.

Reflective Exercise

• How might you adjust your nonverbal communication when conducting a physical therapy interview with a client of Chinese culture?

Reflective Exercise

• How might you best determine if a Chinese client is in pain?

Time Orientation

Most Chinese have a polychromic time orientation, which means that they adhere less rigidly to clock time as a distinct and linear entity. Instead, they focus on the completion of the present tasks. This is in sharp contrast to the typical Western viewpoint, which has a monochromic orientation to time and emphasizes schedules, promptness, standardization of activities, synchronization, and "clock" time (as opposed to "social" time). Because Chinese Americans tend to be more polychromic, which implies that they are present-time oriented, it is important for the physical therapist to remember that some Chinese American clients may not adhere to fixed schedules. They may, in fact, arrive late for appointments, insist on completing one task before moving on to a new task, and start more than one task at a time.

A more modern view emphasizes the importance of punctuality and a more futuristic orientation. Among some Chinese individuals, punctuality is very important, especially with respect to appointments, not only for business meetings but for social occasions as well. Lateness or cancellation is a serious affront. Because tardiness is a sign of disrespect, those who subscribe to this view arrive on time and expect others to do the same. Therefore, it is important for the physical therapist to recognize that far more important than punctuality is the protection of face. If you make a high-ranking person wait for you, both of you have lost face. To Westerners who plan their calendars weeks and even months in advance, this can be frustrating. Therefore, healthcare professionals should be prepared for both concepts of time among Chinese in the United States.

Past temporality for the Chinese is evidenced by their veneration of older people and ancestors. A future orientation is evidenced by their stress on education and the value placed on the younger generation.

Physical Touch
The Chinese do not like to be touched by people they do not know, and they do not ordinarily touch each other during conversation, especially with older people or those in important positions.[12,13] Touching a Chinese person's head is a serious breach of etiquette, especially if that person is a child, whereas touching during an argument indicates shameful loss of control. Children are considered precious, and it is believed that careless touching may damage them. In the same respect, placing one's feet on a desk, table, or chair is regarded as impolite and disrespectful. It is also inadvisable for one to pat a Chinese person on the shoulder or to initiate physical contact. The physical therapist must ask permission and explain the importance and necessity for touch when providing therapeutic interventions.

A public display of affection toward a person of the same sex is acceptable. One may see members of the same sex holding hands to signify friendship, but members of the opposite sex may not. Public displays of affection between people of the opposite gender are considered unacceptable. Chinese point with their open hands, since pointing with a finger is considered rude. Chinese beckon by extending the palm face down and waving the fingers to indicate "Come here." At no time should one put one's hands in his or her mouth (e.g., biting nails, dislodging food from the teeth), as this is considered disgusting. Feet are considered dirty and should not touch things or people. The physical therapist should never sit with his or her legs crossed, lean on a table or desk, or point to anything with the foot when talking with the Chinese client or family.

Reflective Exercise
• Describe the ways that a physical therapist may inadvertently offend someone of Chinese culture with physical touch or gestures.

Name Format and Greetings
Always recognize and greet the most senior or oldest person in a group first. Address the person in a formal manner, and politely inquire about his or her health. Both titles and forms of address are very important. Chinese often avoid identifying themselves precisely, so one should use official and full titles when possible. Calling people by any name except their family name is rude, unless they are close friends or relatives. Physical therapists should address the Chinese client by his or her title and surname, by the whole name, or by family name and title. If a person does not have a professional title (President, Engineer,

Doctor), simply use Mr., Ms., Mrs., or Miss, plus the surname. The family name is stated first and then the given name. If a person's family name is Chu and the given name is Xing-yan, then the proper form of address is Chu Xing-yan.

A Chinese wife does not generally take or use her husband's surname, but maintains her maiden names. Although Westerners commonly address a married woman as Mrs. plus her husband's family name, in the Chinese culture it is more appropriate to call a married female client "Madam" plus her maiden family name. For example, Li Chu-Chin (female) is married to Chang Wu-Jiang (male). Most Westerners would probably call her Mrs. Chang. However, it is more correct and proper to address her as Madam Li. Therefore, unless the woman is from Hong Kong or Taiwan or has lived in a Western country for a prolonged period of time, do not assume that a married woman's name is the same as her husband's.

Most Chinese in the United States adopt an English first name as an additional given name because many Westerners cannot accurately pronounce Chinese names. Some Chinese may give permission to use only the English name. However, if a Chinese client informs the physical therapist that it is acceptable to use the English name, address the client as Miss Mary or Mr. Wally.

Reflective Exercise

• What is the proper way to address a Chinese American child? • A Chinese college student?
• A traditional Chinese physician? • A Taiwanese elder? • A married Chinese female? • A Chinese college professor?

Traditional Chinese nod or bow slightly when greeting each other, although non-firm handshakes are common. When bowing to superiors, one should bow more deeply and allow them to rise first. One shows respect by bowing slightly with the hands at the sides and the feet together. Introductions, which involve a bow, will generally elicit a nod or a slight bow in return. When one is meeting someone from Taiwan for the first time, a nod of the head is sufficient. With younger or for-

eign-educated Taiwanese, a handshake is the most common form of greeting. In Hong Kong, men and women shake hands, and sincere compliments are given. The Chinese appreciate compliments, although the self-effacing nature of the Chinese will not allow them to accept them. It would be poor manners to agree. Traditional Chinese women will rarely shake hands. Western men should not try to shake hands with Chinese women. Western women will have to initiate a handshake with Chinese men. When in doubt, wait for the Chinese person to extend a hand first.

Reflective Exercise

• Compare and contrast Chinese cultural values and practices with Western cultural values and practices in terms of eye contact, touch, punctuality, temporality, and voice volume and tone.

Reflective Exercise

• How might a physical therapist appropriately greet a traditional male Chinese client? • A traditional female Chinese client?

Family Roles and Organization

Head of Household and Gender Roles

Chinese households and kinship traditionally have been organized around the male lines. Fathers, sons, and uncles are the important, recognized leaders between and among families in politics and in business. In this patrilineal culture, father-son relationships are strong. Upon marrying, a woman becomes part of her husband's family. The Chinese view of women is perpetuated to ensure male dominance in a society that has existed for centuries. In 1949, women were given recognition by the Communist Party, which stated that women "hold up half the sky" and are legally equal to men. In China today, over 90% of the women work,[6] and many hold professional positions or are prestigious leaders.

The traditional gender roles of women are changing, but a sense remains that the woman's responsibility is to maintain a happy and efficient home life. However, some Chinese men are beginning to include housework, cooking, and cleaning as their responsibilities when their spouses work. Most Chinese believe that the family is most important, and thus, each family member assumes changes in roles to achieve this harmony.

As a collectivist culture, Chinese consider the family unit more important than the individual. In China, an extended-family pattern has existed for over 2,000 years. This concept—that the Chinese culture emphasizes loyalty to family and devotion to tradition and de-emphasizes individual feelings—is still evident. The family is expected to take care of its members, both immediate and extended. Doing so brings honor to the family; not doing so brings shame.[14,15]

The Chinese perception of family is based on relationships. Each person identifies himself or herself in relation to others in the family.[6] In the Chinese culture, the individual is not lost, but is just defined differently from individuals in Western cultures. For example, personal independence is not valued; rather, Confucian teachings state that true value lies in the relationships a person has with others, especially the family. Kinship relationships are based on the concept of loyalty, and the young experience pressure to improve the family's standing.

Reflective Exercise

• How might the traditional Chinese notion of family and family roles influence a physical therapy program? • How might a physical therapist incorporate these values positively?

Goals and Priorities

To combat its population growth, China has instituted a strict one-child-per-couple policy. As a result of this "one-child law," male children are highly prized because they continue the family line and provide the parents with honor and labor. If a Chinese family desires a second child, they are expected to wait at least 5 years. According to China's laws, couples are not allowed to have three children.

Children are highly valued and loved regardless of their gender. Parents sacrifice luxuries to provide more opportunities for their children to get ahead. Frequently children live with their grandparents or aunts and uncles so that both parents can work, obtain a better education, or advance the family's standing in the community.

Older children have authority over younger children, and all children must show respect and deference to authority figures. The Chinese individual quickly learns to submit to the prevailing opinion rather than disagree.[8,9] Those who experienced the Cultural Revolution may feel some discomfort with their traditional parents. During the Cultural Revolution, many of China's young informed on their elders and their peers who did not espouse the doctrine of the time. Most of those who were reported were sent to "re-education camps," where they did hard labor and were "taught the correct way to think." As a result, many families have been permanently separated. For the Chinese American family, traditional family values risk erosion in the acculturation process. For example, many youngsters do not show respect to the elderly, and many elderly persons cannot count on their children or relatives for help.[13]

Maintaining face is very important to the Chinese and is accomplished by adhering to the rules of society. True equality is not something that exists in the Chinese mind; their history has demonstrated that equality cannot exist. Decisions are made by consensus of the group, which defers to those who have the most ethos—usually the oldest members. The duty of the individual is not to bring shame on any unit of which he or she is a member—family, group, or organization. Individuals must also be very careful not to cause someone else to lose face. Status is acquired through age, job, marriage, and wealth.

Even more important than recognized social status, maintaining face, and corresponding values and beliefs is the Chinese concept of privacy. The Chinese word for privacy has a negative connotation and means something underhanded, furtive, and secret. Urban Chinese grow up in crowded conditions, living and working in small areas, and their value of teamwork and group ideology does not make privacy highly valued. For example, a Chinese client may ask personal questions about salary, life at home, age, and children without considering it offensive. Refusal to answer personal questions is accepted as long as it is done with care and feeling. The one subject that is taboo is sex and anything related to sex.

Privacy is also limited by territorial boundaries. Waiting in an orderly line may not be the Chinese way of doing things. The Chinese may enter rooms without knocking or invade privacy by not allowing a person to be alone. The need to be alone is viewed as "not good" to the Chinese, and they may not understand when a Westerner wants to be alone. A mutual understanding of these beliefs is necessary for harmonious working relationships.[13]

Reflective Exercise

• How does the traditional Chinese concept of privacy differ from the American concept of privacy? • How might these two notions be in conflict in a physical therapy interaction or environment?

Roles of the Aged and Extended Family Members

In Chinese culture, age is revered. Older persons are venerated and have high status. Traditional Chinese view an older person as possessing great wisdom, which replaces physical strength.[16] Chinese children are expected to care for their parents when self-care becomes a concern; in China, this is mandated through law. Devotion to parents includes caring for them physically and psychologically. Older Chinese parents take pride in being supported and cared for by their children. However, the migration of children for better work opportunities, the one-child policy, and a decline in multigenerational families living together may influence this responsibility (Fig. 11-3).

Alternative Lifestyles

Within the Chinese cultures, alternative lifestyles such as homosexuality, lesbianism, bisexualism, transgenderism, and cross-dressing are not commonly expressed. In several provinces in China, alternative lifestyles are illegal and punishable by death. One-parent families are very unusual in China unless a death has occurred. Divorce is legal in China, but is not encouraged. Chinese in

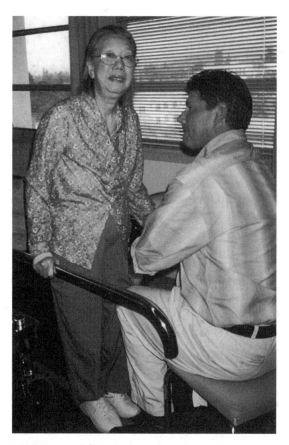

FIGURE 11.3 A Chinese elder. (Photo courtesy of Charng-Shen Wong, AP, MA, PT, and Scott S. Harp, PhD, PT.)

America may espouse many of these same values regarding alternative lifestyles.

Reflective Exercise

• What are the traditional roles of males in Chinese culture? • Of females? • Of children? • Of older people?

Reflective Exercise

• How are the aged viewed in the Chinese culture, and how might this view affect a physical therapist's interaction or physical therapy program with older clients?

Workforce Issues

Culture in the Workplace

In the United States, Chinese Americans have a long history of a strong work ethic, goal orientation, and application of traditional Chinese cultural values. In China, the government assures people a job; therefore, ambition is not as highly valued. In fact, to be noticed for working faster and harder may not be in a person's best interest. Rather, it may cause others to complain or be envious. The Chinese adapt readily to the Western workforce, but the employer needs to be aware of these differences in work-related habits and values because Chinese American workers may appear lazy or slow to U.S. employers. Chinese Americans are not lazy; they believe that working slowly is just as good as working quickly and that quality is more important than quantity. These concepts are in sharp contrast to the typical American workplace, where high productivity is expected.[13]

The Chinese acculturate by learning as much as possible about their new culture and work environment. Recent Chinese immigrants and acculturating Chinese in America watch television and go to movies to learn about Western ways of life. They also read about the new culture in books, newspapers, and magazines. They observe people from the culture in the workplace, listen closely for nuances in language, and watch the interpersonal interactions and connections of others in order to understand how to function effectively in the workplace. In addition, Chinese workers frequently call on other family members, friends, and co-workers to teach them how to fit in more quickly. Chinese Americans are generally supportive of one another in new cultures, help each other find resources, and learn to live effectively and efficiently in the new culture.[13]

Autonomy

Many Chinese Americans do not believe they have control over nature because many Chinese subscribe to a belief in fatalism. Most view people as adjusting to the physical world, not controlling or changing the environment.[9] Moreover, their autonomy is limited and is based on functioning for the good of the group. When a new situation arises that requires independent decision making, the Chinese will typically know what should be done, but do not take action until the person in authority gives permission.[13]

Reflective Exercise

• What challenges might a recent Chinese immigrant encounter in the U.S. workplace? • How do the Chinese see autonomy in the workplace?

Biocultural Ecology

Skin Color and Other Biological Variations

The skin color of Chinese ranges from white with pink or yellow undertones to very dark. Eighty percent of infants have mongolian spots, irregular areas of deep blue pigmentation primarily in the sacral and gluteal regions, and occasionally in other areas. Bilirubin levels are usually higher in Chinese newborns, and neonatal jaundice is seen in 50% of Chinese infants. The bilirubin levels peak on the fifth and sixth days after birth, which is longer than in other groups, whose bilirubin levels peak during the second or third day of life. Breastfeeding increases bilirubin levels; the mother may be encouraged to cease breastfeeding until the infant's bilirubin level returns to normal.[17] Twins and those of the Rh-negative blood group are rare among Chinese.

Chinese Americans tend to be shorter at all ages and tend to complete their growth cycle earlier compared with white ethnic groups,[18] although some Chinese are over 6 feet tall. On the standard growth chart, the mean height and weight of Chinese American children fall in the 10th percentile, compared with the mean height and weight of mainstream American children, which fall in the 50th percentile.[19] On average, Chinese children have longer trunks, shorter limbs, and significantly smaller hip measurements than European American children. Children of Chinese immigrants tend to be taller than native-born Chinese children. Healthcare professionals must consider other factors and not rely solely on the growth chart.

Among the Chinese, the ulnar bone is longer than the radius and bone density is lower than for white Americans,[17] making the Chinese more prone to osteoporosis and fractures. The Chinese also have a high, hard palate, which may cause problems for fitting dentures. Finally, Chinese individuals typically have hair that is black and straight, but some do have naturally curly hair. Most Chinese men do not have much facial or body hair.

Genetic Variations

Three genetic diseases endemic to the Chinese are (a) adult lactose intolerance, (b) alpha-thalassemia, and (c) glucose-6-phosphate dehydrogenase (G-6-PD) deficiency. Lactase deficiency may cause a person who drinks fresh milk to have indigestion, abdominal cramps, bloating, flatus, diarrhea, and vomiting. However, the individual is often able to eat cheese. Thalassemia, of which there are two types, is a genetic disease with a hemoglobin abnormality and is characterized by a high rate of red blood cell destruction. The first type is characterized by an increase in red blood cells, but it generally does not have a major effect on one's health status. The second type, alpha-thalassemia, presents as anemia that necessitates frequent blood transfusions and is associated with an early death.[20]

G-6-PD deficiency, a sex-linked genetic disease, also causes fragility of the red blood cells. In G-6-PD deficiency, an enzyme deficiency results in anemia.[20] Persons with G-6-PD deficiency are prone to anemia when exposed to drugs such as aspirin, phenacetin, nitrofurantoin, chloramphenicol, para-aminosalicylic acid, quinacrine, primaquine, vitamin K, probenecid, quinidine, sulfonamindes, and sulfones.[17] Additionally, many Chinese demonstrate noticeable facial flushing and vasomotor responses when drinking alcohol. This may explain the low alcoholism rate among the Chinese.[17]

Endemics

Diseases endemic to China include chloroquine-resistant malaria, Japanese encephalitis, schistosomiasis, hepatitis B, tuberculosis, and intestinal parasites.[21] Most Asians were vaccinated (bacillus Calmette-Guerin, or BCG) against tuberculosis in their childhood,[17] resulting in positive tuberculin skin tests. Poor living conditions and overcrowd-ing in China contribute to the development of these diseases, which persist after immigrants settle in other countries.

The incidence of cervical, esophageal, liver, lung, nasopharyngeal, pancreatic, and stomach cancers and multiple myelomas is higher among Chinese Americans.[22] The increased incidence of esophageal and liver cancers may be due to fermented and moldy foods and to nitrosamine in bran, corn, millet, and pickled vegetables. Cancers previously considered "low-risk," such as colon, breast, lung, rectal, and leukemia, are gradually increasing among Chinese Americans.[17]

In 1994, mortality data revealed that the four leading causes of death for Chinese Americans were identical to those for European Americans: heart disease; other circulatory diseases, including cerebrovascular disease; accidents; and cancer.[23] However, the proportional mortality rates were different. Studies by the Office of Minority Health Resource Center have found that Chinese American women have a 20% higher rate of pancreatic cancer.[24] In addition, Chinese American females demonstrate higher rates of suicide after the age of 45 years than female European Americans.[25] Healthcare professionals need to screen recent Chinese immigrants from China for the various health conditions discussed here and provide interventions in a culturally congruent manner.

Chinese Americans experience multiple psychosocial stresses when adapting to a new culture and environment, including cultural conflicts, discrimination, language difficulties, and poverty. Several common psychological conditions among the Chinese are depression, social loneliness, anxiety, fear, hypochondria, and somatization. Recently, a modern Chinese psychiatric disorder, neurasthenia (nervous exhaustion), has become more prevalent among Chinese Americans. Unfortunately, few Chinese Americans seek medical help until psychosomatic discomfort is experienced.[26] Typically, a psychiatric condition is manifested by behavior that is out of control and therefore brings shame to both the individual and the family. The family will often attempt to manage the individual on their own. As a result, hospitalized Chinese psychiatric clients appear more disturbed than non-Chinese clients.[27]

Drug Metabolism

Empirical studies have revealed that Asians require lower dosages than white Americans for several psychotropic medications, such as lithium, antidepressants, and neuroleptics. In addition, the plasma levels for desipramine (an antidepressant) are higher and peak earlier among individuals of Asian heritage than for European Americans. Research suggests poor metabolism of mephenytoin (for example, diazepam) in 15% to 20% of Chinese. The plasma levels of diazepam at a given oral dose are higher in Asians than in European Americans. However, Asians tolerate better the sedating effects of diphenhydramine. Research also demonstrates beta-blocker (e.g., propranolol) sensitivity, as evidenced by a decrease in the overall blood levels accompanied by a seemingly more profound response. Also, most Chinese are sensitive to atropine, as evidenced by an increased heart rate. Research has also revealed that analgesics, when given to Chinese Americans, cause increased gastrointestinal side effects, despite a decreased sensitivity to them. In addition, the Chinese have an increased sensitivity to the effects of alcohol.[28]

Reflective Exercise

• What are the common genetic health risks among the Chinese? • To what extent can you impact this outcome? • What approach or steps would you take?

Reflective Exercise

• You suspect that your Chinese American client is suffering from a psychiatric disorder. How would you approach this client and the client's family?

High–Risk Behaviors

Determining the extent of high-risk behaviors such as smoking, alcohol, or other substance abuse among Chinese in the United States is difficult because most of the data is aggregated for all Asian Americans.[21] Even using group data, high-risk behaviors among Asian Americans usually encompass less than 5% of the population. However, among newer immigrants, it appears that more than half (50% to 67%) of the population demonstrate some degree of high-risk behavior.[21,29]

Substance Use

One of the most common high-risk behaviors among men and teenagers in China is cigarette smoking.[30] Most Chinese women do not smoke, but the number of female smokers is steadily increasing, especially among newer immigrants in the United States. Although alcohol consumption among Chinese has been high at times, the level is currently low.[31] Despite these findings, the use of alcohol appears to contribute to a high incidence of vehicular accidents and related trauma.[32]

China also has a long history of illicit recreational drug use. It is a major trans-shipment point for heroin produced in the Golden Triangle. China is currently experiencing a growing domestic drug abuse problem and is also a source country for methamphetamine and hashish. Hong Kong faces serious challenges in controlling the transit of heroin and methamphetamine to regional and world markets, and is also experiencing rising indigenous use of synthetic drugs, especially among young people.

Safety

Individuals in China are susceptible to a variety of environmental toxins, including air pollution, acid rain, water shortages (especially in the north), and water pollution from untreated waste. Because many settle in larger cities in the United States upon immigration, they are at high risk for air pollution and respiratory illnesses. There is no data specific to this group in the United States. Most are compliant with seatbelt and helmet laws. The Asian population in general has low rates of sexually transmitted diseases and HIV/AIDS.

Reflective Exercise

• How would you encourage Chinese American clients to stop smoking?

Nutrition

Meaning of Food

Food and food habits are so significant to the Chinese that food is offered to a guest at any time, day or night. Specific foods are used to promote health and to combat disease. Traditional Chinese medicine uses food and food derivatives to treat diseases and to increase the strength of the weak and the elderly. Each category and type of food selected and presented at a banquet or everyday meal has a distinct purpose, and foods are presented in a specific order—always with the focus on balance, maintaining a healthy body, and combating disease.

Common Foods

Each region in China has its own traditional diet, and all regional diets are low in fat and concentrated sugars. A traditional Chinese meal emphasizes some type of fish or meat with rice, cooked tempura pan style and eaten with chopsticks. Peanuts and soybeans are popular, and common grains include wheat, sorghum, and maize.[13,33] The Chinese eat steamed and fried rice noodles called *bun*. Rice is usually steamed but can be fried with eggs, vegetables, and meats. Rice is considered "filler" and should not be eaten in extensive amounts. Instead of rice, many Chinese eat noodles or beans, especially if they come from the northern part of China. Chinese noodles are usually eaten with a broth base and are served with vegetables and meats. Another staple of the Chinese diet is tofu, which is an excellent source of protein. Tofu is fried, boiled, or served cold like ice cream. Bean products are a common source of protein. The most common meat choice is pork. Other meat preferences include chicken, beef, duck, shrimp, fish, scallops, and mussels. Oil, oil products, and salt are important ingredients in the Chinese diet and play a significant role in the preparation of daily foods. However, sauces and preserved foods contribute to a high sodium intake. Most Chinese do not eat desserts with high sugar content, preferring peeled or sliced fruits or desserts made with bean and bean curd.

Since serving dishes are not passed around the table, it is acceptable to reach in front of others to get to the serving dishes and to use one's chopsticks to obtain food. However, one end of the chopsticks is used for eating and the other for serving. It is considered inappropriate to use the "serving" end of the chopsticks to place food in your mouth. Placing them parallel to the top of your bowl or dropping them is considered bad luck. In addition, one should never stick chopsticks straight up in the rice, as this makes them look very similar to the joss incense sticks used during religious ceremonies and it is considered both disrespectful and bad luck. For soup, a porcelain or ceramic spoon is often provided. Knives are not provided because the food is generally served in bite-sized pieces.

Common drinks include tea, soft drinks, beer, and juice. Traditional Chinese do not like ice in their drinks, as it relates to the concept of cold entering the body, which shocks the body systems out of balance, thereby damaging the body and resulting in illness. Conversely, hot drinks are enjoyed and are believed to be safe for the body. Burping, slurping, and other table noises are not considered offensive and are generally ignored. Moreover, these ingestion-related "actions" are often appreciated. Finally, the serving of fruit typically signals the end of the meal. A very traditional Chinese host or restaurant may not provide napkins. Instead, guests are expected to wipe their hands on the tablecloth. Leaving a messy tablecloth indicates that one has eaten well and enjoyed the food. In the case of a "messy meal" (e.g., Beijing duck) a finger towel may be made available.

Nutritional Deficiencies and Food Limitations

Due to the genetic tendency among the Chinese to be lactose intolerant, most native Chinese individuals do not drink milk or eat milk products. Encourage Chinese clients who are lactose intolerant to use tofu (bean curd) or other protein- and calcium-rich foods to fill the body's need for fresh milk.

Dietary Practices for Health Promotion

Traditional Chinese practitioners view diet and food habits as an area of medicine, and therefore they play a significant and strategic role in health and illness. Foods and beverages are classified as either yin or yang, "cold" or "hot." All food is "yin," "yang," or "neutral" by nature (see Table 11-2).

T A B L E   1 1 . 2

Chinese Yin and Yang Foods

FOOD GROUP	YIN: COLD (THERMAL) FOODS	NEUTRAL	YANG: HOT (THERMAL) FOODS
Vegetables	Bean curds		Bamboo
	Bean sprouts		Chinese dates
	Bland foods		Chiretta (an herb)
	Broccoli		Eggplant
	Broiled foods		Garlic
	Cabbage		Ginger root
	Carrots		Ginseng
	Cauliflower		Green peppers
	Celery		Leeks
	Congee		Mushrooms
	Cucumber		Onions
	Ginkgo		Persimmons
	Most green vegetables		Red beans
	Potatoes		Red peppers
	Seaweed		
	Soybeans		
	Spinach		
	Turnips		
	Watercress		
	Winter melon		
	Winter pumpkin		
	White foods		
	White turnips		
Fruits	Melon		Tangerines
	Pears		Tomatoes
	Some types of fruit		
	Watermelon soup		
Meats	Duck		Beef
	Pork		Broiled meat
	Some types of fish		Catfish
	One type of turtle		Chicken
			Chicken soup
			Eggs
			Fatty meats
			Pig's knuckle soup
			Pork liver
			Shellfish
Nuts			Peanuts
			Roasted peanuts
			Sesame oil

(continued)

TABLE 11.2

Chinese Yin and Yang Foods *(continued)*

FOOD GROUP	YIN: COLD (THERMAL) FOODS	NEUTRAL	YANG: HOT (THERMAL) FOODS
Grains.		Noodles Soft rice	Glutinous rice
Other	Day lily Honey Milk Water	Sugar Sweets	Liquor Fried foods Red foods Sour foods Spicy foods Vinegar Wine

Modified from Ludman, E. K., & Newman, J. M. (1984). Yin and Yang in the health-related food practices of three Chinese groups. *Journal of Nutrition Education, 16*, 4.

Balancing yin and yang foods prevents sudden imbalances and indigestion and maintains physical and emotional harmony. Foods are organized into groups based on their energetic qualities, such as heating, cooling, or moistening. Also, within the Chinese culture, special importance is given to "eating in harmony with seasonal shifts and life activities."

Reflective Exercise

• Explain how "yin" and "yang" are used in dietary practices for health promotion.

Reflective Exercise

• You are a physical therapist in an acute-care environment, and you notice that your Chinese client has not eaten his meals for the past day or so. What actions, if any, would you take? • Why?

Reflective Exercise

• A client has invited you over to his house to celebrate his son's recovery and completion of rehabilitation. How would you respond? • If you did accept the invitation, what different eating practices might you encounter?

Pregnancy and Childbearing Practices

Fertility Practices and Views toward Pregnancy

The most common form of birth control in China is the intrauterine device (IUD), which is used by approximately 50% of women.[16] Chinese mothers with one child are encouraged to use IUDs, and national regulations forbid their removal. Oral contraceptives are also available at no cost to the Chinese citizens and are gaining popularity among younger people. A third option available to Chinese couples is sterilization, which is also common. Although abortion appears to be fairly common, locating specific statistics is difficult. Fertility practices of Chinese in the United States are unknown.

Pregnancy and the birth of a child are seen as important and positive events within both the immediate and extended family. Most Chinese couples wait until the age of 25 to 28 before having a child. If a pregnancy occurs before the couple is ready to have a child, the woman may have an abortion. Once a woman becomes pregnant, special dietary restrictions and prescriptions are practiced. Shellfish may be avoided during the first trimester because it causes allergies.[4] Foods high in iron and iron supplements are avoided because increasing a woman's iron levels will make the delivery more difficult.[13] Pregnant women usually add more meat, especially organ meat, to their diets. In the Chinese culture, amniocentesis may be used to determine the sex of a fetus. The Chinese government's limitation of one child per family causes some to consider abortion if the fetus is female. These practices may continue in the United States.

Birthing and Postpartum Practices

Most Chinese women are very modest and insist on having a female midwife or physician provide their ob-gyn care and deliver their babies. The laboring woman may be silent throughout the entire birthing process, because a loud response and expression of pain will dishonor her and the family.[34] In China, fathers are not allowed in labor rooms, delivery rooms, or postpartum areas. Fathers therefore may need encouragement to attend the birth in the United States. At birth, a Chinese baby is considered to be 1 year old.

In China, the mother typically stays in the hospital for 5 to 7 days after delivery; therefore, the shorter stays in the U.S. healthcare system need to be carefully explained. Some believe that the new mother should not bathe for 7 to 30 days after the delivery. The new mother or her family may voice the need for her to eat only certain foods, such as fish and food that decreases the yin (cold) energy.[4] Fruits and vegetables are avoided because they are considered "cold" foods. Chinese mothers also avoid deep-fried foods, meats in any form of sauce, and spicy foods. Mothers are expected to eat five to six meals a day of highly nutritional foods, such as soups, rice, several eggs (7 or 8 a day), and rice wine. Rice wine is encouraged because it increases the mother's strength and breast milk production. However, it is important for the healthcare professional to caution the "new" mother that drinking rice wine may increase her bleeding time. Brown sugar helps to compensate for blood loss.

In traditional Chinese homes breastfeeding is encouraged, and the mother may continue to breastfeed the child for 4 to 5 years. New mothers refrain from exposing themselves to cold in any form, avoiding the outdoors, bathing, and breezes from fans and air conditioning. In addition, touching or drinking cold water is taboo during the postpartum period. To prevent cold air from entering the body, the mother may wear many layers of clothing and cover herself from head to toe, even in the summer.

Reflective Exercise

• Why do most Chinese couples have only one child?
• What methods of birth control are acceptable?

Reflective Exercise

• What dietary restrictions are practiced during pregnancy? • Postpartum?

Reflective Exercise

• What should a healthcare professional expect with respect to pain responses from a Chinese woman in labor? • Why?

Death Rituals

Most Chinese have an aversion to death and anything concerning death. Life, because of its value, should be preserved at all costs, encouraging healthcare professionals to do everything within their power to save a client.[35] The Chinese also believe that nature should be allowed to run its course, especially when an individual is suffering or dying. To support this position, most Chinese believe that something good happens to them after they die.

The nuclear and extended families are usually involved in the care of the dying patient, providing social support, resources, and tangible aid.[36] Chinese have a deep respect for the body, believing that it is not one's personal possession, but rather is something that is passed down from ancestors. Most believe that a person who is sick or terminally ill should never be left alone. Allow family members to remain with the terminally ill or dying client at all times. The family may also find it disrespectful to make direct eye contact with a Chinese client who is dying.

Because most Chinese fear death, they avoid referring to it and teach their children to avoid referencing death.[37] While white is associated with death, both black and white are considered bad-luck colors. The number 4 is considered unlucky because when pronounced, it sounds like the word for death. Hence, Chinese individuals avoid using it in all aspects of their life. This concept should be familiar to individuals from Western societies, where the number 13 is associated with bad luck. The dead may be viewed in the family's home or in the hospital.

Autopsy and burial practices are left to individual preferences. The eldest son is responsible for all arrangements for the deceased. The family commonly honors the dead by placing objects that signify the life of the dead (e.g., food, spirit money, articles made from paper) around the coffin. In China, cremation is preferred by the state because of a lack of wood for coffins and a lack of space for burial.

Bereavement

Most Chinese do not publicly express grief. Chinese clients feel emotions similar to those of any other group; they just do not overtly express their emotions to strangers. However, some Chinese feel comfortable venting their feelings, even in public, while others may hire professional criers for the funeral. In addition to the relatives present at the funeral, a chief mourner is often present to weep for the individual who has died. Mourners can be recognized by black armbands and white strips of cloth tied around their heads. A few Chinese continue these customs in the United States.

Chinese traditions regarding death are centered on ancestor worship, which is a means by which one may pay respect. Traditional Chinese believe that their spirits can never rest unless living descendants care for the grave and worship the memory of the deceased. The practices associated with ancestor worship were so important to the early Chinese pioneers who came to work

and settled in the West that it was common for them to insist, in their work contracts, that their ashes or bones be returned to China for a proper burial.[3]

Reflective Exercise

• You have a Chinese American client who is terminally ill. What would you expect in terms of the family's assistance with care? • How might they bereave?

Reflective Exercise

• Identify two strategies to ease the terminally ill client's transition to death.

Spirituality

Major Religious Beliefs

Religion does not hold a high place in Chinese society, especially in intellectual circles. In the PRC, the practice of formal religion is minimal. Hong Kong has no official religion. Among the Chinese, the three traditional religions are Buddhism, Taoism, and Confucianism, which influence many aspects of Chinese peoples' lives. See Table 11-3 for the dominant values of these religions. Several folk religions and Islam are practiced by a few in the PRC. Most Chinese are influenced by both an Eastern and a Western religion. Chinese immigrants who practice Christianity have recently become more visible.

Meaning of Life and Individual Sources of Strength

According to the Chinese, life cannot be broken down into simple parts and examined because the parts are all interrelated. Instead, life involves a series of cycles and interrelationships, flowing in accordance with nature and remaining in harmony. The interconnectedness of life provides a source of strength for individuals from before birth to death and beyond. The primary source of strength is the nuclear and extended family. The Chinese frequently draw upon family resources (emotional, financial, mental, physical, or

TABLE 11.3

Comparison of Chinese Spiritual Philosophies

Buddhism teaches	• Harmony/non-confrontation (silence as a virtue) • Respect for life • Moderation in behavior. Self-discipline. Patience. Humility. Modesty. Friendliness. Selflessness. Dedication. Loyalty to others • Individualism devalued

Confucianism teaches	• Achievement of harmony through observing the five basic relationships of society:
	  • Ruler and ruled
	  • Father and son
	  • Husband and wife
	  • Older and younger brother
	  • Between friends
	• Hierarchical roles, social class system, clearly defined behavioral code. Importance of family
	• Filial piety and respect for elders
	• High regard for education and learning

Taoism teaches	• Harmony between humans and nature • Nature is benign because yin (evil) and yang (good) are in balance and harmony. Happiness and a long life • Charity, simplicity, patience, avoidance of confrontation, and an indirect approach to problems

spiritual). However, it is also expected that family members who use the extended family's resources will replace them so that the family remains strong. In addition, some Chinese will call upon their ancestors to provide strength as a resource.

Spirituality and Health

Because Chinese traditionally have a fatalistic outlook on life and often believe that they have no control over nature, they may be hesitant to seek allopathic medical care. In the Chinese culture, spirituality emphasizes balancing mental, physical, and spiritual aspects.

Reflective Exercise

• What are the key aspects of Buddhism, Confucianism, and Taoism? • How might they influence a physical therapy program?

Reflective Exercise

• What are the major sources of strength to the Chinese? • How might these be displayed? • How might they influence a physical therapy program?

Healthcare Practices

Focus of Healthcare

The traditional Chinese focus on prevention, which is a major component of traditional Chinese medicine. Good health depends, to a large extent, on the individual's lifestyle, emotions, and thoughts. Thus, the individual bears much of the responsibility for his or her own health and well-being. The healthcare provider serves as a guide and role model on the client's journey to good health and long life by recommending measures to modify the client's behavior and by offering assistance when needed.

Traditional Practices

Many Chinese do not believe that they have control over nature, especially those with a strong belief in Taoism. A healthy and a happy life can be maintained only if two forces, yang (hot) and yin (cold), are balanced. The terms refer not to temperatures but to attributes or conditions. Yang represents the positive, active, or "male" force while yin represents the negative, inactive, or "female" force. Body organs are categorized into yin and yang groups. A "hot" disease is treated by a "cold" treatment in order to rebalance the patient's condition. On a more ethereal level, heaven and the sun are both considered yang while the earth and the moon are considered yin. The yang force protects the body from outside influences (such as invasion by disease) while the yin force stores the strength of life. An imbalance between the yin and yang forces results in illness. Treatments to restore health focus on the restoration of balance (Fig. 11-4).

Traditional Chinese medicine is a sophisticated and complex system of health that has been practiced for over 3,000 years. Today it is used by approximately one-quarter of the world's population. Within Chinese medicine, there are six evils or excesses (wind, cold, heat, dampness, dryness, and fire) and seven moods (joy, anger, anxiety, obsession, sorrow, horror, and fear). Disease is seen as resulting from the struggle between Qi (energy) and these pathogenic factors. According to Chinese philosophy, if the body has sufficient Qi, it can resist even the most dangerous pathogenic factors.

Some of the more common traditional Chinese medicine practices follow.

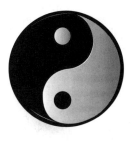

FIGURE 11.4 Yin and yang depiction.

Acupuncture involves inserting thin metal needles at specific points on the body related to the Qi meridians. Meridians are considered a channel system of flow by which Qi moves through the body. Acupuncture's purpose is to treat excesses and restore the balance between yin and yang.

Acupressure is similar to acupuncture; however, instead of needles, pressure using the hands or fingertips is applied at the acupuncture points. Like acupuncture, acupressure restores the balance between yin and yang.

Herbs are an important part of traditional Chinese medicine. Herbs fall into four categories of energy—cold, hot, warm, and cool—and five categories of taste—sour, bitter, sweet, pungent, and salty. There is also a neutral category. Herbs can be applied topically; drunk in the form of a tea, slush, or other drink; eaten; or worn on the body. Each treatment is specific to the underlying problem. Herbal remedies require prescriptions from traditional healers and can be very expensive, partly because it is more difficult for a traditional Chinese practitioner to learn herbology than techniques associated with other forms of traditional Chinese medicine (Fig. 11-5).

Moxibustion involves burning pulverized wormwood or moxa plant on a point near a Qi meridian. There are two techniques used for moxibustion. The first technique involves burning the moxa mound directly on the skin. The second technique involves burning the moxa on acupuncture needles, which are then implanted in the skin around the torso, head, or neck. For example, a traditional Chinese practitioner may place garlic on the distal end of a needle after it is inserted through the skin, and then set the garlic on fire. The heat penetrates deep into the body, stimulating or inhibiting certain target points and restoring the balance of Qi. However, these techniques may produce superficial burns. Moxibustion is used to treat cold or stagnant conditions, such as pain, sore joints, menstrual cramps, diarrhea or abdominal pain as well as to assist in

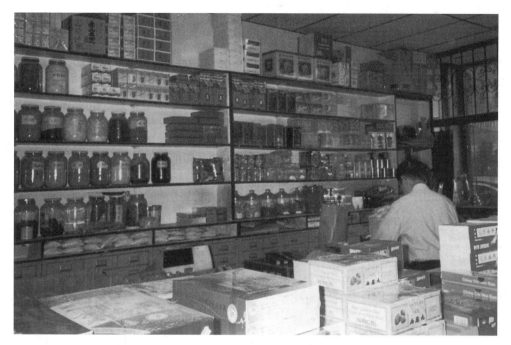

FIGURE 11.5 Herbal medicines. (Photo courtesy of Charng-Shen Wong, AP, MA, PT, and Scott S. Harp, PhD, PT.)

rotating fetuses from breech presentation to the normal delivery position.

Massage therapy and manipulation are practiced on specific body parts associated with meridians in an attempt to restore the balance of Qi in areas where it is blocked, excessive, or lacking. Massage is often used in combination with other therapies. Massage is used to stimulate the circulation, to increase the flexibility of the joints, to reduce tension, and to improve the body's resistance to illnesses. *Tui na* is a combination of massage, acupressure, and manipulation.

Coining, also referred to as skin scraping, is a treatment in which special oil is applied to the symptomatic area. A metal coin is dipped in oil, heated, and then rubbed briskly in a firm downward motion over the skin until welts appear. This treatment is used to treat colds, heatstroke, headaches, and indigestion. After treatment, multiple linear bruises may be observed on the client's skin.

Pinching the skin between the thumb and index finger produces welts, drawing out fever and illness. This procedure leaves long lines of continuous dark bruises over the skin.

Cupping involves creating suction by burning special materials and warming the air inside a glass jar or cup. The cup is then immediately placed over the part of the body requiring treatment. The heat in the cup creates a vacuum, which causes the skin to be drawn up into the cup, producing a negative pressure as it cools. This treatment dispels dampness, warms the Qi, and reduces swelling. Cupping is commonly used to relieve bronchial congestion and to treat headaches, abdominal pain, and certain chronic conditions such as arthritis, joint pain, and bronchitis. This technique results in circular ecchymotic bruise marks approximately 2 inches in diameter.[13]

Qigong, which means "energy work," consists of breathing techniques, repetitive exercises, and meditation involving intense concentration aimed at balancing the Qi.

T'ai chi is a form of exercise that builds on the mind-body connection by combining physical movement, meditation, and breathing to induce relaxation and tranquility of mind, and to improve balance, posture, coordination, endurance, strength, and flexibility. It can even be used for self-defense and has been referred to as the deadliest martial art. Practicing t'ai chi on a daily basis results in a long life, good health, physical and mental vigor, and enhanced creativity. T'ai chi requires total concentration and controlled breathing to ensure the smoothness and rhythmic quality of movement. It is suitable for all age groups, even the very old (Fig. 11–6).

Because some forms of traditional Chinese medicine leave ecchymotic areas, dermabrasion, or welts, some parents whose children have been

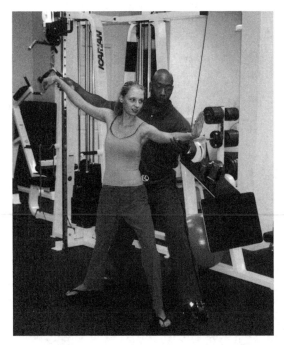

FIGURE 11.6 T'ai chi is used to help improve balance and kinesthetic awareness.

administered these treatments by family members or healers have been charged with child abuse. The marks from some traditional Chinese treatments have also led to reports of spousal abuse by those unfamiliar with the practices of traditional Chinese medicine. Physical therapists must become familiar with these treatments and not mistake them for abuse.

Reflective Exercise

• List the influences that traditional Chinese medicine has had on the modern practice of physical therapy in the United States.

Reflective Exercise

• Describe the skin markings that might be expected from some of the traditional Chinese practices.

Self-Medicating Practices

Many Chinese routinely turn to home remedies, some consisting of nothing more than the use of cooling drinks and foods in hot weather and heating foods and drinks in cold weather. Other folk practices include tonics and herbs, changes in diet, consulting family and friends, and reading home medical manuals that list home remedies. These herbs, patent medicines, and dietary approaches are often a Chinese person's first recourse upon the initial sign of illness. Clients often take herbal medications in combination with prescriptions from Western physicians or even experiment with the dosages prescribed by physicians. Carefully explain the necessity of disclosing all medications and herbs used so that a determination can be made as to whether there are conflicting or potentiating interactions.

Responsibility for Health

Within the Chinese culture, each individual is responsible for his or her own health. Typically, a Chinese American will treat minor or chronic illnesses with Chinese medical services and acute or serious problems with Western medical services.[38] The family provides much of the direct patient care while the healthcare professional is expected to manage the client's care. The family may appear to take over the life of the ill individual, who may appear passive in allowing them the control. If the client is single, one or two family members assume responsibility. If the client is married, one of the two key family members will be the client's spouse. If a family member is hospitalized, other family members traditionally remain with the patient throughout the hospital stay. Education provided by the healthcare professional must include the family members who will be responsible for the client's care once he or she is discharged to the home.

Chinese are reluctant to discuss illness or to comment on the illness of a sick person. Chinese clients, even though they appear to understand a diagnosis and accept a treatment plan, may fail to comply with the prescribed treatment regimen. Because of a cultural respect for harmony, Chinese clients who don't understand a treatment or even disagree with it may avoid conflict and suppress negative thoughts and emotions. This is because nonacceptance of a request, especially one made by a physician (who automatically commands respect), would disrupt harmony. Further, to maintain both their own "face" and the physician's, Chinese clients may avoid admitting that they don't understand the diagnosis or treatment plan, or will pretend to accept it when they disagree with it. Hence, the physical therapist must observe for nonverbal signs that indicate confusion or displeasure about the diagnosis or treatment plan. Periodically ascertain the client's comprehension. Rather than asking a Chinese client, "Do you understand?" ask the patient to describe what he or she has been asked to do or demonstrate what needs to be done.

Blood Transfusions and Organ Donation and Transplantation

In the Chinese culture, there is no overall ethnic or religious belief prohibiting blood transfusions, organ donations, or organ transplants. Within China, blood transfusions are not always safe because of the high incidence of hepatitis B. However, among traditional Chinese, removing body parts is taboo because of a Confucian principle stating that the physical body must be

returned whole at the end of life. In Confucian philosophy, the body is regarded as being loaned to a person during life on earth. Only those who return a "whole" body at death can expect to go to heaven. Hence, a client's strong belief in Confucian ideology can have a profound effect on the client's attitude toward organ donation or the removal of any body part.

Rehabilitation/Chronicity

Studies of children with disabilities indicate that Chinese parents tend to be more pessimistic about the child's outcome than parents from other cultural groups whose children have equivalent disabling conditions.[39] Siblings of disabled and chronically ill Chinese children are frequently admonished that it is their responsibility and obligation to look after the disabled child's education and future. The birth of a disabled child may cause Chinese parents to worry about their own future well-being. Parents may not encourage the use of prostheses such as an artificial arm or hearing aid because they believe it does not really change anything for the child. If the prosthesis is unable to make the child well, why bother with it? Parents may gradually discontinue visits to the physical therapist when they perceive that "nothing is happening" (i.e., the child is not being restored to "normal"). The physical therapist should be cautioned against labeling this behavior as noncompliant or neglectful. The cultural context of the parents' behavior needs to be carefully examined. Overall, the Chinese still view mental and physical disabilities as a part of life that should be hidden.

Reflective Exercise

• How might a physical therapist positively influence the life and the family life of a child with a disability?
• What aspects are important for the physical therapist to consider?

Self-Medication

Most Chinese Americans self-medicate using over-the-counter medications, antibiotics, and tranquilizers in addition to herbal remedies. Some Chinese Americans save part of a prescribed medication and take it at their own discretion at a later time.[13] Additionally, Chinese clients may adjust the dosage downward to as little as a half-dose because they consider most Western medicines overly potent. This is particularly true among individuals who are smaller in stature than Westerners. The client may even discontinue the medication completely without consulting the physician if the symptoms are no longer present or if there has been no relief of the symptoms within a few days. Clients also tend to believe that medication in the form of an injection is more effective than oral medication.

Pain

Chinese are generally quiet in demeanor and vocal expression when experiencing pain[34] and tend to promote a stoical response to pain because a display of emotion is considered a weakness of character.[40] Because it is considered impolite to accept something the first time it is offered, modes of pain relief such as medications and other interventions (e.g., TENS) must be offered more than once. Chinese clients often express their pain in ways that are similar to those of Americans. However, their descriptions of pain differ. For example, the Chinese tend to describe their pain in terms of more diverse body symptoms, whereas Westerners tend to describe pain locally. Also, the Chinese describe pain as dull and more diffuse, whereas Westerners' descriptions include words such as *stabbing* and *localized*. Many explain pain based on the traditional Chinese influence of imbalances in the yang and yin combined with location and cause. Finally, the Chinese tend to cope with pain by using externally applied methods, such as oils, moxibustion, warmth, meditation, sleeping on the area of pain, relaxation, and massage.[13] The preferred pain preparations are topical balms and ointments.[13]

Reflective Exercise

• How might the physical therapist best determine the type and intensity of pain experienced by the Chinese client? • How might the client's experience of pain differ from the physical therapist's perception?

Sick Role

Chinese individuals who have a higher educational level and who have been exposed to Western ideals and cultures are more likely to assume a sick role that is similar to that of Westerners. However, the highly educated and acculturated may also exhibit some of the traditional customs associated with illness. As a result, each client needs to be assessed individually for responses to illness and for expectations of care. Traditionally, the sick person is viewed as being passive and accepting of illness as a part of the life cycle.[13] The Chinese believe that the illness or injury is caused by an imbalance in the Qi or in the yin and yang. Therefore, there should be a medicine or treatment that can restore the balance. If the prescribed medicine or treatment does not seem to do this, then they may refuse to use it.

Mental Health

Chinese have characteristic ways of dealing with mental illness, starting with a protracted period of intrafamilial coping, even for serious psychiatric illness. They obtain advice from friends, older people, and neighbors in the community; consultations from traditional specialists, religious healers, or general physicians; and, finally, treatment from allopathic specialists.

The balance between yang and yin is also used to explain mental health problems. Most Chinese believe that mental illness results from an inability to solve problems, metabolic imbalances, and organic problems; the effects of stress, crises, and recent immigration are inconsequential. Bentelspacher, Chitran, and Rahman[41] found that many use a combination of traditional and Western medicine.

Although Chinese do not readily seek assistance for emotional and nervous disorders, a study of 143 Chinese Americans found that younger, lower-socioeconomic-status, and married Chinese with better language ability seek help more frequently.[42] The researchers recommended that new immigrants be informed that help is available when needed for mental disorders within the healthcare system. A discussion with the Chinese American immigrant family should include the family's perception of the mental condition.

Barriers to Healthcare

Chinese clients face many of the same barriers to healthcare faced by Westerners; however, there are some special concerns. Tan[43] has summarized these as follows:

1. The Chinese have more difficulties facing diagnoses of cancer because families are the main source of support for patients, and many family members are still in China.
2. The Chinese pay less attention to the need for purchasing medical insurance, so any serious illness leads to heavy financial burdens on the family.
3. Once the client responds to the initial treatment, the family tends to stop treatment and the client is lost to follow-up or becomes noncompliant.
4. Chinese families may be reluctant to allow postmortem examinations because of their fear of being "cut up."
5. The most difficult barrier is frequently the reluctance to disclose the patient's diagnosis to the patient or the family.

Reflective Exercise

• What common barriers might the physical therapist encounter when working with a Chinese client?
• How might the physical therapist help overcome the barriers?

Reflective Exercise

• Compare and contrast traditional Chinese medicine and Western allopathic medicine on their approaches to the following: treatment, medications, exercise, prevention, rehabilitation, and practitioners' roles and responsibilities.

Healthcare Practitioners

Traditional versus Biomedical Practitioners

The education of physicians, nurses, and pharmacists in China is similar to Western education and training, although ancillary workers often have increased responsibility in the Chinese healthcare system, especially in rural areas. Most traditional Chinese medical practitioners undergo a rigorous educational curriculum. The practice of midwifery is widely accepted by most Chinese. In China, most nurses are female. Nurses serve in roles that are supplementary to physicians, and social assertiveness is not emphasized. Male nurses usually work in male urology or psychiatric services. Physicians and nurses are seen as people who can be trusted and relied upon for the health needs of a family member.

Perceptions of Practitioners

Traditional Chinese medicine practitioners are shown great respect. In many cases, they are shown equal, if not more, respect compared with Western healthcare professionals. The ideal physician is the one who teaches the client to maximize good health by living correctly. Healthcare providers are usually given the same respect as elders in the family[15] and are recognized as authority figures. In addition, older healthcare providers receive more respect than the younger practitioners. Within the Chinese medical hierarchy, physicians receive the highest respect, followed closely by nurses with a university education. Other nurses with limited education are next in the hierarchy, followed by ancillary personnel. Overall, male practitioners have typically received more respect than female providers. However, this is beginning to change. In China, nurses typically do not provide much direct patient care, except in critical care units, because the family is expected to provide the care. However, most Chinese perceive nurses as caring individuals.[44]

Reflective Exercise

• For which of the following conditions might you expect your Chinese American client to seek traditional Chinese medical treatments? • Arthritis, ankle sprain, post-surgical rotator cuff, cancer, heart disease, epilepsy, back pain, and mental illness.

Most Chinese do not perceive a dichotomy between traditional Chinese medicine and the Western allopathic system. Some illnesses are best treated by traditional Chinese medicine, whereas others are treated more effectively by allopathic medicine. For example, Western physicians should be consulted for problems involving dentistry, fever, allergies, the eyes, heart attacks, strokes, surgery, diabetes, and cancer; traditional Chinese physicians and herbalists should be consulted for asthma, arthritis, bruises, sprains, lumbago, stomach problems, and hypertension. The Chinese frequently do not fully disclose all forms of treatment because they are conscious of saving face. If they inform one healthcare provider about the other, then each of the providers loses face.

Development of a trusting relationship with the Chinese client helps ensure that all information is disclosed. Impress upon the Chinese client and family the importance of disclosing all treatments, because some treatments may have antagonistic effects.[13]

Reflective Exercise

• How might interaction with a client of Chinese culture differ from or be similar to interaction with a client of U.S. culture?

CASE STUDY SCENARIO I

*M*adame Chin Ze is a 48-year-old female with stage IV pancreatic cancer. The cancer has metastasized to her bone and is evident in her pelvis and lumbar spine. She has been discharged to home at the family's request and is undergoing chemotherapy via home infusion. Madame Chin's husband, Bing Lu, is actively involved in her case, as are her mother and her two children. Madame Chin is weak and presents with mobility deficits. She is in a hospital bed in the dining room. She has a commode chair alongside the bed. She is unable to climb stairs to the second-floor bedroom. She transfers to the commode chair with the assistance of a walker and minimal assist of one.

She most likely is in pain, given the nature of her cancer, and yet does not express pain and has denied the initial offer of a TENS unit. The family has requested your services as a female physical therapist for Madame Chin's home physical therapy needs. Madame Chin rarely makes eye contact with you, does not return your handshake, and rarely complains of pain. She most often answers affirmatively and does so when you ask her if she understands her home exercises and if they are going all right.

Upon one visit, you encounter an acupuncturist leaving the house. The family and Madam Chin quickly usher you into the home and seem to be uncomfortable with the encounter.

1. What should a healthcare professional expect with regard to the presence of family members? What roles and responsibilities would the healthcare professional expect the family to demonstrate? Would your expectation change if the client were a visiting Chinese Asian national versus a recent immigrant versus an acculturated Chinese Asian American? If so, why?

2. What gender issues, if any, does the healthcare professional need to be aware of when providing care to Madame Chin? When interacting with the family?

3. What communication issues, either verbal or nonverbal, should be considered in providing care to Madame Chin?

4. How might you accurately assess Madame Chin's level of pain? Should you extend the offer of a TENS unit again?

5. How might you handle the encounter with the acupuncturist? Why might the family and client be uncomfortable discussing it with you?

6. What traditional Chinese interventions, if any, could you incorporate into this client's treatment plan?

7. How might you ensure that Madame Chin's home exercise program is appropriate and agreeable to her?

8. What culturally relevant bereavement and death issues should the physical therapist understand in interacting with Madame Chin or her family?

9. What culturally relevant information should the physical therapist document in this client's chart?

CASE STUDY SCENARIO II

Mr. Zhou, a 35-year-old Chinese male, was referred to your clinic with a diagnosis of unspecified neck pain. His primary care physician (PCP) has requested that you speak with him prior to initiating treatment. During the phone conversation with Mr. Zhou's PCP, the physician informs you that Mr. Zhou was a college student in China during 1989, when the Tiananmen Massacre occurred. As a result of his participation, he was captured, interrogated, imprisoned, and tortured for several years. During his imprisonment, he was isolated, experienced physical abuse, had his family threatened, and underwent mock executions. His physical torture included nonsystematic beatings, including falange (beating of the feet), suspension by the upper extremities (with the arms tied behind the back), strapping with claws, suffocation in water filled with human waste, and being forced to maintain unusual positions for prolonged periods (e.g, flexed spinal thoracic stretch position in a cage that allows no movement). Eventually he was released after being "re-educated." His family in China arranged for him to be transported to Hong Kong, where he was smuggled out of the country on a freighter. Four months later he arrived in the United States and immediately sought political asylum.

1. What, if any, precautions would you observe in treating this client?

2. What *culturally relevant* problems, if any, did you identify in treating this client?

3. What are your short-term goals for this client, and when would you expect to achieve them?

(continued)

Case Study Scenario II Continued

4. What *culturally relevant* interventions would you consider incorporating into this client's program? Provide a comprehensive rationale for each of your decisions.

5. What interventions, if any, would you avoid incorporating into this client's treatment plan? Provide a comprehensive rationale for each of your decisions.

6. What communication-related issues, either verbal or nonverbal, if any, might you need to consider when interacting with this client? Why?

7. When providing care to this client, what would you expect in terms of chief complaints, attitudes, behaviors, and participation level?

8. What, if any, traditional Chinese "treatment" approaches would you include in this client's program? Why?

9. What *culturally relevant* expected outcomes, if any, would you document?

10. What *culturally relevant factors*, if any, would you incorporate into this client's treatment or training sessions over the next week? Two weeks? Month?

REFERENCES

1. CIA. The world factbook: China. Available at: http://www.cia.gov/cia/publications/factbook/print/ch.html. Accessed April 15, 2003.
2. CIA. The world factbook: Hong Kong. Available at: http://www.cia.gov/cia/publications/factbook/print/hk.html. Accessed March 19, 2003.
3. Halporn R. Introduction. In: Chel CL, Lowe WC, Ryan D, Kutscher AH, Halporn R, Wang H, eds. *Chinese Americans in Loss and Separation.* New York, NY: Foundation of Thanatology; 1992:v-xii.
4. Campbell T, Chang BC. Health care of the Chinese in America. In: Henderson G, Primeaux M, eds. *Transcultural Health Care.* Reading, Mass: Addison-Wesley; 1981:162–171.
5. Chang B. Asian-American patient care. In: Henderson G, Primeaux M, eds. *Transcultural Health Care.* Reading, Mass: Addison-Wesley; 1981:255–278.
6. Chin A. *Children of China: Voices from Recent Years.* New York, NY: Alfred A. Knopf; 1988.
7. Liu C. From *san gu po* to Caring Scholar: The Chinese Nurse in Perspective. *Int J Nurs Stud.* 1991;28:315–324.
8. Anderson JM. Ethnicity and illness experience: Ideological structures and the health care delivery system. *Soc Sci Med.* 1986;22:1277–1283.

9. Gudykunst WB, Stewart LP, Toorney ST. *Communication, Culture, and Organizational Process.* Newbury Park, Calif: Sage; 1985.
10. Argyle M. Intercultural communication. In: Samovar LA, Porter, RE, eds. *Intercultural Communication: A Reader.* 5th ed. Belmont, Calif: Wadsworth; 1982:31–44.
11. Samovar LA, Porter RE. *Intercultural Communication: A Reader.* 5th ed. Belmont, Calif: Wadsworth; 1988.
12. Fisher NL. *Culture and Ethnic Diversity: A Guide for Genetic Professionals.* Baltimore, Md: Johns Hopkins University Press; 1996.
13. Wang Y. People of Chinese ancestry. In: Purnell L, Paulanka B, eds. *Transcultural Health Care: A Culturally Competent Approach.* 2nd ed. Philadelphia, Pa: FA Davis; 2003:106–122.
14. Kim YY. Intercultural personhood: An integration of Eastern and Western perspectives. In: Samovar LA, Porter RE, eds. *Intercultural Communication: A Reader.* 5th ed. Belmont, Calif: Wadsworth; 1988:344–351.
15. Louie KB. Providing health care to Chinese clients. *Top Clin Nurs.* 1985;7:118–125.
16. Butterfield F. *China: Alive in the Bitter Sea.* Rev ed. New York, NY: Random House; 1990.
17. Overfield T. *Biological Variations in Health and Illness.* Reading, Mass: Addison-Wesley; 1995.

18. Molnar SC. *Human Variation: Races, Types, and Ethnic Groups.* 2nd ed. Englewood Cliffs, NJ: Prentice-Hall; 1983.

19. Boyle JS, Andrews MM. *Transcultural Concepts on Nursing Care.* Glenview, Ill: Scott, Foresman; 1989.

20. Gaspard KJ. The red blood cell and alterations in oxygen transport. In: Porth CM, ed. *Pathophysiology: Concepts of Altered States.* 4th ed. Philadelphia, Pa: JB Lippincott; 1994:323–339.

21. Chin JL. Health care issues for Asian-Americans. *J Multicult Community Health.* 1991;1:17–22.

22. Office of Minority Health Resource Center. Cancers of cervix, stomach, and esophagus run high for some. In: *Closing the Gap: Cancer and Minorities.* Washington, DC: Author; 1994:1.

23. National Center for Health Statistics, Healthy People 2000 Review. *Health, United States, 1992.* Hyattsville, Md: Public Health Service; 1993.

24. Office of Minority Health Resource Center. *Closing the Gap: Health and Minorities in the U.S.* Washington, DC: Author; 1994:1.

25. Office of Minority Health Resource Center. Older Chinese women at high risk for suicide. In: *Closing the Gap: Homicide, Suicide, Unintentional Injuries, and Minorities.* Washington, DC: Author; 1994:1.

26. Hsu LR, Hailey BJ, Range LM. Cultural and emotional components of loneliness and depression. *J Psychol.* 1987;121:61–70.

27. Binder RL. Cultural factors complicating the treatment of psychosis caused by B12 deficiency. *Hosp Community Psychiatr.* 1983;34:67–69.

28. Levy RA. Ethnic and racial differences in response to medicines: Preserving individualized therapy in managed pharmaceutical programmes. *Pharm Med.* 1993;7: 139–165.

29. Sue D, Sue DW. Counseling strategies for Chinese Americans. In: Lee CC, Richardson BL, eds. *Multicultural Issues in Counseling: New Approaches to Diversity.* Alexandria, Va: American Association for Counseling and Development; 1992:79–90.

30. Yang P, Lawson JS. Health care for a thousand million. *World Health Forum.* 1991;12:151–155.

31. Weatherspoon AJ, Danko GP, Johnson RC. Alcohol consumption and use norms among Chinese Americans and Korean Americans. *J Stud Alcohol.* March 1994: 203–206.

32. Lawson JS, Lin V. Health status differentials in the People's Republic of China. *Am J Public Health.* 1994;84:737–741.

33. Worcester N. Diet and nutrition in the People's Republic of China. In: Hillier SM, Jewell JA, eds. *Health Care and Traditional Medicine in China, 1809–1982.* London: Routledge & Kegan Paul; 1983:408–425.

34. Weber SE. Cultural aspects of pain in childbearing women. *J Obstet Gynecol Neonatal Nurs.* 1996;25:67–72.

35. Coor CA, Nabe CM, Corr DM. *Death and Dying, Life and Living.* Pacific Grove, Calif: Brooks/Cole; 1994:73–121.

36. Luckmann J. *Transcultural Communication in Health Care.* Albany, NY: Delmar Thomson; 2000.

37. Huang W. Attitudes toward death: Chinese perspectives from the past. In Chen CL, Lowe WC, Ryan D, Kutscher AH, Halporn R, Wang H, eds. *Chinese Americans in Loss and Separation.* New York, NY: Foundation of Thanatology; 1992:1–5.

38. Liu WT. Health services for Asian elderly. *Res Aging.* 1986;8:156–175.

39. Reilly J. Health survey for England. Available at: http://www.data-archive.ac.uk/findingData/snDescription.asp?sn=3886. Accessed May 30, 2004.

40. Thiederman S. Stoic or shouter: The pain is real. *RN.* 1989;52:49–55.

41. Bentelspacher CE, Chitran S, Rahman MA. Coping and adaptation patterns among Chinese, Indian, and Malay families caring for mentally ill relatives. *J Contemporary Hum Serv.* 1994;4:287–294.

42. Ying Y, Miller LS. Help-seeking behavior and attitude of Chinese Americans regarding psychological problems. *Am J Community Psychol.* 1992;20:549–556.

43. Tan CM. Treating life-threatening illness in children. In: Chen CL, Lowe WC, Ryan D, Kutscher AH, Halporn R, Wang H, eds. *Chinese Americans in Loss and Separation.* New York, NY: Foundation of Thanatology; 1992: 26–33.

44. Morales ET, Jiang SL. Applicability of Orem's conceptual framework: A cross-cultural point of view. *J Adv Nurs.* 1993;18:737–741.

Chapter 12

Cultural Considerations for the Latino/Hispanic Client

● Florence Thillet-Bice, PT, DPT, MA, PCS

Señora Maria Hidalgo recently emigrated from Mexico to live with her two sons and daughter in a rural Arizona town. She speaks very little English and lives within a Spanish-speaking community. When she suffered a right cerebrovascular accident, she underwent rehabilitation at the local hospital. The staff encountered difficulties in treating Señora Hidalgo because of the language barrier and other, nonverbal miscommunications. The staff also had difficulty with the family members, as they were often present beyond visiting hours and tried to assist Señora Hidalgo more than the staff believed they should have.

Overview

The United States 2000 census defines Spanish/Hispanic/Latino as "a person of Cuban, Mexican, Puerto Rican, South or Central American, or other Spanish culture or origin regardless of race."[1] For the purpose of this chapter, the designation "Hispanic" will be used for brevity. "Hispanic" refers to a conglomerate of groups and races that the U.S. Office of Management and Budget have clustered together for the purpose of statistical tracking and to augment the precision of the demographics of the U.S. population. Even though members share many characteristics, the Hispanic population is very heterogeneous. Therefore, one must be careful not to stereotype or expect that all the members in this group are and act the same. One must address members of this group as individuals without losing perspective of the cultural characteristics they share. Most of the studies currently available about Hispanics are based on the three largest Hispanic subgroups—Cubans, Mexicans, and Puerto Ricans.

Although the U.S. census has defined a category for Hispanics, great variability exists among the many groups that fall under this umbrella.[2] In the 2000 U.S. census, Hispanics described themselves as *criollo*, *mestizo*, mulatto, *Latinegro*, *indigena* (indigenous), white, and/or black.[3] In the 2000 census, approximately 48% of the Hispanics identified themselves as white, less than 4% identified themselves as black, and 6% identified themselves as having two or more races.[4] Most Hispanics identify themselves by their country of origin.

The Hispanic population is one of the fastest growing and largest minority groups in the United States. According to the U.S. census of

2000, over 35 million people identified themselves as Hispanic, up from 22.4 million in 1990, an increase of 57.9%.[1] In 1997, one in two foreign-born residents of the United States was from Latin America, compared with one in five in 1970. By 2003, two in five (15 million) Hispanics were foreign born and two-thirds were born in the United States. Hispanics are also more likely to have children under age 18 years compared with non-Hispanic whites.[5]

The median age of Hispanics in the United States is 26.5 years, and approximately 41% of the population is under 21 years old. The fertility rate is 56% higher than that for non-Hispanic white groups. Thus, the Census Bureau estimates that by the year 2050, one-third of those under age 18 will be Hispanic. As of 2002, the Current Population Survey listed 37.4 million Hispanics, with Mexicans being the largest group (66.9%), followed by Central and South Americans (14%), Puerto Ricans (8.6%), and Cubans (3.7%).[2,5] In recent years, a new wave of Hispanic emigrants has arrived to the United States from the Dominican Republic, Spain, and other countries, accounting for an additional 6.5% of the total Hispanic population[1] (Fig. 12-1). The numbers of Hispanics may be greater because many undocumented persons may not have been included in the census. The poverty level is higher among Hispanics compared with other groups.[5]

Heritage and Residence
Not all Hispanics are descendants of Spaniards, and not all of them have Spanish as their native tongue. The majority of Hispanics in the United States live in the West (44.2%) and the South (34.8%), with fewer in the Northeast (13.3%) and the Midwest (7.7%). Cubans comprise 75% of the southern residents and are clustered mainly in the state of Florida[5] (Fig. 12-2).

Reflective Exercise

• Why is it impossible to draw an accurate depiction of the Hispanic culture?

Hispanics can be found in urban areas, in rural areas, and, to a lesser extent, in the suburbs.[5] In many Hispanic neighborhoods, or "barrios," they can purchase their native foods and products. Additionally, the Spanish language is strongly preserved in such areas as Little Havana in Miami, East Los Angeles in California, and East Harlem in New York City, to name a few. Many rent houses in poor neighborhoods because they are undocumented immigrants and/or are below the poverty level. Some encounter abusive landlords who threaten to report them to immigration; thus, tenants often do not complain about their poor living and sanitary conditions. Many lack transportation because they do not know enough English to take the written test to obtain a driver's license or do not have enough income to purchase a car. Others live in areas where there is no local public transportation. They may be uncomfortable having healthcare professionals enter their homes to provide services because of their poor housing conditions and undocumented status.

Reflective Exercise

• How might one's undocumented status affect physical therapy services?

Migration and Associated Economic Factors
Hispanics migrate to the United States to seek better economical opportunities, to escape from political oppression, to study at universities, and to escape from environmental disasters.[6] Others come to seek medical care.[5] The first Hispanic settlement in the United States was in St. Augustine, Florida, in 1565; however, Mexicans have been in the lands now known as the West before they were annexed to the United States.[7] Mestizos of Indian and Spanish descent settled on land that today is New Mexico (Fig. 12-3). The first group of Hispanics to come to the United States were Mexicans, and they were followed by Cubans, Puerto Ricans, and people of other Latin American countries. Mexicans came in early 1900 during the Mexican Revolution because of political persecution.[5] Currently, most come for improved economic opportunities and work in farming and other low-paying jobs, such as housekeeping and day work. Many arrive illegally

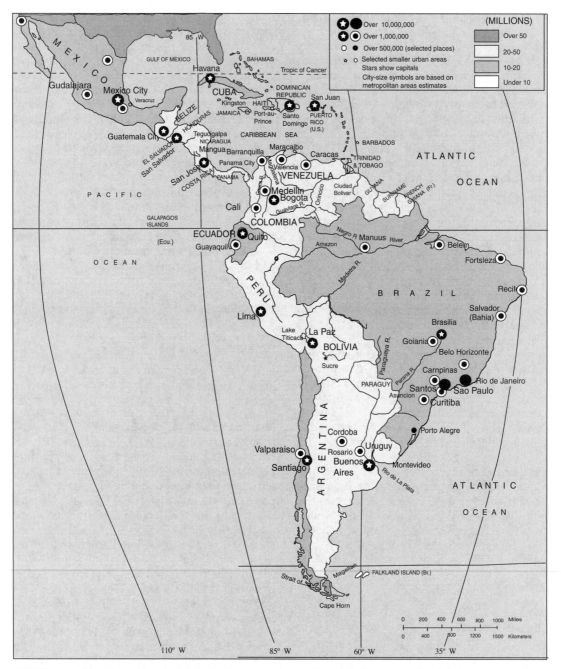

FIGURE 12.1 Map of countries of origin for the largest numbers of Hispanic/Latin American immigrants to the United States.

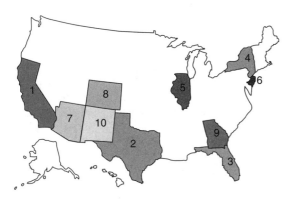

FIGURE 12.2 Map of top 10 states of residence for Hispanic immigrants in the United States.

and are sometimes referred to in derogatory terms such as "mojados" or "wetbacks" (because they "cross the Rio Grande River").

Cubans have immigrated in distinct waves. The first group, most of whom were wealthy individuals and/or professionals, came after Fidel Castro became president. They joined a group of wealthy Cubans who were already in Florida.[8] Between 1965 and 1978, many came directly from Cuba while others came through Spain, Mexico, and Jamaica to the United States. In the late 1970s and early 1980s, Cubans came when Castro allowed political prisoners to meet their families in the United States. The last large group arrived in the United States in the early 1980s and were derogatorily called "Marielitos" because they left from the Mariel port in Havana, Cuba. This group was very different from the initial groups of Cuban émigrés; they were of lower socioeconomic status,

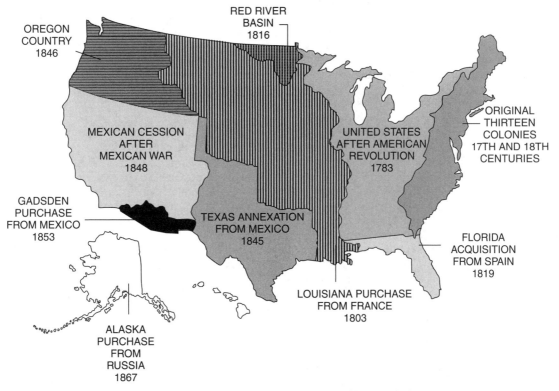

FIGURE 12.3 Map showing areas of the United States formerly governed by Mexico and other countries.

had criminal records, were less educated, and were more likely to live in poverty.[9]

Contrary to other Hispanics not born in the mainland United States, Puerto Ricans are U.S. citizens. In the Spanish-American War in 1898, Puerto Rico became a U.S. colony; in 1917, Puerto Ricans became U.S. citizens, and in 1952 Puerto Rico became a commonwealth of the United States. Many Puerto Ricans came to the mainland United States and some migrated to Hawaii to work on the farms.[10] Their descendants have kept many Puerto Rican traditions and have integrated with the local Hawaiian cultures and U.S. mainland cultures. Currently, most Puerto Ricans emigrate in search of better job opportunities in the northeastern United States.[5] Many Puerto Rican professionals are leaving the island to seek better employment opportunities and additional education. Puerto Ricans call themselves "Boricuas," a name derived from the word *Boriquen*, which is the name given the island by the Taino Indians. The Spanish invasion of Puerto Rico led to the demise of the Taino Indians, and those who remained intermarried with the Spaniards.[10]

Because of the relationship between the United States and Puerto Rico, Puerto Ricans can move back and forth freely between the mainland and the island. Many of them receive major medical services on the mainland. Unlike many other Hispanic immigrants, Puerto Ricans maintain many cultural, family, and social connections with the island even after many years in the mainland United States.

Oropesa and Landale[11] found that when Puerto Ricans migrate to the mainland United States, child poverty decreases but does not improve to the level of non-Hispanic white children. They also noted that when Puerto Rican children return to the island, they do not fare as well as the children who remained on the island, perhaps because of employment disruption or unstable living arrangements upon their return. They also found that more highly acculturated Puerto Ricans did not have the same difficulty upon return to the island.

People from Central and South American countries, including Colombia, Nicaragua, Guatemala, and Venezuela, have come to the United States over the last 25 years because of political instability (civil wars) and natural disasters such as landslides, earthquakes, and tropical storms.[6]

Reflective Exercise

• How might someone's reason for migration alter his or her acculturation to the United States? • How might the reason for migration influence the physical therapy program?

Education

According to Therien and Ramirez,[12] Hispanics have the lowest educational levels of any group in the United States, resulting in limited economic opportunities. Many Hispanic children are positively affected by Head Start programs, probably as a result of increased opportunities to speak English. Hispanics are more likely to drop out of school than non-Hispanics. As of 1997, only 45% of adult Hispanics age 25 years and older had completed high school. The percentage who completed high school and had some college increased from 31% in 1971 to 54% in 1997. Hispanics born in the United States have higher rates of high school graduation than non-natives, and Cubans have the highest level of education among the Hispanic subgroups.[13]

Many Hispanic immigrants are not familiar with the model of education practiced in the United States. With the exception of Puerto Rico, most come from an educational system that follows the European practice of oral instruction. Schools in most Central and South American countries divide levels into primary, secondary, and *preparatoria* (preparatory), which is similar to a junior college or a vocational/technical program in the United States. Once the students finish *preparatoria*, some continue study of professional disciplines at a university.

Learning styles also vary from those of traditional white European Americans. Griggs and Dunn[14] found that Hispanic children prefer to work in groups, like colder environments, and do not like to eat while they are in class. The majority prefer (a) to learn later in the day, (b) a more structured method of learning, and (c) a more mobile and kinesthetic style of learning. Mexican American students prefer to learn in groups rather than in isolation.[15] Typical educational practices in the United States are geared to the convergent thinker, whereas Hispanics may have problems because they tend to be divergent thinkers.[15,16] Differences in learning styles, cooperation vs. competition, and other methodological differences affect learning.

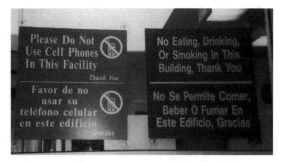

FIGURE 12.4 Bilingual signage in a physical therapy clinic waiting room.

Reflective Exercise

• How might the educational differences discussed above affect a physical therapy intervention? • What considerations might the physical therapist make?

Communication

Dominant Language and Dialects

Spanish is the primary language spoken by most Hispanics; however, not all households use Spanish as their first language. In many cases, Spanish is spoken at home by the parents but not by the children. Sometimes only the first generation, or grandparents, read, write, and speak Spanish; the second generation may speak Spanish but not read or write it; and the third generation may understand Spanish but only speak, read, and write English. In many instances, children of immigrants understand only Spanish words associated with home and use English for vocabulary associated with the school and community. Bilingual signage can be useful in the physical therapy clinic (Fig. 12-4).

Linguistic diversity in the Spanish language exists in terms of pitch, vocabulary, accent, pronunciation, dialect, and grammar rules, depending on the country of origin. For example, people from the Caribbean have a higher pitch and different accent compared with the people in Central and South America. Puerto Ricans do not pronounce the last "s" and pronounce the double "r" with a guttural sound; the Spaniards pronounce the "c" with a "z" sound.[17] The same word can be offensive in one country but not in another; therefore, it is important to know the difference when the healthcare provider uses Spanish to communicate with the patient.[7] Likewise, the Spanish language has verb tenses and pronoun construction that are different from the English language, and the physical therapist should consider that miscommunications with mistranslations might easily occur. When in doubt, always obtain a qualified interpreter (Table 12-1).

Reflective Exercise

• A physical therapist called the grandmother of a pediatric client to inquire about the status of the client's orthotics. The grandmother spoke limited English, so the physical therapist assumed that the family would prefer written instructions in Spanish. She translated the instructions into Spanish and sent them home with her client. The next day, the physical therapist received a phone call from the grandmother requesting the instructions in English because she did not know how to read Spanish. How should the physical therapist have handled the communication initially? • What can she learn?

In addition to Castilian Spanish, Spain has four other semiofficial languages—Basque, Catalán, Valenciano, and Gallego—and 16 other languages and dialects.[17] Although all these groups speak Spanish, they have different accents and customs. There are over 50 different languages and dialects in Mexico and over 15 in Central and South America.[18]

(text continues on page 217)

TABLE 12.1

Medical Words and Phrases in Spanish

1. ¿Cómo está usted?—How are you? (formal)
2. ¿Cómo tu estas?—How are you? (informal; used with children and youth and in more familiar situations)
3. ¿Donde le duele?—Where does it hurt? (formal)
4. ¿Donde te duele?—Where does it hurt? (informal)
5. Me duele la/el _____.—I have pain in the ___.
6. ¿Cómo es el dolor?—How is the pain?
   a. Fuerte—Strong
   b. Agudo—Acute
   c. Afilado—Sharp
   d. Apagado/No agudo—Dull
   e. Débil/flojo—Weak
   f. Constante—Constant
   g. Intermitente—Throbbing
7. ¿Con quién vive?—Whom do you live with?
8. ¿Dónde vive/reside?—Where do you live?
9. ¿Su casa tiene escaleras? Escalones?—Does your house have stairs? Steps?
10. ¿Cuantos escalones/escaleras?—How many steps/stairs?
11. ¿Usted fuma, bebe, usa drogas?—Do you drink, smoke, use drugs?
12. ¿Cómo se llama?—What's your name? (formal)
13. ¿Cómo té llamas?—What's your name? (informal)
14. Volteese boca arriba—Turn on your back (formal)
15. Volteate boca arriba—Turn on your back (informal)
16. Volteese boca abajo—Turn on your abdomen (formal)
17. Volteate boca abajo—Turn on your abdomen (informal)
18. Levante—Raise/Lift
    a. Su (el) brazo—Your (the) arm
    b. Su (la) cabeza—Your (the) head
    c. Su (el) hombro—Your (the) shoulder
    d. Su (la) pierna—Your (the) leg
    e. Su (la) rodilla—Your (the) knee
    f. Su (el) pie—Your (the) foot
    g. Sus (los) pies—Your (the) feet
    h. Su (el) muslo—Your (the) thigh
19. Levante el brazo hacia el lado—Lift your arm to the side
20. Levante la pierna para el lado—Lift your leg to the side
21. Arrriba—Up
22. Abajo—Down
23. Hacia el lado—To the side
24. Baño—Bath
25. Bañera—Bathtub
26. Inodoro—Commode
27. Excusado/Baño—Bathroom
28. Dentaduras—Dentures

29. *Body parts*
    a. Cabeza—Head
    b. Cara—Face
    c. Ojos—Eyes
    d. Nariz—Nose
    e. Dientes—Teeth
    f. Orejas—Ear lobes
    g. Oidos—Ears
    h. Boca—Mouth
    i. Lengua—Tongue
    j. Cuello—Neck
    k. Senos (female)/Mamilas (male)—Breasts
    l. Hombro—Shoulder
    m. Codo—Elbow
    n. Antebrazo—Forearm
    o. Muñeca—Wrist
    p. Mano—Hand
    q. Dedos—Fingers/toes
    r. Tronco—Trunk
    s. Estómago—Stomach
    t. Abdomen/Vientre—Abdomen
    u. Espalda—Back
    v. Barriga—Belly
    w. Tórax—Thorax
    x. Torácica—Thoracic
    y. Lumbar—Lumbar
    z. Cintura—Waistline
    aa. Nalgas/Sentaderas—Buttocks
    bb. Cadera—Hips
    cc. Ombligo—Belly button
    dd. Pelvis—Pelvis
    ee. Rodilla—Knee
    ff. Canilla—Shin
    gg. Pie—Foot
    hh. Dedo indice—Index finger
    ii. Dedo meñique—Pinky finger
    jj. Dedo anular—Ring finger
    kk. Dedo del corazón—Heart finger
    ll. Dedo gordo—Big toe

Other expressions/words
 1. Botella——Bottle
 2. Mamila/bobo/chupete—Pacifier
 3. Arco de movimiento—Range of motion
 4. Fuerza—Strength
 5. Fuerte—Strong

(continued)

TABLE 12.1

Medical Words and Phrases in Spanish *(continued)*

6. Débil/flojo——Weak
7. Aguante/Sostenga—Hold (formal)
8. Fuerza muscular—Muscle strength
9. De rodillas—Kneel
10. De media rodilla—Half-kneel
11. Hydrocefálico—Hydrocephalic
12. Convulciones—Seizures
13. Hipertonia—Hypertonic
14. Hipotonia—Hypotonic
15. Espástico(a)—Spastic
16. Perlesia cerebral—Cerebral palsy
17. Impedido/discapacitado—Handicapped/disabled
18. El lado derecho—The right side
19. El lado izquierdo—The left side
20. ¿Tiene dificultad para respirar?—Do you have difficulty breathing?
21. ¿Cuantos años tiene?—How old are you?
22. ¿Cuantos hijos(as) tiene?—How many children do you have?
23. ¿Tiene el niño o la niña ____?—Does the boy or girl have ____?
24. Vuelva a la clinica/ clase ____ —Return to the clinic/class ____
    El lunes—Monday
    El martes—Tuesday
    El miércoles—Wednesday
    El jueves—Thursday
    El viernes—Friday
    El sábado—Saturday
    El domingo—Sunday
25. Ejercicios—Exercises
26. Agarre de pinza—Pincer grasp
27. Férulas—Orthotics
28. Abrazaderas—Braces
29. Movimiento—Movement
30. Terapia física—Physical therapy
31. Terapia ocupacional—Occupational therapy
32. Terapia del habla y lenguaje——Speech and language therapy
33. Camine—Walk
34. Camine derecho/a—Walk straight
35. Corra/corre—Run
36. Rápido—Fast
37. Despacio—Slow
38. El niño (hombre) es lento—The boy (man) is slow
39. La niña (mujer) es lenta—The girl (woman) is slow
40. Parece en un solo pie—Stand on one foot only
41. ¿Cuanto pesa?—How much do you weigh?
42. ¿Cuanto mide?—What is your height?

43. Doble la/el—Bend the____
44. ¿Quién es su doctor(a)?—Who is your doctor?
45. Diabetes—Diabetes
46. Enfermedades del corazón—Heart diseases
47. Enfermedades de cáncer—Cancer diseases
48. Enfermedades del pulmón—Lung diseases
49. Respire—Breath
50. Tosa—Cough (verb)
51. Toz—Cough (noun)
52. Asistencia técnologica—Assistive technology
53. Sordo(a)—Deaf
54. Ciego(a)—Blind

Reflective Exercise

• A 5-year-old Mexican boy was taken to the emergency room by his mother. The mother had very limited English skills. The staff physician diagnosed a dislocated shoulder. The mother told them that "el niño se pegó." This phrase was interpreted as the child was hit. The child was immediately removed from the mother and placed in protective police custody. Upon the arrival of a relative, the relative clarified the situation by saying that the child "se pegó," or hit himself, when he fell from a swing. How did this misunderstanding occur? • How should the situation have been handled?

Nonverbal Communication

Most Hispanics maintain a closer personal space than non-Hispanic whites when conversing or interacting with family, friends, and healthcare providers. If the physical therapist maintains an increased spatial distance, the Hispanic client may perceive it as denoting a lack of interest, detachment from the patient's needs, or insensitivity.[19] Not only do most Hispanics stand in close proximity, but they also often touch the person as they talk, which connotes interest in what is being communicated.

An issue of importance for many Hispanics is the demonstration of respect (*respeto*) for others, particularly persons in authority, such as physical therapists and older people.[7,19,20] Always address a person formally with a title such as Mr., Mrs., Miss, Ms., or Dr. when meeting him or her for the first time. Do not use the first name alone until told to do so. Use the equivalent Spanish title (*Señor, Señora, Señorita, Doctor,* or *Doctora*) when appropriate (Fig. 12-5).

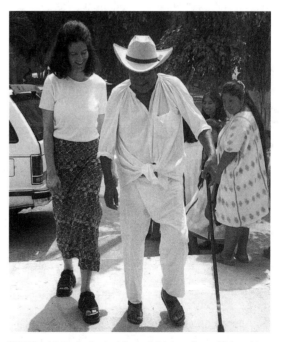

FIGURE 12.5 A physical therapist interacting with an elderly Hispanic client.

Many Hispanics "talk with their hands" and become animated when expressing emotions and giving emphasis to a personal conversation or topic of interest such as politics. Furthermore, voice inflections may be perceived as overly emotional or "out of control."[7] Some Hispanics do not maintain eye contact when conversing, especially with someone in a hierarchical position, considering it disrespectful.[16] Many use limited verbal expression toward authority, nodding the head when a person speaks; however, a nod of the head does not necessarily mean agreement with the speaker, only that the message has been heard or understood.

Women greet each other with a kiss on the cheek, and a male may kiss his father, son, or grandfather. Men also kiss female relatives and familiar acquaintances on the cheek. *Personalismo*, the establishment of a personal, respectful relationship with a person of authority, is done through a handshake or embrace.[7,21,22]

Reflective Exercise

• What aspects of nonverbal communication might make you uncomfortable? • What do you think about the Hispanic value of personalismo?

Format for Names

In most Hispanic countries, individuals use both the mother's and father's last names—for example, Maria Elena Rodriguez Colón. Colón is the mother's last name and Rodriguez is the father's last name. When the woman marries, for all legal purposes she keeps her maiden name; if she takes the husband's last name, the word *de* is added (e.g., Maria Elena Rodriguez de Rivera González) or she simply uses both her name and her husband's last name (Maria Elena Rodriguez de Rivera).[23] In formal situations, such as in writing and in conversation, the title *Doña* or *Don* is used (*Doña* Maria). *Señora* or *Señor* can also be used when addressing an older person. Do not use only the first name of an older person unless the person specifically asks to be addressed with the more familiar form. Children commonly have more than one name; at times up to three names are used. Many times the oldest son carries the father's name.

Family Roles and Organization

Head of Household and Gender Roles

Most Hispanic families are traditional and extended, with a mother, father, children, and grandparents living in the same household. The Hispanic family is usually patriarchal; however the mother cares for the children and older relatives and possesses power within the family. Mothers within the Mexican American community enjoy a high social status. Lagana[24] found that Mexican American women considered motherhood a desirable and respectable role and were more likely to leave job and career to take care of themselves during pregnancy and their children as they grew.

Mendelson[25] interviewed Mexican American mothers regarding their values and found that their role as mothers came second in importance only to God. *Familismo,* or commitment to family members, is a traditional value of the Hispanic culture.[7] As Hispanic families become more and more acculturated to the American value of individualism and autonomy, family support may become less certain, creating a cultural struggle within Mexican American mothers.[25]

Family extends beyond the nuclear family to include the extended family and often non–blood relatives. The role of the *compadre/comadre,* or godparent, is highly valued. *Compadres* participate in major rites of passage, such as infant baptism and marriage ceremonies (Fig. 12-6). The importance of family is manifested in the interdependence of family welfare. Two or three generations may live together in the same household or in close proximity. Many times the entire family unit moves as a group, which may include aunts, uncles, parents, children, and grandparents. Even second and third cousins are considered family and may accompany a relative to a health appointment to assist with translation or provide transportation.

In recent studies of Cuban and Puerto Rican families, researchers found that family proximity is changing because of the need for many families to move in order to find suitable jobs.[26,27] This is also evident in Mexican American families.[28] Moreover, as a result of acculturation, the number of older people who live alone has increased, par-

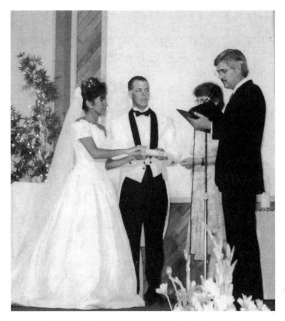

FIGURE 12.6 Godparents or *compadres* taking part in a wedding ceremony.

ticularly among Cubans and Puerto Ricans.[26,27] The divorce rate has also increased among Cubans, increasing the number of single older women living by themselves.[26,28] Fourteen percent of Hispanic households consist of one person, compared with 30% of black households.[5]

Machismo, or a male's manhood, is a concept prevalent among Hispanics and is seen as an expression of honor and dignity—a way to protect the family name. Machismo is both a positive and a negative concept. In positive terms, men are responsible for providing for the family, and display physical strength and virility. In negative terms, male strength is "in control" of the household, implying that men have greater decision-making ability than women.[29] Therefore, in some Hispanic families, men feel they have to protect women and be respected by women.[7]

Although the mother is the primary caregiver and cares for the sick, and the entire family is involved in the decision-making process, most fathers make the final decision, although recent research reports that one-third of the time men are the primary decision makers, one-third of the time the women are the primary decision makers,

and one-third of the time the decisions are egalitarian.[30,31] The father is also responsible for obtaining social assistance and networking.[32] In many families, the oldest daughter is the one responsible for the parents' care when self-care becomes a concern.[33] Children, in particular female children, are expected to live at home with the parents until they marry. Because new immigrants are accustomed to having family nearby, children are not usually left alone with older siblings while parents work. Siblings are responsible for taking care of their younger brothers and sisters. If one sibling has a disability, other siblings are expected to assist with his or her care. In the case of an adult with a disability, the remaining adult siblings are expected to provide care rather than place the person in a long-term care facility.[34]

Reflective Exercise

• How might the concept of *familismo* conflict with a physical therapy program? • How might it enhance a physical therapy program?

Reflective Exercise

• How might the concept of *machismo* conflict with a physical therapy program? • How might it enhance a physical therapy program?.

Developmental Tasks and Roles of the Aged

Hispanic children as old as 5 years of age may use a bottle or pacifier. One commonly hears a 5-year-old child referred to as "Bebé," which translates as "baby." Children are highly valued, and parents take pride in keeping their children clean, a sign of the child's well-being. In addition, many parents don't like to see their child cry, and it is not unusual for a parent to take the child away from the physical therapist if the child cries while receiving medical attention.[35]

Puerto Rican newborns are more alert than white non-Hispanic babies, while their muscle tone is the same as that of non-Hispanic whites.[36] A study of Puerto Rican children reported that they attain functional skills at a slower pace than white non-Hispanic children. Parents of Puerto

Rican children had different expectations as to when their children should be able to accomplish tasks such as using the fork, performing chores, and independent car transfers.[37] Another study demonstrated that the more acculturated the child and family, the closer the functional skill score was to that for a non-Hispanic white child.[38] Kolobe[39] studied the child-rearing practices and developmental expectations of Mexican American mothers and found they emphasized the child's development of proper behaviors and a sense of dignity over early achievement of developmental milestones. They exhibited strong nurturing behaviors (Fig. 12-7).

Anthropological studies reported that some Hispanic children did not engage in gross motor activities, social or symbolic play, or verbal play beyond the minimal level before the age of 2 years. After the age of 2, children began to spend more time with their older siblings engaged in motor activities. Between the ages of 2 and 5, children in the studies were observed climbing trees, chasing each other, chasing bugs, and twirling around to get dizzy.[40]

Reflective Exercise

• Hector is a 2-year-old diagnosed with developmental delay. He recently learned to walk and was referred to the assessment team for an arena assessment. Once the assessment begins, the mother remains close by but does not get on the floor with Hector. As the team begins the assessment, Hector begins to cry and reaches out to his mom. His mother quickly gets down on the floor and holds him. Once Hector's mother is on the floor with him, she cuddles him and holds him close to her until he stops crying. What should the team have known about the child-parent relationship among Hispanic families that could have prevented the cultural misalignment?

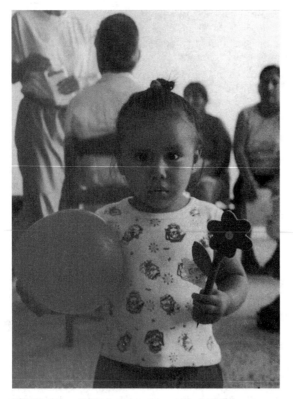

FIGURE 12.7 A Mexican American child at a family gathering.

According to Riojas-Cortez,[41] Mexican American children create stories in dual language during "free play" by applying their cultural background to create complex language experiences during their sociodramatic play. Similar findings were made by Saracho.[42] Many Hispanic girls play with dolls that resemble popular Hispanic TV performers, and boys from Latin America, Central America, and Spain play football/soccer more than they play American football. Riojas-Cortez[41] suggests that children be allowed to use their cultural background to enhance their sociodramatic play rather than being given a sketch to follow. The latter could be accomplished by modifying the environment to impact the child's play behavior.[42] Therefore, physical therapists working with Mexican American children should provide creative "play" opportunities during the intervention. Hispanic children are valued and are often pampered and protected by the adults.[43]

Hispanic parents expect their children to follow orders and tend to be more authoritarian than non-Hispanic whites and blacks. Because *familismo* is the basis for self-importance in the community at large, children are expected to respect their parents' authority and behave well in public, thus representing the family well. If the child acts inappropriately or disrespectfully to others, the child may be corrected or reprimanded verbally or physically, which may expose the parents to scrutiny by child protective services.[43]

Hispanic culture values honor, *respeto* (respect), and the role of elders as authorities.[7] With a very important role in the family, elders are protected and cared for by family members. Professionals are also regarded as authority figures and therefore treated with respect.[22]

Reflective Exercise

• What would be important for a pediatric physical therapist to know about Hispanic family roles and organization? • What would be important for a geriatric physical therapist to know?

Traditions are important in Hispanic communities. Rites of passage such as baptism, *quinceañeras* (sweet 15), weddings, and funerals are celebrated with traditional rituals. A party usually follows baptism. In some families, children may have two sets of godparents. One set of godparents is used for the *bautismo de agua* (baptism of water), when infants are symbolically baptized soon after birth in case they die before they are baptized in the church. The second set of godparents is chosen when the child is baptized in the church. The compadres, or godparents, are expected to be involved in caregiving and rearing of their godchildren. *Quinceañeras* is a common festivity in many Latin American countries. It is considered the young woman's introduction to society and womanhood.[44] The *quinceañera* is celebrated with a mass followed by a party. This custom is celebrated differently in each country.[44] Box 12-1 lists other important holidays celebrated by Hispanics from different countries.

Reflective Exercise

• Have you heard of 5 de Mayo? • Have you heard of 16 de Septiembre as Mexico's Independence Day? • Which would you think is more important to your client from Mexico? • Why?

Social status is considered important to people in many Hispanic families. Families may not like to socialize with other families or individuals they do not consider to be of their social stratum. In

BOX 12-1

PATRIOTIC HOLIDAYS		
5 May	Cinco de Mayo/Battle of Puebla	This holiday commemorates the French invasion of Mexico.
16 September	National Mexican Independence Day	This holiday is more important to Mexicans than Cinco de Mayo.
25 July	Puerto Rico celebrates commonwealth with the United States	
19 November	Discovery of Puerto Rico	
RELIGIOUS CELEBRATIONS		
6 January	Three Kings Day/Epiphany	
1 November	Dia de los Muertos—The day of the dead	
	Viernes Santo—Good Friday	
12 December	Our Lady of Guadalupe	

Other important dates include specific celebrations to commemorate particular religious patron saints in various Latin American countries and, in some cases, the patron saint of the city, and the celebration of the Independence Day of each Latin American country.

many countries, indigenous groups are considered to be of a lower class and are treated as such. They may work as housekeepers, nannies, and other low-paying positions.

Reflective Exercise

• A physical therapist visited the home of a 75-year-old Cuban American woman, Señora Perez, who had suffered a stroke. The physical therapist learned that other family members lived with her. The physical therapist asks Señora Perez to make sure that her children are present during her next visit to learn the exercise program. Señora Perez states that her children cannot possibly attend. The physical therapist finds this hard to believe. She had attended a cultural competency workshop and knows that Hispanic families are interdependent. What assumptions did the physical therapist make? • What other options could she have offered Señora Perez?

Alternative Lifestyles

Divorce among newer immigrants is not common; however, the divorce rate increases with assimilation.[45] Homosexuality is considered taboo for many Hispanics. Because of the concept of *machismo* and the Catholic Church's view of homosexuality as a sin, many gays and lesbians remain closeted to their relatives and co-workers or move away from their families so that they can express their sexuality.

Workforce Issues

Hispanics have experienced a decline in economic status over the past 30 years. Issues such as discrimination, language barriers, and lower educational levels negatively impact employment opportunities. Overall, Hispanics earn less than non-Hispanic whites, more often working in blue-collar and less skilled jobs. Compared with non-Hispanic women, Hispanic women have higher rates of employment in service industries.[46] Cubans represent the highest percentage of professionals among the three larger subgroups of Hispanics. Although one can encounter Hispanics in all areas of the labor force, many Hispanics come to the United States to be migrant workers.

Cubans have the highest income level of all Hispanic subgroups, averaging $39,530 in earnings per year. In comparison, Puerto Ricans average $28,953 and Mexicans $27,883 annually.[5] The unemployment rate among individuals age 16 years and older is 7% for Puerto Ricans and Mexicans and 5% for Cubans. Cubans' economic advantage most likely relates to their reason for migration. Those who migrated to flee Fidel Castro's regime were of the elite class. In addition, these Cuban immigrants received financial assistance due to their status as political refugees.[8]

Acculturation and Autonomy

Hispanics relate better to a cooperative working model than to a competitive model, preferring to work in groups rather than in isolation. They have a more relaxed work ethic than non-Hispanic whites. In business dealings, Hispanics tend to be more casual and prefer to converse about personal issues prior to dealing with "business" issues.[7] Issues such as differences in the concept of time, *familismo,* and cooperation pose potential conflicts in the U.S. workforce.

Punctuality may not be as important to Hispanics as it is to their non-Hispanic white counterparts, and in fact may conflict with the important concept of *personalismo.*[7] A flexible consideration of time allows for more attention to relationships with others and opportunities to establish *confianza* (trust) in one's healthcare provider. Hispanics may prefer to engage in familiar conversations before they discuss medical issues.[7,22] Many Hispanics place more importance on a family event or issue than on punctuality with appointments. A present time orientation, common in Hispanic cultures, contributes to a more relaxed attitude about punctuality. Many live for the moment, and goals are for immediate action. *Mañana* (tomorrow) is a prominent concept among many Hispanics and it should be considered when planning visits; the patient may not perform an exercise program today because there will be another day when conflicting needs are not as great. Another concept of time that may impact the provision of services is the perception of "crisis orientation."[47] Here the client follows the regimen during a crisis, and once the client perceives that the crisis is past, the motivation to attend therapy ends or diminishes.

Reflective Exercise

• How might time orientation and time concepts negatively or positively impact physical therapy programs? • How might a physical therapist deal with challenges related to punctuality and temporality?

Language in the Workplace

Many Hispanics, particularly first-generation and recent immigrants, prefer to speak Spanish when at work. Recently, the Department of Labor reported that the English-only rule could be discriminatory.[48] The inability of many workers to speak English well could cause safety hazards, in particular accidents as a result of not understanding instructions, labels, or safety alerts. Therefore, the physical therapy supervisor should access the U.S. Department of Labor and Occupational Safety and Health Administration (OSHA) to obtain translated information to help in prevention of accidents.

Biocultural Ecology

Skin Color and Biological Variations

With a multiracial heritage, Hispanics' skin coloring varies from white to light olive or dark brown to black. Hair color can also vary from blonde or red to dark brown or black. Hispanic infants frequently have mongolian spots (dark blue-green discoloration) or "birth marks" on the back or the thighs. In individuals with dark eye color, it may be difficult to assess the size of the pupils when testing dilation.

Diseases and Health Conditions

Diseases endemic to Central and South America include Hansen's disease (leprosy), cholera, yellow fever, malaria, ascariasis, and roundworm. Dengue fever and hemorrhagic dengue fever are endemic in the Caribbean and have been found in border towns and in Central America.[49,50] Another condition often seen in migrant workers is tuberculosis.[49–51] Ciguatera is a tropical disease

that affects the neurological system of humans who have eaten infected fish.[49] A physical therapist working with newer immigrants should be alert for symptoms of diseases common in the patient's home country and make referrals as necessary.

With the exception of Cubans, only about 60% of Hispanics initiate prenatal care in the first trimester, and Hispanics are three times less likely than non-Hispanic whites to receive prenatal care at all. Hispanic infants born in the United States are less likely to be breastfed compared with infants born in Latin American countries.[52,53] Babies born to Hispanic women tend to have high birth weights despite socioeconomic disadvantages; however, the longer Hispanic women are in the United States, the greater the risk of giving birth to low-birth-weight babies, resulting in increased morbidity of mothers and infants.[24,52,54] According to the National Institutes of Health, Hispanic women are at risk for osteoporosis, although no statistics exist on the incidence of fracture.[55] Hispanic women also have a higher risk of death associated with pregnancy; however, the causes of death were not clear, other than an increase in pregnancy-induced hypertension.[56]

Common childhood illnesses and diseases among Hispanics include lead poisoning and anencephaly/spina bifida in the southwestern border towns. Spina bifida is more prevalent in Hispanics compared with non-Hispanic whites[57] (Fig. 12-8). Lead poisoning may result from eating out of lead-painted pottery, from living in housing with lead paint, or from drinking folk remedies containing lead. Poisoning due to ingestion of mercury is found among some Mexican children whose parents give them *azogue,* a type of mercury, to treat "empacho" (upset stomach).[35,58]

According to the analysis of the National Longitudinal Mortality Study of 1993, the rate of cancer is lower in Puerto Ricans and Mexican immigrants than in non-Hispanic whites.[59] The most common sites for cancer are the stomach, esophagus, pancreas, and cervix; the least common sites are lungs, bladder, colon, and rectum.[7,60] Although the risk of breast cancer among Hispanics is the same as for non-Hispanic whites, the likelihood of cervical cancer is twice

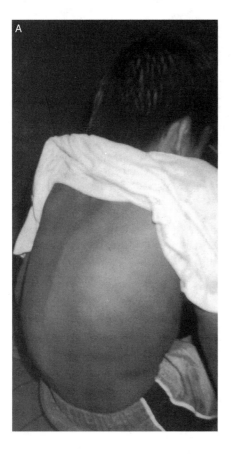

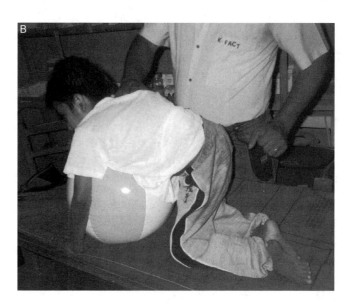

FIGURE 12.8 Child with spina bifida.

that for white women and is associated with a 5-year survival rate, slightly higher than for whites.[55] Death due to stomach cancer is twice as likely for Hispanics as for whites. Skin cancer is most commonly detected in Hispanics on the mucosal areas of the body, under the nails, and on the palms of the hands and soles of the feet.[60] Chronic obstructive pulmonary disease (COPD) is lower in Hispanic immigrants compared with whites and non-immigrant Hispanics.

Heart disease risk is lower in non-Hispanic whites, yet is higher in Mexican American women than in non-Hispanic women.[7,55] Hispanics are more likely to have diabetes and more complications from diabetes than their white counterparts. A positive correlation exists between obesity and hyperinsulinemia and a higher risk of neural tube defects in women along the Texas-Mexico border.[61] Approximately 30% of males and 39% of females of Mexican American descent are overweight.[7] Obesity is also seen in 29% of Cuban males and 34% of Cuban females. Of Puerto Ricans, 25% of males and 37% of females are obese.[7]

Mental illness is considered a stigma and may lead to denial, anxiety, or fear among the Hispanic population.[62–65] Studies on the effect of drugs for the treatment of mental health problems in Hispanics are inconclusive due to the lack of conclusive research data on specific Hispanic subgroups.[63] Drug interactions must be carefully monitored in work with this population because many use herbal remedies and over-the-counter medications, which may interfere with prescription medicines. Always ask clients if they are taking over-the-counter medicines, herbs, or teas.

High–Risk Behaviors

Among Hispanics, the more common high-risk health behaviors are illicit drug use, HIV/AIDS, alcoholism, and teenage pregnancy. The drug of choice for many men is alcohol, followed by cocaine. Women use marijuana. The longer Hispanics are in the United States, the greater their risk of using recreational drugs. Puerto Rican women have a greater incidence of drug problems than other Hispanic subgroups. Hispanic youth have a preference for inhalants.[7]

Alcoholism and cirrhosis are prevalent among Hispanics, particularly Mexican Americans and Puerto Ricans. Mexican-born men have a 40% higher risk of death due to cirrhosis than their European American counterparts. Deaths due to violence account for higher mortality rates among male adolescents and young adults of Mexican Americans, Puerto Ricans, and Cuban Americans than among the white subpopulation.[7,66]

HIV/AIDS is more common in men than in women. Puerto Ricans have a high incidence of HIV/AIDS compared with other subgroups.[7,66] Hispanic women are five times more likely to die from AIDS than white non-Hispanics; this is probably due to the lack of early intervention and treatment and the aversion to using condoms. Reasons for not using condoms include the following: (a) Condoms are not accepted by the Catholic Church because they promote promiscuity and are an unnatural method of birth control. (b) Men may not like to use condoms because they feel that they decrease their satisfaction. (c) Women may not like men to use condoms, believing it implies that they are infected with a venereal disease.[67] Because sex is a taboo topic, many women and men are embarrassed to discuss sexuality with healthcare professionals in order to clarify misconceptions about sexually transmitted diseases.[7] Moreover, the concept of *machismo* may encourage males to be more aggressive and pursue numerous sexual encounters; likewise, some women may have been conditioned to acquiesce.[67] Teenage pregnancy rates are higher in native-born Hispanics than in immigrants.[7]

In recent years, cigarette smoking has increased among women.[7,66] Cigarette smoking among Hispanics plays a part in their risk for cardiovascular disease.[7] Men who are less acculturated have higher smoking rates, whereas women who are more acculturated are more likely to smoke than their non-acculturated counterparts.[66]

National survey data show that 65% of Mexican American men and 74% of Mexican American women engage in little or no leisure activity.[68] In a study of health-promoting lifestyle behaviors of Spanish-speaking Hispanic adults, physical activity received the lowest rating.[69]

Juarbe, Lipson, and Turok[70] interviewed 51 married Mexican American women regarding their physical activity beliefs and behaviors. Seventy-eight percent were not involved in regular physical fitness despite the fact that 93% acknowledged its benefits in health promotion. Reasons given for not exercising were rooted in the cultural beliefs and values of spouses and family. For instance, 89% of the women mentioned that their husbands and/or other family members discourage them from exercising to avoid harming the woman's reproductive health. Moreover, some family members and spouses convey the notion that exercise is not for women or that exercise leads to a physical image incongruent with motherhood. Other reasons given included concerns regarding safety in the community, proximity to a place of exercise, cost of the exercise facility, and lack of personal knowledge. A number of women reported that they had not engaged in an exercise program due to many consecutive pregnancies, which also accounted for significant weight gain.

Reflective Exercise

• How might a physical therapist introduce and encourage physical activity to a client in a culturally appropriate manner? • What considerations must he or she make?

Hispanic children are less physically active than non-Hispanic whites.[71] Children prefer nonstructured games. How long the family has been in the United States determines whether they play football or soccer (also known as football outside the United States). Hispanic adults walk less and engage in less vigorous activities than European Americans.[7,72,73]

Nutrition

Meaning of Food, Common Foods, and Food Rituals

For Hispanics, food is the center of formal and informal socialization and helps celebrate births, baptisms, weddings, and funerals. Food is typically offered when one visits a home; to refuse the offer is impolite. Food also contributes to improved health and wellness.

Although commonalities exist in food choices across Hispanic groups, preparation differs depending on the availability of products, ancestral background, and customs as well as the topography (mountainous, farmland, seashore) of their country of origin. For example, Mexicans and Mexican Americans consume more corn products.[74] Puerto Ricans consume more pork[75] while Argentineans and Chileans generally prefer red meat.[76] Horse meat, iguana, calamari, oysters, and other types of seafood are staples among some Hispanic groups, depending on the country of origin.

Deficiencies and Limitations

Overall, the Hispanic diet is rich in complex carbohydrates such as corn, rice, bread, beans, and root plants. Due to the abundance of fresh fruits in Latin America, many eat mangos, papayas, guavas, citreous, avocados, plantains, and bananas regularly. In contrast, many Hispanic diets are low in vegetables. Studies show that as Hispanic immigrants acculturate to the U.S. diet, they tend to develop high cholesterol.[7]

Foods for Health Promotion

Many Hispanics use a variety of foods to enhance health, believing in the theory of "hot" and "cold" food classifications to maintain the balance between health and illness.[19,49,77] Many do not eat certain foods during pregnancy or menstruation. Chamomile (*manzanilla*) is used to treat colic and to relieve menstrual cramps. Cinnamon (canela) is used to stop vomiting, to control spasms, and to

treat upper respiratory tract infections.[19,49,77–79] Clove (*clavo*) is given for toothaches and teething pain.[78]

Cumin (*comino*) is commonly used for diarrhea and ginger (*jengibre*) for vomiting and *empacho* (upset stomach). Other fruits and herbs used are lemon/lime, tangelo, sábila, catsclaw, garlic, grapefruit, salvia, plantain, and mangrove.[30,31,49,77] Box 12-2 lists other common herbal remedies.

Death Rituals

Most Hispanics show emotion during funerals and observe a longer grieving period than is the U.S. custom.[29,79] They also expect others to acknowledge their grief. Funeral services vary among subgroups and according to acculturation status. Many will have a wake (*velorio*) and will wait for the family to come from other states. Many take the body back to their birthplace.[29] Dressing in black or dark colors for as long as a year after the passing is common.

Pregnancy and the Childbearing Family

Fertility Practices and Views toward Pregnancy

Birth rates among Hispanics are higher than in non-Hispanic groups. There are also differences among Hispanic subgroups. Religious beliefs have an impact on the fertility practices of many Hispanic women; however, many Hispanic women use contraceptives or sterilization, and may also get abortions.

Because pregnancy is associated with good health and well-being, many Hispanic women do not see the need for prenatal care. Some women may associate taking medications while pregnant with increased risk of a birth defect. Because weight gain is considered healthy, many women gain more weight than is advised during pregnancy. The "Mexican paradox" is documented in the literature. Hispanic infants, with the exception of Puerto Rican infants,[7,29,66,80] are healthier than other minority infants despite their lack of prenatal care and lower economic status. The longer the mother lives in the United States, however, the worse the outcome. This paradox is attributed to the close attention and care given

BOX 12.2

Common Herbal Remedies

Anise—antispasmodic

Agua maravilla (wonder water)—a witch hazel (*Hamamelis virginiana*) compound; often added to a mixture containing juice of the aloe vera leaf, honey, cod liver oil, egg white, garlic, and onion; ingested for asthma and upper respiratory tract infection (URTI)

Alcanfor (camphor rub)

Castor oil (*Ricinus comminis*)—asthma, URTI

Chamomile (manzanilla)—colic

Cinnamon (canela)—vomiting, antispasmodic, URTI

Clove oil (clavo)—toothache, teething

Cumin (comino)—diarrhea

Eucalyptus (eucalipto)—URTI, asthma

Ginger (jengibre)—vomiting, empacho

Lemon (plant leaves or fruit) (limon)—asthma, URTI, antispasmodic

Spearmint ("hierba buena" or "yerba buena")—antispasmodic

Tangelo (naranja)—antispasmodic, empacho

Seven syrups (siete jarabes)

Maguey syrup (jarabe maguey)

Sweet almond oil (*Prunus amygdalus*)

Tolu (*Myroxylon balsamum*)—asthma, URTI

Wild cherry (*Prunus serotina*)—asthma, URTI

Licorice (*Glycyrrhiza glabra*), cocillana (*Guarea rusbyi*), and honey

Other remedies and spiritual/religious beliefs:

Vicks VapoRub and alcanfor (camphor rubs)—rubbing ointments

Bracelet with azabache (black stone)

Eyes of Saint Lucia (*Ojos de Santa Lucia*)—eye diseases

God's hand (Mano de Dios)—for protection

Olive oil—ear infection (placed on cotton directly into the ear)

Garlic clove—ear infection, colic

Guava—teething

Adapted from Autotte (1995),[83] De Stefano (2002),[78] and Purnell (1999, 2000).[30,31]

the mother and the newborn from their mothers and or other women in the Hispanic family.[24,80]

Puerto Ricans experience a higher infant mortality rate compared with other Hispanic groups, and the longer the mother lives on the mainland, the worse the potential outcomes. Newborn infants of Central and South American mothers have a higher survival rate than Puerto Rican infants.[81,82]

Prescriptive practices during pregnancy include restrictions on certain foods (varies by subgroup), special baths, and massages by *sobadoras*. Exercise is perceived as dangerous to the baby and is therefore discouraged during the pregnancy as well as immediately postpartum, when the woman is still weak from the delivery (Fig. 12-9). Some women may carry a safety pin or other metal object on the abdomen to prevent the baby's early arrival. Others do not go out during a full moon or an eclipse because it may cause deformities. Others satisfy cravings during the pregnancy and have *antojos* (cravings) for food or other substances. Some Puerto Rican women do not eat crab during pregnancy because it may cause the child to be born with very curly hair. Many women believe that the shape of the

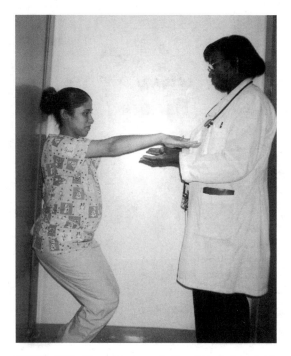

FIGURE 12.9 Exercise is generally thought to be beneficial during pregnancy, but in Hispanic culture exercise is sometimes discouraged during pregnancy.

abdomen can determine the sex of the child. Women may refrain from sexual intercourse during their pregnancy, as they believe it may cause an abortion or premature delivery; however, if the delivery is expected to be post-term, they may have intercourse to accelerate the delivery.

The theory of "hot and cold" carries over to pregnancy. The classification of diseases and illnesses as "hot" or "cold" is based on the belief that the body needs to be in harmony between hot and cold forces and environments.[83–86] Pregnant women are considered to be in a "hot" state and therefore need warm or cold food to maintain the balance.

Birthing and Postpartum Practices
As in many other groups, some women prefer to deliver at home with a *partera* (midwife) while others prefer the hospital. Fathers do not usually participate in the labor and delivery, as it is considered a "woman's activity." Many may not feel comfortable participating if asked.[27,75,79]

After the delivery, the baby may sleep in the same bed or the same room with the parents for up to 2 years. A belt made of soft cotton is wrapped abound the infant's umbilicus to prevent hernias. Some mothers add a coin or key to maintain pressure on the umbilicus. An herbal medication may be applied around the umbilical stump to keep it "clean."

Many women participate in *cuarentena*, a 40-day postpartum lying-in period. During his time, women are not supposed to do hard work, do heavy lifting, wash their hair, or take showers or sitz baths. They are permitted, however, to take sponge baths and to wash their hair with a wet towel. After delivery, the mother traditionally receives help from her mother, sisters, or *comadre*.

Spirituality

Religious Practices and Use of Prayer
The majority of the Hispanics self-identify as Catholic.[23] Other religions common among this group are Protestantism, Santeria/*Espiritismo*,[87] shamanism, Judaism, Buddhism, and Islam. Many believe that illnesses are due to God's will and that fate controls life and health. Spirituality and religiosity can be manifested by a fatalistic feeling in which individuals are seen as having little control over their health and lives, or by an optimistic belief that divine trust can conquer any possible adverse events.[23,87,88]

The Meaning of Life and Individual Sources of Strength
In studies on Mexican American,[69] Panamanian, and Guatemalan[30,31] mothers' health beliefs and values, the authors found spirituality and belief in God as a primary source of strength. In another study the researchers found that Mexican American women relied heavily on prayer to God, the Virgin of Guadalupe, or St. Francis to maintain peace and physical and emotional strength.[25] Family and church are a great source of strength for Hispanics[88] (Fig. 12-10).

Many Hispanics do not have life directives, believing that God will determine one's time to die and that one should not make that decision on one's own.[89] Likewise, most Hispanics

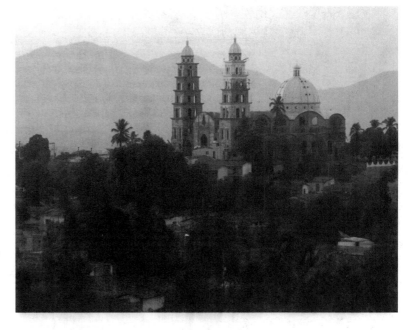

FIGURE 12.10 Churches are an important aspect of Hispanic culture. Many small towns in Central and South America boast grand Catholic cathedrals that dwarf the local residences.

believe they possess a soul and a spirit and must tend to their spiritual needs, particularly in times of physical infirmities and needs.[23,88] Indeed, Mendelson[25] found that perceptions of health among Mexican American women were grounded in spiritual or soul-related issues.

Healthcare Practices

Focus of Healthcare
Although health beliefs vary among individuals and Hispanic subgroups, most believe that illnesses and disabilities are God's will or a gift from God. Common phrases are *"pobrecito"* (poor thing) or *"Ay bendito"* (Oh, blessed) when a person is ill.[75] Children with illnesses or disabilities are "angels protected by God" and should be loved and cherished in this life (Fig. 12-11).

When illness occurs, it may be seen from a fatalistic viewpoint: *"Que sea lo que Dios quiera"* (Let it be what God wants) or *"Si Dios quiere"* (If God wills). As a result, many may not seek immediate medical care. In the case of children with disabilities, the parents may not consent to surgery if they feel the child is going to "suffer" more as a result of the intervention. On the other hand, if

an adult has a terminal illness, he or she may encourage the medical team to intervene as much as possible, including total resuscitation if necessary.[89] The concept of *conformismo*,[7] to accept the situation as it is, is part of the belief system of many Hispanics. Thus, some may have difficulty challenging medical authorities or fighting an illness or disability.

Familismo, familism, is a concept that includes providing material and emotional support to family members. Hispanics value a healthcare system that turns to the family for help and support in solving problems and making decisions. The healthcare provider should consult with family members for informed consent, intubation and extubation, and end-of-life decisions.

Reflective Exercise

• How might the physical therapist work with someone who embraces the concept of conformismo?

Traditional Practices
Hispanic folk medicine is derived from the ancient Greek belief that illnesses arise from dis-

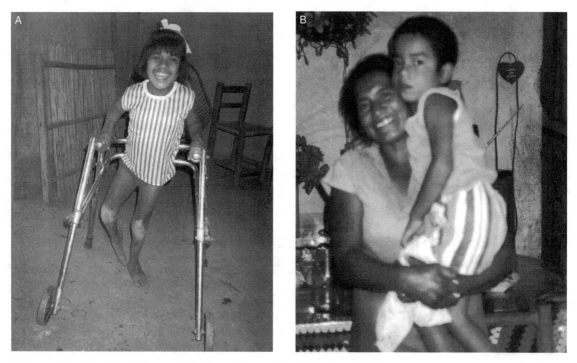

FIGURE 12.11 (*A*) A child with a disability. (*B*) A mother and her child with a disability.

harmony between the hot and cold forces of nature.[83-86,90] Exposure to excessive changes in temperature can cause illness; therefore, one must avoid extremes of hot or cold. Low metabolic diseases are cold diseases, while hot diseases are high metabolic. Cold diseases and conditions include menstrual cramps, "*frio de la matriz*" (cold of the cervix), and colic. *Fatiga* (fatigue) and asthma are also considered cold diseases. Hot diseases and conditions are *susto* (magical fright/stress, fright-induced illness),[91] diabetes, hypertension, and pregnancy. Hot diseases are treated with cold remedies and cold diseases are treated with hot remedies in order to restore the balance.

Other common folk illnesses include "*caida de la mollera*," or fallen fontanelle of infants, usually associated with infant dehydration. *Empacho*, or constipation or "ate too much," may occur if a child swallows saliva during teething, or when a parent changes the baby formula or changes from formula to regular milk. The belief is that the different formulas or the formula and milk mix and produce a *pelota*, or ball of material, that sticks to the walls of the stomach.[85] *Mal de ojo* or "evil eye" is a spell cast as a result of someone looking at an infant and complimenting the child without physically touching the child[90] (see Fig. 4-9). *Susto* (fright) is described as the experience of the spirit leaving the body as a result of a traumatic event and is associated with panic attacks and panic disorders.[64,91] *Ataque de nervios* (attack of the nerves) occurs when a person is not able to deal with stress.[29,58,79]

Families may treat the folk conditions in more than one way. Some may do *promesas* (promises), let the hair grow long, dress the child or oneself in robes or white clothes, kneel-walk to church, or offer extra tidings to a specific church. Others use amulets such as *Ojos de Santa Lucia*, or Saint Lucy's eyes (to care for eye diseases), or *mano de azabache*, a small, black hand carried by newborn infants for good luck and to keep them healthy.[92,93]

Household remedies used by many Hispanics include teas made from various tree leaves (chamomile, mint, lemon, tangelo, and ginger), *santigüos* by masajistas (massage blessings), *alba-yarde* (contains lead), *siete jarabes* (seven syrups), and *el huevo* (the egg) treatment, where an egg is rubbed against the body of a child with a fever and is then placed under the bed. If in the morning the egg is deemed to be cooked, the child is healed. Others use mercury, called *azogue,* for santeria purposes; used as an amulet, it speeds magical spells, although the users may not know the negative effects.[29,58,79]

Reflective Exercise

• A therapist visited a patient at home. Upon arriving at the house he noticed a bucket of water with leaves; the floor was recently mopped. The mother noticed that the therapist appeared to be uncomfortable and explained that she had washed the house to get rid of the "evil eyes." What should the therapist do in the initial assessment of this patient? • How does the therapist deal with this issue? • What should the therapist do with this information?

Rehabilitation and Chronicity

Many Hispanics believe that a disability can occur because of a past transgression or can be inherited. Some believe a disability is due to the mother's rejection of a pregnancy, lack of faith in God, an eclipse, a spell on the mother, the mother making fun of a person with a disability, or the type of job the mother had.[30,31,78,85] Individuals with disabilities are often considered a "gift from God," or the disability is "God's will."[34,94] In either case, families may overprotect (by Western standards) the person with a disability (Fig. 12-12). Bailey and colleagues[94] found that mothers denied a child's disability and took extra effort in raising the child. Mothers interviewed in the study also described themselves as extraordinary because of their ability and the sacrifices they made to raise a child with a disability. They referred to their children as special children and "angels."[94]

In many cases, children with disabilities are regarded as "normal" because they were not born

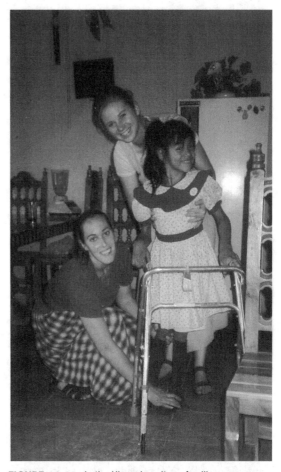

FIGURE 12.12 In the Hispanic culture, families may overprotect children with disabilities, which might prevent them from improving and becoming more independent.

sick or "crazy" and are able to attend to activities of daily living.[94,95] Few studies describe beliefs regarding rehabilitation among Hispanics, but the literature does find that the nuclear family, extended family, neighbors, and friends are an important component in caring for people with disabilities. Group support decreased the sense of isolation and stigmatization and promoted acceptance.[92,96,97]

Elderly Hispanics do not use skilled nursing facilities as often as do non-Hispanic whites. Familism, preference for traditional remedies, lack of insurance, lack of knowledge about skilled nursing facilities, and concerns about discrimination are among the reasons given by Mexican American elderly and their families for not seeking skilled nursing facilities.[98]

Familismo often factors into a rehabilitation program when the physical therapist is trying to teach the client to perform independently, and the family in attendance repeatedly tries to do everything for their loved one. This is a clash between the values of independence and autonomy promoted by the physical therapist and the interdependent, supportive role mandated by *familismo.*

Reflective Exercise

• How might a physical therapist best handle the situation where the client's family desires to help in ways that interfere with the client's independence?
• How might the situation be handled in a culturally sensitive manner?

Barriers

Hispanics in the United States face many barriers to accessing healthcare. Lack of insurance, language barriers, cultural differences, and lack of transportation are just a few.[5,43] Many Hispanic immigrants are not covered by health insurance and do not know about available healthcare services. Most are not used to health maintenance organizations (HMOs), and some believe that health insurance is only for the rich.[99] Additional barriers include (a) fear of deportation if they go to see a healthcare provider, (b) distance to the closest healthcare facility, (c) preference for a *curandero,* and (d) sharing medications and herbal remedies with relatives.[43,100] If primary interventions fail and the condition worsens, clients often go to the hospital emergency room.[32] The inability to access healthcare and to understand prescriptions, appointment schedules, and home programs causes anxiety and stress for many. Barriers to healthcare may hinder adherence to therapy either at home or at a clinic.[47]

Many Hispanics practice traditional medicine along with allopathic medicine. One's level of acculturation, level of education, and socioeconomic status determine the intensity of this duality. Although many Hispanics practice traditional medicine, studies suggest that Hispanics tend to trust the Western medical system.[84]

Pain and the Sick Role

To most Hispanics, pain is accepted as part of life, a fate that one is obligated to endure as a human duty.[101] Pain accepted without complaint is a sign of courage and strength. Pain may also signify immoral behavior, a punishment from God. Finally, pain represents disharmony between the person and the environment and, therefore, must be managed in order to restore balance.[101] When Hispanics describe pain, they do so with emotional terms that may not be easy to quantify, such as *terrible, doloroso,* or *fatal.*[101] Because of *machismo,* some males may exhibit a high tolerance for pain and not complain.[102] Studies have shown that Hispanics are less likely to receive pain medication or to have their pain acknowledged by medical staff than are white ethnic groups.[33,103]

Healthcare Practitioners

In general, Hispanic clients appreciate kindness, respect, and a positive attitude from their healthcare providers. A very serious and distant healthcare provider may be perceived as uncaring, and the client might view the provider with distrust. Lack of trust may mean that the client will not give complete, accurate information or may not follow through with the recommended program.

Personalismo, or professional friendship, is an important quality expected from healthcare workers. In addition, physicians and other healthcare personnel are treated with a higher level of authority and respect; they are not to be questioned. Patients expect healthcare workers to be "friendly" and ask questions not necessarily associated with the illness. However, if the healthcare provider is too friendly or asks too many personal questions, the patient may interpret this as lack of knowledge. Many Hispanic patients may not feel comfortable answering personal, intimate questions put to them by a member of the opposite sex.

Many Hispanics visit *curanderos* (folk healers), *masajistas* (masseuses), *hierberos* (herbalists), or *sobadores* (faith healer masseuses) to treat illnesses. Mexican Americans also practice "cupping." Cupping consists of placing a heated glass or cup onto the skin; as it cools it creates negative pressure, and this produces an area of ecchymosis when the cup is pulled from the skin.[93] *Curanderismo* is a folk healing method based on the belief that disease is caused by bad forces beyond one's control and that disruption in the peace of the soul causes illness. *Curanderismo* includes the use of herbs, diet, massage, prayer, and rituals.[92,93]

Reflective Exercise

• A 10-year-old boy is having physical therapy for rehabilitation after a torn anterior cruciate ligament. The parents were reluctant to bring the child more than once a week. The mother felt that he could be treated at home with a *sobo* (massage) once the grandmother arrived from Puerto Rico. Both parents were born in Puerto Rico but came to New York as children. How should the therapist address *sobo*?
• Should the therapist determine if there is someone else in the community who can perform the same skill and ask the family if they can bring that person?
• Should the therapist tell the family the *sobo* will not do anything for the child? • Of what issues about *sobo* should the therapist be aware?

Gender and Healthcare

Many Hispanic women prefer to be treated by another woman, whereas some men may see women professionals as less knowledgeable and prefer a male practitioner. These characteristics are not necessarily seen among younger generations and more acculturated individuals. Because healthcare providers are seen as authority figures, they are treated with respect and their authority not questioned. Older people may also have difficulty receiving care from younger professionals because they may be considered "too young to have any wisdom."[29]

Conclusion

In summary, Hispanics are a heterogeneous group with many similarities, yet many differences. Each client must be seen within the context of his or her circumstances, his or her family, and his or her subgroup. Acculturation, level of education, socioeconomic status, and country of origin must be considered in working with Hispanic clients.

CASE STUDY SCENARIO

A 56-year-old Panamanian, Mr. Rivera, is referred to physical therapy after an amputation secondary to type II diabetes mellitus. The patient seems depressed and does not want to comply with the physical therapist's requests because he will no longer be able to provide for his family. The patient lives 50 miles from the treatment center, and the family is not able to come every day to see him. The therapist makes arrangements through the social worker for visits. The wife, children, and *compadres* come to see the patient, bringing him a medication from the local *curandero*. He asks his wife to show the therapist how to use the medication, which consists of lotion (composed of medicinal plants). The therapist did not believe there would be any negative effects and told the patient to use the lotion prior to bandaging the amputation site. The patient seemed pleased and asked the therapist to show his family how to perform the exercise program. Next, through interviewing the family, the therapist found that Mr. Rivera could work at his *compadre*'s grocery store because he would no longer be able to do farm work. The therapist showed the family different activities that Mr. Rivera could do while working at the grocery store to prevent him from having problems with the amputation and uninvolved leg. Mr. Rivera felt that he could now go home with his family, and help as much as he could.

(continued)

1. What should the physical therapist have done when the patient asked him to learn to use the lotion? Should he have used it?

2. What impact does the family/*compadres* have?

3. How could the rehabilitation goals be accomplished in the environment to which Mr. Rivera was to return?

4. How did the family see Mr. Rivera's ability to function?

5. What nontraditional and spirituality arenas should the therapist explore to improve the quality of life for this patient?

WEBSITES

http://cdc.gov/ncns	National Center for Health Statistics
http://hispanichealth.org	National Alliance for Hispanic Health
http://dhhs.gov	Department of Health and Human Services
http://oas.org	Organization of American States—health statistics of Central and South American countries and Caribbean islands
http://census.gov	U.S.Bureau of the Census
http://www.dol.gov	Department of Labor—has a section of publications written in Spanish or specifically for migrant workers

In addition, the Minority and International Affairs Department of APTA has a large reference list of Websites, videos, and organizations.

REFERENCES

1. US Bureau of the Census. Race and ethnicity classification. Available at: http://www.census.gov/population/www/documentation/twp17contents.html. Accessed June 2, 2004.

2. US Bureau of the Census. Coming from the Americas: A profile of the nation's foreign-born population from Latin America. Available at: http://www.census.gov/prod/2002pubs/cenbr01–3.pdf. Accessed June 2, 2004.

3. Amaro H, Zambrana R. Criollo, Mestizo, Mulato, Latinegro, Indigena, White, or Black? The US Hispanic/Latino population and multiple responses in the 2000 census. *Am J Public Health*. 2000;90: 1724–1727.

4. Grieco EM, Cassidy RC. Overview of race and Hispanic origin, Census 2000 brief, United States Department of Commerce, Census Bureau. Available at: www.census.gov/population/www/socdemo/race/html. Accessed June 2, 2004.

5. Ramirez RR, de la Cruz GP. *The Hispanic Population in the United States: March 2002, Current Population Reports, P20–245*. Washington, DC: US Bureau of the Census; 2002.

6. Korzeniewicz RP, Smith WC. Poverty, inequality and growth in Latin America: Searching for the high road of globalization. *Latin Am Res Rev*. 2000;35:7–54.

7. Duran DG, Pacheco G, eds. *Quality Health Services for Hispanics: The Cultural Competency Component*. Washington, DC: Department of Health and Human Services, Health Resources and Services Administration Bureau of Primary Health Care Office of Minority Health. Substance Abuse and Mental Health Services Administration; 2000. DHHS publication 99–21.

8. Portes A, Truelove C. Making sense of diversity: Recent research of minorities in the United States. *Annu Rev Sociol*. 1987;13:359–385.

9. Queralt M. Understanding Cuban immigrants: A cultural perspective. In: *National Association of Social Workers*:115–121. Available at: http://cirrie.buffalo.edu/cuba.html. Accessed June 2, 2004.

10. Scarano FA. La política y cultura en dos frentes. In: *Puerto Rico: Cinco Siglos de Historia*. Columbus, Ohio: McGraw–Hill; 1993.

11. Oropesa RS, Landale NS. From austerity to prosperity? Migration and child poverty among mainland and island Puerto Ricans: Demography. Available at: http://athens.pop.psu.edu/allen/prmihs-bib.cfm. Accessed June 2, 2004.
12. Therien M, Ramirez R. *The Hispanic Population in the United States: Current Population Reports, P20–535.* Washington, DC: US Bureau of the Census; 2000.
13. Day J, Newberger E. Educational attainment. Available at: http://www.census.gov/prod/2002pubs/p23–210.pdf. Accessed June 2, 2004.
14. Griggs SL, Dunn R. Hispanic-American students and learning styles. Available at: http://www.ericfacility.net/databases/ERIC_Digests/ed393607.html. Accessed June 2, 2004.
15. Creason P. Changing demographics and the importance of culture in student learning styles. Available at: http://www.newschool.edu/milano/cdrc/pubs/r.2002.4b.pdf. Accessed June 2, 2004.
16. Norman KI, Keating JF. Barriers for Hispanics and American Indians entering science and mathematics: Cultural dilemmas. Available at: www.ed.psu.edu/ci/Journals/97pap22.htm. Accessed August 17, 2003.
17. Ethnologue. Languages of Spain. Available at: http://www.ethnologue.com/show_country.asp?name=Spain. Accessed June 2, 2004.
18. Instituto Nacional Indigenista. Plan Nacional de Desarrollo, 2001–2006, Foros de Consulta Ciudadana a los Pueblos Indígenas de México, Memoria INI. Available at: http://www.unilini.gob.mx/. Accessed June 2, 2003.
19. Flores G, Abreu M, Schwartz I, Hill M. The importance of language in pediatric care: Case studies from the Latino community. *J Pediatr.* 2000;137:842–848.
20. Office of Minority Health. Latino/Hispanic culture & health, Rhode Island Department of Health. Available at: www.healthri.org/chicc/minority/lat_cul.htm. Accessed August 25, 2003.
21. Burk ME, Wieser PC, Keegan L. Cultural beliefs and health behaviors of pregnant Mexican-American women: Implications for primary care. *Adv Nurs Sci.* 1994;17:37–52.
22. Galant GA. The Hispanic family and male-female relationships: An overview. *J Transcult Nurs.* 2003;14:180–185.
23. Castex GM. Providing services to Hispanic/Latino populations: Profiles in diversity. *Soc Work.* 1994;39:288–296.
24. Lagana K. Come bien, camina y no se preocupe—Eat right, walk, and do not worry: Selective biculturalism during pregnancy in a Mexican American community. *J Transcult Nurs.* 2003;14:117–124.
25. Mendelson C. Health perceptions of Mexican American workers. *J Transcult Nurs.* 2002;13:210–217.
26. Martinez I. The elder in the Cuban American family: Making senses of the real and ideal. *J Comp Fam Stud.* 2002;33:359–379.
27. Zsembik BA, Bonilla Z. Eldercare and the changing family in Puerto Rico. *J Fam Issues.* 2000;5:652–674.
28. De Vos S, Arias E. A note on the living of elders 1970–2000, with special emphasis on Hispanic subgroup differentials. *Popul Res Policy Rev.* 2003;22:91–101.
29. Zoucha R, Purnell L. People of Mexican heritage. In: Purnell L, Paulanka B, eds. *Transcultural Health Care: A Culturally Competent Approach.* 2nd ed. Philadelphia, Pa: FA Davis; 2003:264–278.
30. Purnell L. Panamanians' practices for health promotion and the meaning of respect afforded them by healthcare providers. *J Transcult Nurs.* 1999;10:333–340.
31. Purnell L. Guatemalans' practices for health promotion and wellness and the meaning of respect afforded them by healthcare providers. *J Transcult Nurs.* 2000;11:40–46.
32. Derose KP. Networks of care: How Latina immigrants find their way to and through a county hospital. *J Immigr Health.* 2000;2:79–87.
33. Berger JT. Culture and ethnicity in clinical care. *Arch Intern Med.* 1998;158:2085–2086.
34. Salas-Provance MB, Erickson JG, Reed J. Disabilities as viewed by four generations of one Hispanic family. *Am J Speech Lang Pathol.* 2002;11:151–162.
35. Zambrana RE, Greenberg R, Weitzman M. The health of Latino children: Urgent priorities, unanswered questions, and a research agenda. *JAMA.* 2002;288:82–90.
36. Coll C, Sepkoski C, Lester BM. Differences in the Brazelton Scale performance between Puerto Rican and mainland white and black newborns. In: Lester BM, *A panorama of uses and misuses of the Brazelton Neonatal Behavioral Assessment Scale.* Symposium presented at the meeting of the Society for Child Development; March 1977; New Orleans, La.
37. Gannotti M, Cruz C. Content and construct validity of a Spanish translation of the Pediatric Evaluation of Disability Inventory for children living in Puerto Rico. *Phys Occup Ther Pediatr.* 2001;20:7–24.
38. Gannotti ME, Handwerker WP, Groce NE, Cruz C. Sociocultural influences on disability status in Puerto Rican children. *Phys Ther.* 2001;81:2093–2015.
39. Kolobe THA. Childbearing practices and developmental expectations for Mexican-American mothers and the developmental status of their infants. *Phys Ther.* 2004;8:439–453.
40. Gaskins S. Children's daily lives in a Mayan village: A case study of culturally constructed roles and activities. In: Göncü A, ed. *Children's Engagements in the world: Sociocultural Perspectives.* Cambridge, UK: Cambridge University Press; 1999:25–61.
41. Riojas-Cortez M. Mexican-American preschoolers create stories: Socio-dramatic play in a dual language. *Bilingual Res J.* 2000;24:295–309.
42. Saracho ON. Cognitive style and social behavior in young Mexican American children. *Int J Early Child.* 1991;23:21–38.

43. Flores G, Fuentes-Afflick E, Barbot O, et al. Child discipline and physical abuse in immigrant Latino families: Reducing violence and misunderstandings. *J Couns Dev.* 2002;80:31–40.

44. Napolitano V. Becoming a mujercita: Rituals, fiestas, and religious discourse. *J R Anthropol Inst.* 1997;3:279–296.

45. Landale NS, Oropesa RS, Llanes D, Gorman BK. Does Americanization have adverse effects on health? Stress health habits, and infant health outcomes among Puerto Ricans. *Social Forces.* 1999;78:613–641.

46. Council of Economic Advisers for the President's Initiative on Race. Changing America: Indicators of social and economic well-being by race and Hispanic origin. Available at: http://w3.access.gpo.gov/eop/ca/pdfs/dcs.pdf. Accessed June 2, 2004.

47. Antshel KM. Integrating culture as a means of improving treatment adherence in the Latino population. *Psychol Health Med.* 2002;17:435–450.

48. Facts about National Origin Discrimination. Available at: www. eeoc.gov/facts/fs-nator.html. Accessed June 2, 2004.

49. Kemp C. Mexican & Mexican-Americans: Health beliefs & practices. Available at: www.baylor.edu/~Kemp/hispanic_health.htm. Accessed July 20, 2003.

50. White C, Atmar RL. Infections in Hispanic immigrants. *Clin Infect Dis.* 2002;34:1627–1633.

51. Much DH, Martin J, Gegner I. Tuberculosis among Pennsylvania migrant farm workers: Brief report. *J Immigr Health.* 2000;2:115–117.

52. Higgins PG, Learn CD. Health practices of adult Hispanic women—Issues and innovations in nursing practice. *J Adv Nurs.* 1999;29:1105–1112.

53. National Women's Health Information Center. Women of color health data book: Factors affecting the health of women of color, Hispanics. Available at: www.4women.gov/owh/pub/woc/hispanic/htm. Accessed September 17, 2003.

54. Van Hanswijck DJ, Waller G, Stettler N. Ethnicity modifies seasonal variations in birth weight and weight gain. *J Nutr.* 2003;133:1415–1418.

55. National Institutes of Health. Osteoporosis and Related Bone Diseases National Resource Center Fact Sheet: Latino women and osteoporosis. Available at: www.osteo.org. Accessed September 17, 2003.

56. Hopkins FW, MacKay AP, Koonin LM, Berg CJ, Irwin M, Atrash HK. Pregnancy related mortality in Hispanic women in the United States—Part I. *Obstet Gynecol.* 1999;94:747–752.

57. Larry JM, Edmonds LD. Prevalence of spina bifida, at birth—United States, 1983–1990: A comparison of two surveillance systems, surveillance summaries. Available at: www.cdc.gov/mmwr/preview/mmwrhtml/00040954.htm. Accessed August 27, 2003.

58. Riley DM, Newby CA, Leal-Almeraz TO, Thomas VM. Assessing elemental mercury vapor exposure from cultural and religious practices. *Environ Health Perspect.* 2001;109:779–785.

59. Sorlie PD, Backlund E, Johnson N, Rogot E. Mortality by Hispanic status in the United States. *JAMA.* 1993;270:2464–2468.

60. Franz R. Skin cancer update. *Dermatol Nurs.* 2001;3:236.

61. Hendricks KA, Nuno OM, Suarez L, Larsen R. Effects of hyperinsulinemia and obesity on risk of neural tube defects among Mexican-Americans. *Epidemiology.* 2001;12:630–635.

62. Vega WA, Lopez SR. Priority in Latino mental health services research. *Ment Health Serv Res.* 2001;3:189–200.

63. Office of the Surgeon General. Mental health care for Hispanic Americans. Available at: http://www.mental-health.org/cre/ch6_current_status.asp. Accessed December 10, 2003.

64. Lewis-Fernández R, Guarnaccia PJ, Martinez IE, Salmán E, Schmidt A, Liebowitz M. Comparative phenomenology of ataque de nervios, panic attacks and panic disorder. *Cult Med Psychiatr.* 2002;26:199–223.

65. Guarnaccia PJ, Lewis-Fernández R, Rivera Marano, M. Toward a Puerto Rican popular nosology: Nervios and ataque de nervios. *Cult Med Psychiatr.* 2003;27:339–366.

66. Williams DR, Collins C. US socioeconomic and racial differences in health: Patterns and explanations. *Annu Rev Sociol.* 1995;21:349–386.

67. VanOss B. HIV prevention in the Hispanic community: Sex, culture, and empowerment. *J Transcult Nurs.* 2003;14:186–192.

68. Crespo CJ, Keteyian SJ, Heath GW, Sempos CT. Leisure-time physical activity among US adults. *Arch Intern Med.* 1996;156:93–98.

69. Hulme PA, Walker SN, Effle KJ, et al. Health-promoting lifestyle behaviors of Spanish-speaking Hispanic adults. *J Transcult Nurs.* 2003;14:244–254.

70. Juarbe TC, Lipson JG, Turok X. Physical activity beliefs, behaviors, and cardiovascular fitness of Mexican immigrant women. *J Transcult Nurs.* 2003;14:108–116.

71. Simons-Morton BG, McKenzie TJ, Stone E, et al. Physical activity in a multiethnic population of third graders in four states. *Am J Public Health.* 1997;87:45–50.

72. Hayward MD, Heron M. Racial inequality in active life among adult Americans. *Demography.* 1999;36:77–91.

73. Juniu S. The impact of immigration: Leisure experience in the lives of South American immigrants. *J Leisure Res.* 2000;32:358–381.

74. Pareo-Tubbeh LJ, Romero L, Baumgartner RN, Garry PJ, Lindeman RD, Koehlr KM. Comparison of energy and nutrient sources of elderly Hispanics and non-Hispanic whites in New Mexico. *J Am Diet Assn.* 1999;99:572–577.

75. Juarbe T. People of Puerto Rican heritage. In: Purnell L, Paulanka B, eds. *Transcultural Health Care: A Culturally*

Competent Approach. 2nd ed. Philadelphia, Pa: FA Davis; 2003:307–326.

76. Stephenson S. *Understanding Spanish-Speaking South Americans.* Thousand Oaks, Calif: Sage; 2003.

77. Risser AL, Mazur LJ. Use of folk remedies in a Hispanic population. *Arch Pediatr Adolesc Med.* 1995;149:978–981.

78. De Stefano AM. *Hierbas Buenas: La Guia Imprescindible de las Hierbas y Plantas Medicinales Hispanas y Sus Usos Tradicionales.* New York, NY: Random House Español; 2002.

79. Purnell L. People of Cuban heritage. In: Purnell L, Paulanka B, eds. *Transcultural Health Care: A Culturally Competent Approach.* 2nd ed. Philadelphia, Pa: FA Davis; 2003:122–137.

80. Fuentes-Afflick E, Lurie P. Low birth weight and Latino ethnicity: Examining the epidemiologic paradox. *Arch Pediatr Adolesc Med.* 1997;151:665–674.

81. Parker-Frisbie W, Song S. Hispanic pregnancy outcomes: Differentials over time and current risk factors effects. *Pol Stud J.* 2003;33:237.

82. Centers for Disease Control and Prevention. Reproductive Health Information Source, Surveillance and Research Fact Sheet: Increased risk of dying among Hispanic women in the United States. Available at: www.cdc.gov/nccdphp/drh/surv_hispanicswus.htm. Accessed June 2, 2004.

83. Autotte PA. Folk medicine [editorial]. *Arch Pediatr Adoles Med.* 1995;149:949–950.

84. Flores G. Culture and the patient-physician relationship: Achieving cultural competency in health care. *J Pediatr.* 2000;136:14–23.

85. Pachter LM. Culture and clinical care: Folk illness beliefs and behaviors and their implications for health care delivery: Special communication. *JAMA.* 1994;271:690–710.

86. Worsley P. Non-Western medical systems. *Annu Rev Anthropol.* 1982;11:315–348.

87. Moreno-Vega M. Espiritismo in the Puerto Rican community: A new world recreation with the elements of Kongo ancestor worship. *J Black Stud.* 1999;29:325–353.

88. Rehm RS. Religious faith in Mexican-American families dealing with chronic childhood illness. *J Nurs Sch.* 2000;131:33.

89. Romero LJ, Lindeman RD, Koeheler KM, Allen A, Andrew MS. Influence of ethnicity on advance directives and end-of-life decisions. *JAMA.* 1997;277:298–299.

90. Neff N. Folk medicine in southwestern United States. Available at: http://www.rice.edu/projects/Hispanic Health/Courses/mod7/mod7.html. Accessed June 2, 2004.

91. Weller SC, Baer RD, De Alba Gracia JG, et al. Regional variations in Latino descriptions of susto. *Cult Med Psychiatr.* 2002;26:449–472.

92. Harris ML. *Curanderismo and the DSM-IV: Diagnostic and Treatment Implications for the Mexican-American Client.* Julian Zamora Research Institute, Michigan State University; September 1998. Latino Studies Series Occasional Paper 45.

93. Padilla R, Gomez V, Biggerstaff SL, Mehler P. Use of *curanderismo* in public health care systems. *Arch Intern Med.* 2001;161:1336–1341.

94. Bailey DB, Skinner D, Rodriguez P, Gut D, Correa V. Awareness, use, and satisfaction with services for Latino parents of young children with disabilities. *Excep Child.* 1999;65:367–381.

95. Harry B. Making sense of disability: Low income Puerto Rican parents' theories of the problem. *Excep Child.* 1998;59:27–40.

96. Smart J, Smart DW. Cultural issues in rehabilitation of Hispanics. *J Rehabil.* 1992;58:29–38.

97. Smart J, Smart DW. Acculturative stress of Hispanics: Loss and challenge. *J Couns Dev.* 1995;73:390–397.

98. Crist JD. Mexican American elders' use of skilled home care nursing services. *Public Health Nurs.* 2002; 19:366–376.

99. Ross J. Hispanic Americans. *Hosp Health Networks.* 1995;69:65.

100. Harrell J, Carrasquillo O. The Latino disparity in health coverage. *JAMA.* 2003;289:1167.

101. Dubberly W. Helping Hispanic/Latino population home health patients manage their pain. *Home Healthcare Nurs.* 2003;21:174–179.

102. Gilkey DP, Keefe TJ, Hautaluoma JE, Bigelow PL, Sweere JJ. Low-back pain in residential construction carpenters: Hispanic and non-Hispanic chiropractic patient differences. *Top Gen Chiro.* 2002;9:26–27.

103. Bonham VL. Race, ethnicity, and pain treatment: Striving to understand the causes and solutions to the disparities in pain treatment. *J Law Med Ethics.* 2001;29:52.

Chapter 13

Cultural Considerations for American Indian Cultures

- Teresa M. Cochran, PT, DPT, GCS, MA
- Patrick S. Cross, PT, DPT

Thomas Hodgins, a 72-year-old Navajo Indian, lives with his wife, age 70, on the Navajo reservation. He suffered a cerebrovascular accident (CVA) last month and had a complication of pneumonia. He was also diagnosed with non–insulin-dependent diabetes mellitus. While in the hospital, he started a rehabilitation program for aphasia secondary to his CVA and decubitus ulcers on his sacrum and right ankle. He is still unable to use a walker safely without assistance from his wife. His wife has decreased pulmonary capacity resulting from tuberculosis. She is now responsible for caring for her husband as well as taking care of the house and goats. They do not have running water in the house, requiring her to carry water from a nearby well.

American Indians and Alaska Natives (AIANs) make up 0.9% of the U.S. population, representing just over 2 million people.[1] While their population is small in comparison with other ethnic groups, over 500 recognized tribes exist, creating tremendous diversity in languages, histories, worldviews, sociopolitical organizations, religions, and healthcare practices.[2] The term *Native American* includes native Hawaiians, Samoans, and other Pacific Islanders.[3] Recognition of specific tribal identities, such as Navajo, Cherokee, Omaha, and so on, is preferred by most Native communities. Acceptable terminology is a matter of personal choice, varying across tribes and across members within tribes. If doubt exists at the level of the individual, the patient should be asked his or her preference. Even the title American Indian or Native American is controversial. For the purposes of this chapter, the term *American Indian* is used, mainly because it is consistent with the federal designation.

Overview/Heritage

Origins and Residence

The American Indian population approximated 2 million members prior to Columbus's arrival in 1492. Diverse Indian cultures flourished, with agriculture being the dominant occupation. The introduction of diseases such as typhoid, small-pox, measles, and tuberculosis decimated the Indian population, reducing the number to fewer than 200,000 and extinguishing over 200 tribes.[4] Currently, AIANs have approximated their pre-Columbian numbers. Indian political endeavors have been influenced by U.S. federal policy over the past century and are delineated by four major time periods: (a) assimilation and incorporation, 1880–1932; (b) indirect rule, 1933–1945; (c) termination, 1946–1960; and (d) economic development and self-determination, 1961–1990s.[5] The first period was characterized by attempts to acculturate and educate Indians in boarding schools for entry into mainstream society. Later, attempts were made to reorganize traditional Indian leadership groups to facilitate adoption of Western policies and rules. The failure of such attempts resulted in the termination of Indian status through denial of services and removal of Indian tribal designation and land. The fourth period represents the time when individual tribes began to exert control over the distribution of services and programs originally administered by the Bureau of Indian Affairs.[4]

Residence/Economics

Since 1955, the Indian Health Service (IHS), an entity under the jurisdiction of the U.S. Department of Health and Human Services, has coordinated federally mandated health-related services for AIANs. The administration of IHS activities is monitored through 12 regional area offices. The 12 regions are further divided into service areas, composed of counties on and near federal Indian reservations.[6] Approximately 60% of all Indians reside in these service areas.[6] Depending on an area's size and proximity to other service areas, available health resources may include hospitals, health centers, school health centers, or health stations. Health services may be directly administered through IHS departments, tribal programs, or contracts with private entities.[2] The 1975 Indian Self-Determination Act (P.L.93–638) allows tribes to manage health services independently and permits flexibility in addressing specific community needs via networks with other government agencies or nongovernmental partners such as private foundations or academic medical centers.[2]

The U.S. Census identifies 310 federally recognized Indian reservations, 228 Alaska Native villages and regional corporations, and 50 Indian trust lands. Reservations are located in 35 states—half of them in the West, followed by the South, Midwest, and East—and provide opportunities for communities to practice and celebrate tribal customs (Fig. 13-1). Oklahoma is home to 38 distinct tribes.[2] Over half of American Indians reside in large metropolitan areas,[4] having migrated from reservations. Urbanization originated as part of the government's relocation strategy for Indians during the 1950s and 1960s and was later reinforced by economic needs.[7] The historical locations of various tribes across the United States are shown in Figure 13-2.

Today, a generation of urban-dwelling Indians exist who have been distanced from their tribal heritage, having never visited their native reservations, spoken their native language, or listened to their tribal elders.[4] Today, diversity within and among tribes also depends on age, economic resources, rural versus urban residence, and other primary and secondary characteristics of culture as identified in Chapter 1. While it is recom-

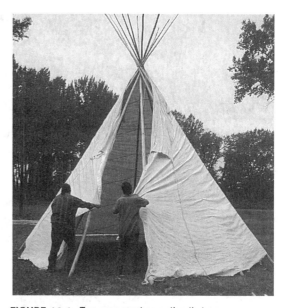

FIGURE 13.1 Two men erect an authentic teepee on a Midwestern reservation. (Photo courtesy of Patrick S. Cross.)

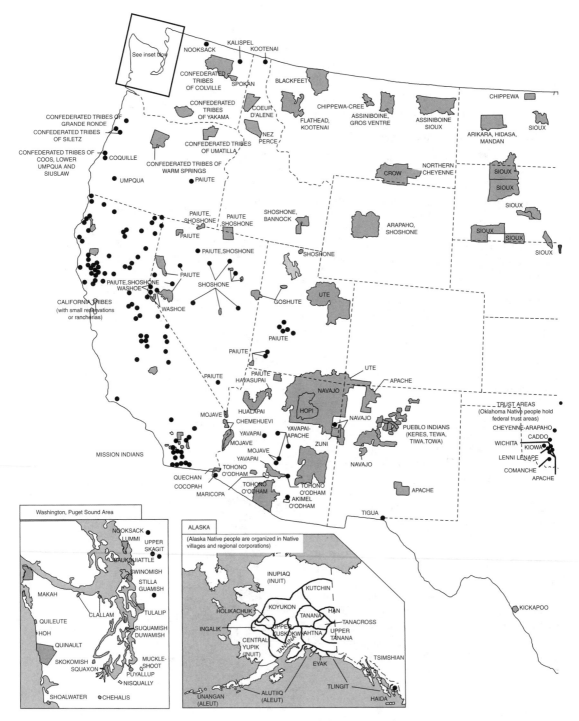

FIGURE 13.2 Map showing U.S. Indian reservations.

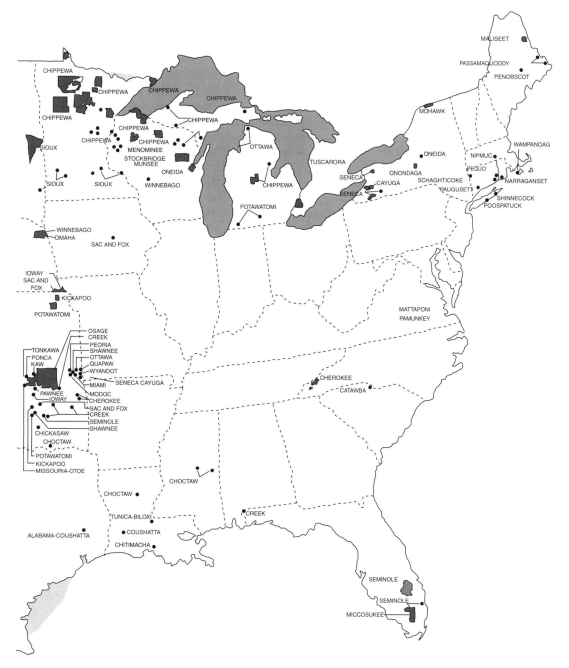

FIGURE 13.2 Continued

241

mended that physical therapists become familiar with specific cultural characteristics of the tribe with which they work, it is almost impossible to become familiar with the range of clinically relevant cultural differences across all tribes.[8] Literature does, however, support several core themes central to many AIAN groups, which are especially apparent among individuals less influenced by acculturation into the dominant society.[9] Insight into cultural characteristics conflicting with Western beliefs is essential for effective cross-cultural healthcare.

Education and Employment

"The American Indian of today can be described as the poorest, least educated, and most neglected minority group in the United States"[4] (pp. 278–279). Only 20% of American Indians age 25 years or older have earned high school diplomas, with 32% of these individuals receiving less than a ninth-grade education. Just 8.9% of Indians (versus 20.3% of the general population) earn baccalaureate degrees.[10] Consistent with lower educational achievement, American Indians are more likely to be unemployed than other groups and experience higher rates of poverty.

Reflective Exercise

• As the physical therapist responsible for Mr. Hodgins's rehabilitation program, what additional services do you envision him and his wife needing? • What role should the Indian Health Service have in his rehabilitation program?

Communication

A contract physical therapist received a referral to evaluate and recommend a restorative care plan secondary to end-stage renal disease for an 82-year-old man, Mr. Bodner, in a tribe-run skilled nursing facility (SNF). Upon review of the client's chart, it was noted that the person could communicate only in his native language and was hard of hearing. Once an interpreter was found (one of the other SNF residents) and consent was given to conduct the evaluation and use the internal interpreter, the evaluation began.

The physical therapist guided the subjective examination, using simple language for the interpreter to translate into the native language. After the first question was asked, the client looked at the door, away from the physical therapist. After a minute went by, there was still no answer, nor had the interpreter asked the question again with the thought that the client did not comprehend or hear the question. Suddenly, the client answered without interrupting his stare at the door, and the communication was translated to the therapist in English. The subjective exam continued in this manner. The physical therapist did not ask the client about awareness of his condition, knowing that speaking of death was a taboo in this culture. The therapist also did not stare at the elder while waiting for an answer, because respect is shown by not interrupting a period of silence.

Following the subjective evaluation, a thorough objective evaluation was conducted. Interpreting how the tests would be performed was very difficult, so the therapist showed what he was going to do through demonstration on the interpreter. Through the interpreter, the therapist was able to explain why certain tests were being performed, after which the client shook his head in approval.

At the end of the session, the therapist used the interpreter to explain his recommendations and gain support for them from the client. The client seemed content with what was being told to him, but no verbal agreement was given. As the therapist was about to leave the room, concluding the evaluation, the elderly client put out his hand to shake the therapist's hand and said, in his native language, "Thank you for helping me and my people."

Dominant Language and Communication Practices

More than 300 Indian languages exist among the tribes in the United States.[7] One out of every 20 AIANs lives in a home where no adult or adolescent speaks English.[11] Although tribes differ in their dominant language, other verbal and nonverbal communications are remarkably similar across tribes.

Traditional American Indian culture is highly contextualized,[12] being more implicit and indirect. The unspoken message may not readily be clear to those unaccustomed to the culture. The principle of noninterference facilitates uncoerced interpersonal interaction, preventing the development of individual dominance in a relationship.[9] The non-Indian physical therapist who is unaware of the behavioral norm of noninterference may find some interactions confusing. Direct questioning and forthright responses are expected by Western health practitioners; however, many AIANs, especially elders, perceive such discourse as aggressive, authoritarian, and in violation of patient dignity.[13]

Reflective Exercise

• What is the recommended method of obtaining an interpreter? • How might the interpretation have been affected if the interpreter was not acceptable to Mr. Bodner in terms of understanding his culture?

Be extremely careful when attempting to use American Indian language because minor variations in pronunciation may change the entire meaning of a word or phrase. Differences in pronunciation, particularly while speaking with an older Navajo, may cause a misunderstanding.

Such misunderstandings make subsequent care for the individual difficult. Using an interpreter is safer and meets federal guidelines. Failing to allow adequate time for information processing may result in an inaccurate response or no response. Allow time for people to respond to questions.

Nonverbal Communication

Most traditional AIANs do not maintain steady eye contact when conversing; rather, they exhibit peripheral gaze or engage in eye contact for very brief periods of time.[14] Diversion of gaze is considered respectful, especially with elders, for whom sustained direct eye contact may be perceived as impolite or even threatening.[15] The degree of acculturation contributes to variability in eye contact.

Communication is often filled with thoughtful periods of silence, which the physical therapist should avoid interrupting. Allowing prolonged periods of silence (prolonged by European American standards) is considered respectful.[16] A conversation during a physical therapy examination proceeds at its own pace. Moreover, attempts to persuade or advise may be undesirable until a sufficient level of trust has been established.[17]

Reflective Exercise

• In what ways is Mr. Bodner's behavior congruent with his American Indian culture? • Why did he not maintain eye contact with the physical therapist?

While Western culture emphasizes a linear movement of time from past to future, the American Indian concept of time is intuitive, personal, and flexible.[9] Indian references to time include relationships to naturally occurring phenomena such as daily cycles; morning, afternoon, or night; moons rather than months; and seasons rather than years.[18] Cultural norms for arrival to an event, appropriate length of time to wait, and duration of "pre-event" socialization all vary depending on cultural norms,[9] which vary by individual and tribe.

Mirroring a patient's nonverbal behaviors may be helpful when communicating with AIANs.

Because wide variation exists in communication style both within and across tribes, it is desirable to reciprocate eye contact, nonverbal cues, and physical contact consistent with patient modeling.[13] As in any healthcare setting, patients should always be asked for permission to be touched or for removal of clothing.

Temporality

For most traditional American Indians, the temporality sequence is present, past, and future in that order, especially for those of lower socioeconomic status. Very little planning is done for the future because their view is that many things are outside one's control and may affect or change the future. In fact, the Navajo language does not have a future tense. Time is viewed as something that is always with the individual. To plan for the future is sometimes viewed as foolish. Events do not always start on time, but rather time starts when the group gathers. To help prevent frustration in scheduling events, time factors need to be taken into consideration and the speaker made aware of these unique time perceptions. Appointments may not always be kept, especially if someone else in the clan needs help.[16]

Reflective Exercise

• Do you think the physical therapist has gained the trust of Mr. Bodner? • Why or why not? • What evidence exists demonstrating that he may be agreeable to complete a rehabilitation program? • Was mutual trust established? • What evidence do you see for Mr. Bodner being part of a collectivist culture?

Format for Names

Most AIANs follow the dominant American tradition of having a first, middle, and last name used in that order. Physical therapists upon meeting a client for the first time should be more formal until told to do otherwise. Thus, address the person as Mr., Mrs., or Ms. Older people are addressed as grandmother or grandfather, or as mother or father by members of their clan. Otherwise, they are called by a nickname. A physical therapist can call an older client "grand-mother" or "grandfather" as a sign of respect once a therapeutic relationship is established.[16]

Family Roles and Organization

Decision Making and Gender Roles

Traditionally, gender roles were determined by survival needs such as procuring food, child rearing, and physical protection. Division of responsibilities varied widely among tribes; thus, generalizations of gender roles would be inaccurate. For example, Iroquois women traditionally maintained responsibility for property, possessions, and child and crop development, and could even subvert war efforts by controlling men's participation in war.[19,20] Currently, responsibilities appear to be more evenly distributed between men and women, suggesting that gender roles in AIAN cultures are similar to those found in the dominant American culture.[20] Over the past 30 years, the number of American Indian households headed by females has increased to 30%.[21]

Grandbois and Schadt[22] found that urban-dwelling American Indian females experienced increased feelings of isolation and loss of power compared with women living on reservation lands. A "more bleak and stressful" lifestyle is often experienced by Indians residing in metropolitan areas.[23]

Roles of the Aged and Extended Family

An important dynamic in AIAN cultures is the relationship between youth and elders. One encounters tremendous respect for elders, a respect that appears common across the majority of tribes.[20] Elder designation is revered and conferred out of respect and wisdom, not necessarily chronological age. Elders are the living historians, guarding and teaching traditional language and beliefs (Fig. 13-3). The successful physical therapist recognizes the role of elders as a powerful link with the community.[24] Many consider it an honor to care for an aging elder, an opportunity for adult children to reciprocate for their own care earlier in life.[13]

When making decisions about acceptable interventions, it is important to note that no

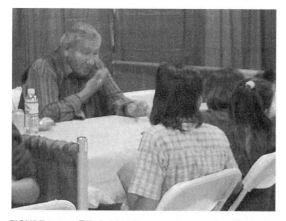

FIGURE 13.3 Tribal elder discusses the negative effect of alcohol abuse with school children. (Photo courtesy of Patrick S. Cross.)

decision is made until the appropriate decision maker (frequently an elderly woman) is present. Find the appropriate gatekeeper; otherwise time is lost and the problem must be addressed again at a later time.

The importance of the extended family is also emphasized in Indian culture.[17] AIAN cultures recognize the value of collectivism, the importance of group needs superseding individual needs. The family network has been fundamental to the social and economic organization of Indian communities. The status of the extended family, once critical to the survival of the community, is not as integral as in the past. Urbanization has resulted in dispersion and isolation of AIANs, limiting contact with the family. Acculturation, marriage within and across ethnic groups, and poverty have negatively modified the structure of and support by the extended family.[25]

Alternative Lifestyles
Alternative lifestyles are not usually discussed among AIANs. However, special individuals exist who are not looked on with disfavor, but rather are accepted as being different. In Zuni society and some northern tribes, some men take on women's roles. There are no pressures for them to change. Single-parent households are becoming more prevalent and are an accepted practice, with family members providing assistance with child

rearing. It is common for a mother to have children from different fathers.[16]

Biocultural Ecology

Skin Color and Biological Variations
Skin color of AIAN populations varies from light brown to very dark brown. Most have epithelial folds over the eyes. To assess for oxygenation in darker-skinned people, examine the mucous membranes and nail beds for capillary refill. Anemia is detected by examining the mucous membranes for pallor and the skin for a grayish hue. To assess for jaundice, examine the sclera rather than relying on skin hue. Newborns and infants commonly have mongolian spots on the sacral area. One should not mistake these spots for bruises and suspect child abuse.

The Navajo, Shawnee, and Apache are generally taller and thinner than members of other American Indian tribes. Remember that these characteristics are not seen with everyone; variations in this population do exist. The Navajo have traditionally been good runners and excel in relay races and long-distance running.

Endemic, Hereditary, and Genetic Diseases
Type II diabetes mellitus is reaching epidemic proportions in the American Indian population, with increased mortality.[26] In some communities, particularly in the southwestern United States, 40% to 50% of American Indian adults have diabetes,[27] with complications including retinopathy, renal disease,[29] and lower-extremity amputation.[28]

In concert with high rates of diabetes mellitus, acanthosis nigricans (AN) also occurs frequently in the native population. Acanthosis (hyperplasia) nigricans (hyperpigmentation) is characterized by a darkened (brown or black), velvety appearance of the skin of the neck, groin, and axillae and sometimes other areas of the body[30,34] (Fig. 13-4). The condition is labeled "hyperpigmentation" of skin, but according to Kurzrock and Cohen,[31] this term is a misnomer because light microscopy reveals hyperkeratosis rather than changes in melanin deposition. Although several forms of AN exist, a malignant form is associated

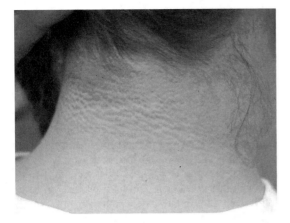

FIGURE 13.4 Grade 2 acanthosis marking on the nape of the neck of an American Indian youth. (Photo courtesy of Patrick S. Cross.)

with carcinoma in middle-aged adults. Others exhibit the benign form of AN, which is correlated with an endocrinopathy such as diabetes mellitus. The exact etiology of AN is unclear,[32] but according to Matsuoka, Wortsman, and Gavin,[33] hyperinsulinemia and insulin resistance are implicated. High levels of insulin cross-bind with insulin-like growth factor receptors, resulting in abnormal cellular growth.[34] The presence of AN has become a reliable clinical indicator of hyperinsulinemia in individuals who are obese.[35] While topical intervention is often ineffective, increased exercise and weight loss frequently result in diminished cutaneous markings.[36]

Diseases and Health Conditions

American Indians historically died of acute infectious diseases such as smallpox, measles, and diphtheria, but currently die of chronic diseases associated with alcoholism, heart disease, cancer, and diabetes.

A shorter life expectancy and overall younger population are evident among American Indians compared with all other races in the United States. For example, American Indian elders, defined by the IHS as age 55 years and older,[37] represent 11% of the American Indian population, compared with 21% for all other races.[38] The average life expectancy at birth for American Indian males is 67.4 years, compared with 73.6 years for males nationally; for American Indian females, it

is 74.2 years, compared with 79.4 years for females nationally.[39] Collectively, the average life expectancy for American Indians is 70.6 years, compared with the national average life expectancy of 76.5 years.[39] As a group, Indians are younger, with a median age of 24.2 years, compared with 32.9 years nationally.[21]

The most common causes of death among American Indians include diseases of the circulatory system; accidents, violence, and poisoning; neoplasms; and diseases of the respiratory system. These conditions account for nearly 80% of Indian deaths and have changed little in order of importance over the years.[37] In addition, the Indian age-adjusted mortality rates for the following causes are considerably higher than those for all races: tuberculosis, 440%; alcoholism, 430%; diabetes mellitus, 154%; and pneumonia and influenza, 46%.[21]

The two main causes of American Indian infant deaths are sudden infant death syndrome (SIDS) and congenital anomalies.[40] Four and one-half percent of American Indian mothers consume alcohol, a rate three times higher than that for non-Indian women in the United States.[40] Bagheri, Burd, Martsolf, and Klug[41] found that 80.3% of children diagnosed with fetal alcohol syndrome (FAS) in North Dakota were American Indian. According to Kaskutas,[42] women may not understand the consequences of FAS or the value of reducing alcohol intake during pregnancy.

Reflective Exercise

• What diseases and other health problems exist with the Hodgins and Bodner families that are common among American Indians? • What strategies can physical therapists use to decrease the incidence of these diseases among American Indians? • How might these approaches be different from those used with other ethnocultural groups?

Research has not yet conclusively identified the reasons for the prevalence of alcohol abuse by American Indians. Genetic theories have been proposed (e.g., inactivity of at least one ALDH2*2 allele, resulting in slowed oxidation of acetaldehyde in blood serum[43]), but no single theory has been supported unequivocally. Poverty, lower educational levels, and financial stressors associated with large families influence the high rate of alcoholism.[44]

The rate of SIDS among American Indian infants is consistently above the U.S. average. Grossman, Putsch, and Inui[45] reported 11 deaths out of every 1,000 urban American Indian live births from 1989 to 1991. Twenty percent of Indian women report smoking during pregnancy.[40] Once risk factors for SIDS such as age, parity, and smoking during pregnancy are removed, the risk for SIDS decreases to a level similar to that for the general U.S. population.[46] Binge drinking during pregnancy has also been found to be a correlated high-risk factor for SIDS among Northern Plains Indians.[47]

High-Risk Behaviors

Alcoholism among AIANs is epidemic and is a leading cause of health and social problems, including cirrhosis of the liver, accidents, and homicide. The federal government estimates that the alcoholism mortality rate among this group is more than five times greater than for all other races combined: 37.2 versus 6.8 per 100,000.[48] Similarly, the alcohol-related death rate for males ages 55 to 64 years is five times the rate for other races of the same age category. Although the death rate associated with alcoholism in female Indians in the same age range is less than one-half the rate for males, it remains over nine times higher than for females of other races.[40] The death rate from liver cirrhosis, often associated with alcohol abuse, is five times higher among AIANs ages 25–44 years than for the general population. In addition, alcohol use has been associated with at least 80% of homicides, suicides, and motor vehicle accidents in the American Indian population.[4] American Indians are more likely to die in accidents than are members of the general U.S. population. The IHS estimates that American Indian elders are more likely to die from traumatic accidents and homicide than elders from other races, with males at greater risk than females.[49] In fact, the homicide rate for Indian males ages 75 to 84 years is nearly triple

that of the same age cohort for other races.[49] Motor vehicle crashes account for a major portion of accidental deaths and hospitalizations.[37]

Reflective Exercise

• What strategies can physical therapists use to decrease high-risk health behaviors specific to AIAN populations?

High fertility rates, high birth weight, diabetes, inadequate prenatal care, and high-risk behaviors are concerns associated with American Indian pregnancies. Only about two-thirds of American Indian women begin prenatal care in the first trimester.[40] Of those who receive prenatal care, 14.4% in urban settings receive inadequate care.[50]

Nutrition

Meaning of Food
In many AIAN cultures, food symbolizes generosity.[51] Unfortunately, limited financial resources or access to healthy foods may lead to difficulty in maintaining adequate nutritional status for many. In some communities, more than 65% of adults are considered obese,[52] compared with 33% of adults of all other races.[53] Poor diet and insufficient levels of activity are associated with cardiovascular disease, specific cancers, liver cirrhosis, and non–insulin-dependent diabetes mellitus, 4 of the 10 leading causes of adult mortality and morbidity for Indians.[51,54]

Deficiencies and Limitations
Based on the recommended daily allowances developed by the National Research Council, nutritional problems exhibited by American Indians include excessive caloric intake, increased fat, and insufficient intake of fiber, iron, calcium, and vitamins A and C.[51] In addition to nutritional deficiencies, AIANs' lifestyles have become more sedentary. The reduced need for walking and outdoor physical activities has resulted in diminished levels of physical exercise.[51]

AIAN communities have been impacted by the dependence of many members on nonnative food allocations from federal distribution programs such as the Women, Infants, and Children's Program, the U.S. Department of Agriculture (USDA) Food Commodity Program, and the USDA Food Stamp Program.[55] Rural reservations are usually located some distance from markets that offer healthy food choices, and transportation to such facilities may be irregular or nonexistent for some Indian families. Additionally, the taste of water in rural supplies on some reservations is poor due to high mineral content, contributing to the frequent use of sugared beverage powders to improve palatability.[55] Although tribal members may be knowledgeable about dietary requirements, some communities have insufficient resources for changing social, economic, and environmental conditions to support improved nutritional status.[51] Table 13-1 lists factors influencing AIAN food choices and nutrient intake.

Reflective Exercise

• If the Hodgins family needed assistance with meeting their nutritional needs, what might the physical therapist do? • What might the physical therapist do if Mr. Bodner does not eat well because he dislikes the food in the SNF?

TABLE 13.1

Factors Influencing Native American Food Choices and Nutrient Intake

Income level relative to household size

Access to food stores, including
    Proximity to stores
    Access to reliable transportation

Food stores vary from trading posts and small convenience stores that carry predominantly canned foods, soft drinks, prepackaged snack foods, and other items having a long shelf life to supermarkets offering a wide selection of fresh and frozen foods, as well as "designer foods"

Reliance on food assistance programs, such as
    Supplemental Food Program for Women, Infants, and Children (WIC)
    United States Department of Agriculture (USDA) Food Commodity Program
    USDA Food Stamp Program
    Tribal feeding and food assistance programs

Availability of cooking facilities, which is influenced by
    Access to electricity and gas to maintain a functional oven and range
    Reliance on wood cooking stoves
    Access to and use of other appliances (hot plate, microwave)

Availability of reliable refrigerators

Adherence to traditional food practices, including
    Use and availability of wild food sources
    Use of and familiarity with traditional food preparation techniques
    Cultural food preferences and ideas of "healthy" foods

Historical experience with food insecurity, undernutrition, and starvation, which influences cultural perspectives of appropriate body size and food restriction

Impact of local nutrition education and intervention programs

Reprinted from *Primary Care of Native American Patients: Diagnosis, Therapy, and Epidemiology*, Galloway. Table 38-1, copyright 1999, with permission from Elsevier.

Pregnancy and the Childbearing Family

Fertility Practices and Views toward Pregnancy

American Indian women on average bear children at a younger age than women in the general U.S. population.[40] Adolescent childbearing is twice as common among American Indians compared with all other races combined.[56] Horn[57] found that American Indian women believe contraception should not be used until after the first baby is born and that value is placed on becoming pregnant at an early age, validating one's feminine role.

Although value may be placed on early childbearing, in a qualitative study by Liu, Slap, Kinsman, and Khalid[56] of 25 American Indian adolescents who became pregnant, 13 were afraid to tell their families about the pregnancy. In addition, 3 of the participants used alcohol and 3 used tobacco during pregnancy. Fifteen became pregnant because they failed to use contraception, and half reported barriers to obtaining prenatal care due to lack of transportation, family problems, and/or missing school.

In a study of rural teenage Indian adolescents, Chewning and colleagues[58] found that lower perceived health-risk behavior of friends, higher perceived parental support, higher perceived parental knowledge and monitoring of activities and friends, and higher value placed on scholastic achievement are all factors correlated with abstention from intercourse or with consistent use of birth control. Through community prevention programs, modifiable factors can be addressed.

Reflective Exercise

• Fifteen-year-old Alaskan Native Marissa Debon is seeing the physical therapist for gait training after reconstructive surgery following knee injuries. She is pregnant and 60 pounds overweight. She tells you that her parents do not know she is pregnant and that she does not want them to know. What should you as a physical therapist do?

Pre- and postnatal care must include education of young women and their families. Education should incorporate beliefs specific to a clan or tribe because of the wide variance in values, beliefs, lifestyles, and rituals among tribes. Traditional storytelling and talking circles can be used to assist in the education.[59]

Death Rituals

Galloway and colleagues[60] report that open discussions of death and dying among many American Indians are viewed as "willing it on oneself" (p. 327). Adhering to the ethical principle of nonmaleficence, a physical therapist must not cause harm to the patient physically or mentally by speaking of death as freely as is common in Western medicine. The patient must understand the disease process and treatment recommendations and share information in a way that he or she understands. Moreover, the message must be handled in a manner that is not perceived by the patient as taboo.[60]

One death taboo among the Navajo involves talking with clients concerning a fatal disease or illness. Effective discussions require that the issue be presented in the third person, as if the illness or disorder occurred with someone else. Never suggest that the client is dying. To do so may imply that the provider wishes the client dead. If the client does die, it may imply that the provider might have evil powers.

Reflective Exercise

• Janny James, a 55-year-old American Indian, has severe contractures resulting from being in bed for several months at home. She has multiple systemic health problems in addition to the contractures. The visiting health nurse has suggested that she enter a hospice. The physical therapist is working with Mrs. James to help reduce the contractures. Mrs. James tells the physical therapist that she is very upset over the nurse's suggestion that she is dying and that she never wants to see that nurse again. What might the physical therapist do to provide emotional support to Mrs. James?

Bereavement

Healing of the community after a death may include the use of traditional healing and religious ceremonies and counseling services.[45] Some use humor as a form of healing to "erase, cleanse, or change what was embarrassing, oppressive, sorrowful, or painful"[61] (pp. 67–68). Group activities, including storytelling and prayers for good health, may also be an acceptable outlet during a time of bereavement.[62]

After a personal loss, some American Indians have dreams and hallucinations about the deceased. Dreams of the dead may represent illness or death or that the spirit has laid claim to the dreamer.[62] Grossman and colleagues[45] describe a phenomenon known as Spirit Sickness, an illness with features of depression that results from a loss of a guardian spirit to connect with deceased family members and acquaintances. The belief is that if Spirit Sickness is untreated, it could lead to "soul loss" and death. Thus, it is important to understand the importance of body, mind, and spirit; recognize local native traditions after the loss of a family member; know the individual on a personal level; provide empathy; monitor for signs of depression; and know what community interventions are available to help in the bereavement process.

Spirituality

Dominant Religions and Use of Prayer

In AIAN cultures, spiritual and healthcare practices cannot be separated.[63] The American Indian Church or peyote religion predominates in many tribes. The focus of this religion is the revival of American Indian culture and beliefs (Fig. 13-5).[64] Sometimes hospital admissions are accompanied by traditional ceremonies and consultation with a pastor. Spirituality and wellness are often intertwined, and events such as death may be viewed as steps in a natural, inevitable progression along the life cycle.[15,63]

Although individual American Indian tribes have distinct belief systems and practices, Locust[65] and Andrews and Boyle[64] summarize core spiritual beliefs related to health that are shared by many tribes: (a) A Supreme Creator exists;

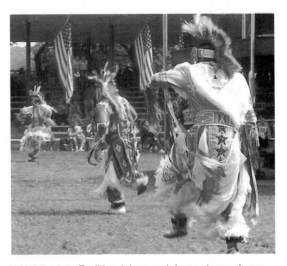

FIGURE 13.5 Traditional dress and dance at annual pow wow. (Photo courtesy of Patrick S. Cross.)

(b) individuals possess mind, body, and spirit, and wellness represents harmony among all;

Reflective Exercise

• A 40-year-old female American Indian, Mrs. Davies, had been attending physical therapy for adhesive capsulitis consistently for 3 weeks. The patient had made large improvements in active range of motion and strength, and was pleased that she could now do her activities of daily living and help with household activities for her family with limited discomfort. She was also pleased that she no longer had to take medications to resolve pain, previously fearing addiction to pain medications. Suddenly, the client stopped coming. The therapist tried to call the client, but no phone number was present for her. Community health nurses also tried to establish contact with the client through family members, but without success.

Three weeks later, the client came into the physical therapy clinic. She stated that her father had died and she had to cope with his death before returning to the reservation. She told the therapist that the time had come for her to restart her life and do what was necessary to be well physically, mentally, and spiritually.

(c) all physical things, living and nonliving, are part of the spirit world; (d) the spirit existed before it came into a body and it will exist after death; therefore, medicine men and women strive to restore harmony rather than prolong life; (e) illness affects body, mind, and spirit and results in disharmony; (f) natural unwellness may be caused by violation of a sacred or tribal taboo; (g) witchcraft may produce unnatural wellness; (h) individuals are responsible for their own health, as opposed to sickness being related to external organisms or abnormalities as espoused in Western medicine.[65]

Reflective Exercise

• From what you know about Indian cultural beliefs, what do you think Mrs. Davies means when she says she needed to be well physically, mentally, and spiritually? • How might the physical therapist help her in each of these areas?

Maugan[66] has developed an assessment tool to assist health practitioners in determining a patient's spiritual history as related to health interventions. This assessment may be used for any religious affiliation and is represented by the mnemonic SPIRIT (see Table 13-2).

TABLE 13.2

SPIRITual History: Interviewing Tool for Spiritual History Assessment

S—spiritual belief system

P—personal spirituality

I—integration and involvement in a spiritual community

R—ritualized practices and restrictions

I—implications for medical care

T—terminal events planning (advance directives)

Healthcare Practices

Focus of Healthcare

Among AIANs good health results from following certain lifeways that promote harmony between self and universe.[63] Although tribal beliefs vary widely, many AIAN cultures respect the natural world order and recognize the importance of earth and sky elements.[20] Imbalances in or disruptions of harmony may result in illness. Depending on cultural beliefs, correction of an imbalance and restoration of health may involve ceremonies including but not limited to rituals, prayers, chants, songs, herbal substances, sweats, smokes, body adornments, sand paintings, and physical manipulations.[67]

Traditional Practices

AIANs access a dual healthcare system, using traditional healers and Western allopathic medicine. Approximately 38–74% of urban-dwelling Indians seek assistance from traditional healers, and rates may be as high as 70–90% for Indians residing on reservations.[68] Prior to European influence, traditional practices served as the only source of intervention for health maintenance.[67] With approval of the Dawes Act, the U.S. Congress rendered traditional practices illegal from 1887 until 1978, when passage of the Indian Religious Freedom Act legalized their use.[67] No quantitative data exists comparing the effectiveness of traditional practices with Western medicine, and according to Hollow,[67] this data may never be generated "given the current mistrust Indian people have toward scientific research, secondary to their historic maltreatment, the breaking of treaties, and the Western scientific labeling of traditional Indian medicine as 'savage' and 'uncivilized'" (p. 31). Descriptive data from case studies illustrates the positive effect of traditional practices when coupled with Western allopathic medicine. Improvements have been documented for patients with depression, stroke and aphasia, and arthritis,[69–71] and a governmental task force has formally recognized the importance of both Western and traditional medicine in the maintenance of health for AIANs[68] (Fig. 13-6).

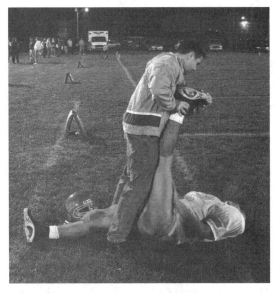

FIGURE 13.6 Community physical therapist assists an athlete with pregame stretches. (Photo courtesy of Patrick S. Cross.)

*F*redrick, an 18-year-old American Indian football player, is tackled out of bounds and gets his foot and ankle caught in an inverted position. Fredrick has immediate pain, rated as 10/10 on a visual analog scale (VAS). He also reports experiencing an audible "pop." Upon examination of the ankle by the athletic trainer and physical therapist, it was determined that the patient was tender to palpation with withdrawal over the anterior tibial fibular ligament, and the anterior drawer test was positive. Fredrick was sent to the hospital, where radiographs ruled out a fracture. The physician at the hospital diagnosed the injury as a grade 2 or 3 ankle sprain. Fredrick was to be on crutches for at least one week, to wear an immobilizer, to elevate and ice the ankle, to follow up with his local physician, and to attend physical therapy. The doctor told Fredrick he would not be able to participate in his last football game, which was scheduled a week from the date of injury.

When the therapist saw Fredrick four days after the injury occurred, he still experienced 6/10 pain on a VAS, had a moderate amount of swelling at the lateral ankle region, was able to perform only weight bearing as tolerated (WBAT), and had minimal ankle active range of motion (AROM) in all planes. During physical therapy treatment, Fredrick stated that he was going to try some native healing rituals so that he could play in his final game. At first, the therapist was skeptical and hoped that the rituals would not give the athlete false hope; he did not feel that the rituals would harm the individual's physical progress, nor did he feel that he should be the one determining if the individual should participate in culturally accepted rituals.

Two days later, one day prior to the game, Fredrick did not attend his physical therapy appointment. The coaches had not seen him at school that day. On Friday, the therapist went to provide coverage at the football game. To the therapist's amazement, the first person he saw was Frederick dressed in full gear. Observing Fredrick's gait pattern, the physical therapist noted no abnormalities or antalgic gait pattern. The coaches said he had spent two days doing sweats and other local traditional healing rituals and had come back saying he was 100%. Skeptical, the therapist and coaches agreed they would not let him play unless he was given clearance by the therapist and athletic trainer.

Fredrick underwent a thorough physical therapy examination, including functional athletic field tests. He had full ankle AROM and 5/5 strength, and was able to cut, jump, and sprint at full speed without reported or observed pain or signs of weakness. Fredrick was given clearance to play. Not only did he start, but he played every second of the game as a starter on offense, defense, and special teams.

Responsibility for Health

Unlike the situation for other minority groups in the United States, the federal government is obligated through treaty and statute to provide healthcare to recognized AIAN tribes through the IHS.[72] Dependence on federal rather than state government may contribute, in part, to diminished access to assistance and increase the risk of substandard housing, poverty, malnutrition, and poor health.

In Western healthcare, the practitioner asks the client what he or she thinks is wrong and then prescribes a treatment. This practice is sometimes interpreted by American Indians as ignorance on the part of the non-Native healer.

Reflective Exercise

• How is Fredrick taking responsibility for his health?
• From your perspective as a physical therapist, is this consistent with standard therapy?

Pain and Sick Role

Obtaining adequate pain control is of concern for American Indians who receive care within the context of Western medicine. Frequently, attempts at pain control are ineffective because the actual intensity of the pain is not obvious to the physical therapist and because clients do not request pain medication. The traditional view of pain is as something that is to be endured; thus, patients do not ask for analgesics and may not even understand that pain medication is available. Other times, herbal medicines are preferred and used without the knowledge of the physical therapist. Not sharing the use of herbal

medicine with the Western healthcare provider is a carryover from the times when individuals were not allowed to practice their native medicine. Establishing trust will encourage clients to fully disclose the herbal treatments used for pain control. The physical therapist may explain that the pain medicine will promote healing.

Reflective Exercise

• Do you see any contradictions in therapy with Fredrick using traditional healing practices? • What might they be? • Do you think Fredrick has a high pain threshold?

Cultural perceptions of the sick role for the American Indian are based on the ideal of maintaining harmony with nature and with others. Ill people have obviously done something to place themselves out of harmony or have had a curse placed on them. In either case, support of the sick role is not generally accepted; rather, support is directed at assisting the person to regain harmony. Elderly people frequently work even when seriously ill and may need to be encouraged to rest.

Reflective Exercise

• Is Fredrick's behavior consistent or inconsistent with American Indian practices? • Provide a rationale for your belief. What might the physical therapist do to ensure that further injury does not occur with Fredrick's sports participation?

Mental Health

Mental illness is perceived as resulting from witches or witching (placing a curse) on a person. In these instances, a healer who deals with dreams or a crystal gazer is consulted. Among the Navajo, individuals may wear turquoise to ward off evil; however, a person who wears too much turquoise is sometimes thought to be an evil person and, thus, someone to avoid. In some tribes, mental illness may mean that the affected person has special powers.[16]

Many AIAN cultures consider illness as resulting from imbalances in mind, body, and spirit. Traditional healers are capable of understanding illness from a perspective that includes spirituality and symptom etiology in the context of a patient's specific culture. Awareness of the patient's cultural beliefs and background is particularly important in the management of mental health. As an example, Roubideaux[73] describes circumstances in which symptoms of depression are present but etiology is culture dependent. A patient may present with depressive symptoms closely aligned with DSM-IV classification criteria.[74] In other circumstances, hallucinations may be present, usually following a relative's death.[75] Other specific conditions, such as Spirit Sickness[45] and ghost illness,[76] may include depressive symptoms. Depending on a patient's level of acculturation, Western counseling or pharmacological interventions may be culturally congruent, but some patients or illnesses may respond only to traditional ceremonies or strategies. The healthcare practitioner must be aware that mental health issues must be interpreted in the context of the patient's cultural beliefs.

Barriers to Healthcare

Multiple barriers to receiving healthcare exist for AIANs. Some credit the health challenges faced by AIANs to poor quality of care and long waits associated with the IHS.[73] Others note that the IHS was originally designed as a hospital-based, acute-care system and it is poorly equipped to deal with the predominantly chronic problems of today. Most agree that the IHS is severely underfunded.[13] In 2001, American Indians received one-third as much in healthcare expenditure per capita as individuals in the general population.[73]

In addition to profound financial constraints, many reservations are located in rural regions geographically isolated from clinical facilities, do not have adequate transportation and communication facilities, and lack an overall sufficient infrastructure. The inadequate number of healthcare practitioners to meet the needs of the 1.46 million eligible patients hinders their ability to receive adequate care.[37] Those living in urban areas are not eligible for healthcare provided by the IHS.

Reflective Exercise

• Identify barriers to healthcare in each of the following case scenarios in this chapter: the Hodgins family, Mr. Bodner, Marissa Debon, Mrs. James, Mrs. Davies, and Fredrick. What might the physical therapist do in each case to decrease these barriers and promote more effective interventions?

Rehabilitation and Chronicity

The concept of rehabilitation is relatively new to American Indians because in years past they did not survive to an age where chronic diseases became an issue. Because life expectancy is increasing, an additional stress is placed on families who are expected to care for elderly relatives. Many families do not have the resources to assume this responsibility. Home healthcare is occasionally available, but this is a recent development that tribes are just beginning to accept. Federal public health nursing is also available to assist with home care.

The increased prevalence of chronic diseases and the associated burden of care among American Indians are profoundly challenging IHS resources.[73] The IHS healthcare delivery system was created using an acute-care paradigm, but shifting demographics of chronic disease and functional limitations of elders increase the need for rehabilitation professionals.[73] In addition, the highest rates of disability for any ethnic group in the United States are claimed by American Indians.[77] IHS priorities have historically provided for maintenance of "life and limb," so emergent cases obviously demanded priority for scarce financial resources. The role of rehabilitation in restoring functional mobility and independence is gaining acceptance as benefits of regular exercise are recognized by American Indian patients and physical therapists.

Healthcare Practitioners

Most AIANs have traditional healers of some kind and use them to varying degrees depending on the primary and secondary characteristics of culture as presented in Chapter 1. In general, na-

Reflective Exercise

Andrew, a 25-year-old obese American Indian male, is referred to physical therapy from the general medical clinic for degenerative disc disease of L3-S1. Andrew gives consent for the physical therapist to perform the evaluation and ensuing care. During the subjective evaluation, Andrew states that his goals are to lose weight, reduce pain, and be in good enough shape to pass physical fitness tests for admission into the Army. He states he is able to work only manual labor jobs because he did not graduate from high school. He is currently trying to complete his GED but has been having difficulty finding reliable transportation. Andrew also notes that he has a learning disability, resulting in difficulty with reading. He also states that although his friends stay up late and are into drugs and alcohol, he does not partake in the festivities and socializes with them only because his friends are "all he has left." In addition, during the subjective evaluation, the therapist found that Andrew had not been tested for diabetes since high school. Grade IV cutaneous markings associated with acanthosis nigricans were present on the nape of his neck.

Following the objective portion of the evaluation, a significant amount of time was spent talking with Andrew—providing education about his medical problem and home exercise program (giving the client pictures, instead of written instructions, to facilitate memory), establishing realistic goals, and discussing how the therapist could help him in accomplishing his personal goals through therapy and other services available in the community. Andrew agreed to meet with the diabetes educator. He also stated he would like the physical therapist to contact local agencies about transportation and extra help with reading. The therapist replied that he would talk to the military recruiter once Andrew was ready for him to do so. While Andrew was present, the therapist called the agencies and even had the diabetes educator come over to introduce herself and make an appointment with him.

Andrew is hesitant to begin a program at the local wellness center once he is discharged from skilled physical therapy services. He tells the therapist he does not like to be seen going into and out of the wellness center because his friends might "make fun of him" and "might think that he is trying to be better than them." He voices his desire to attend therapy at the clinic. The therapist agrees and tells him that once he is discharged from skilled therapy, he will arrange for him to use the clinic's equipment when other clients are not there. Through significant patient advocacy and interprofessional collaboration, therapeutic rapport was established with the patient, appropriate services were accessed, and the patient was empowered to achieve his established goals.

---

tive healers are divided primarily into three categories: those working with the power of good, those working with the power of evil, and those working with both. Generally, they are divinely chosen and promote activities that encourage self-discipline and self-control and that involve acute body awareness. Some practitioners are endowed with supernatural powers, whereas others have knowledge only of herbs and specific manipulations.

The acceptance of Western medicine is variable, with a blending of traditional healthcare beliefs. Many individuals are suspicious of American Indian physicians. Many health concerns of American Indians can be treated by both traditional and Western healers in a culturally congruent manner when practitioners are willing to work together and respect each other's differences.

Western practitioners, traditional medicine men, and herbal healers receive respect on the reservation. However, not all individuals accord equal respect to these groups, and many prefer one group over the other, while others use all three. Navajo tribal practitioners divide their knowledge into preventive measures, treatment regimens, and health maintenance. An example

BOX 13.1

Traditional American Indian Healthcare Practitioners

1. People who can use their power only for good, can transform themselves into other forms of life, and can maintain cultural integration in times of stress.
2. People who can use their power for both evil and good and are expected to do evil against someone's enemies. People in this group know witchcraft, poisons, and ceremonies designed to afflict the enemy.
3. The diviner diagnostician, such as a crystal gazer, who can see what caused the problem but cannot implement a treatment. Another example of this type is a hand trembler, who, rather than using crystals, practices hand trembling over the sick person to determine the cause of an illness.
4. Specialist medicine people treat the disease after it has been diagnosed and specialize in the use of herbs, massage, or midwifery.
5. Those who care for the soul and send guardian spirits to restore a lost soul.
6. Singers, who are considered to be the most special, cure through the power of their song. These healers use laying on of hands and usually remove objects or draw disease-causing objects from the body while singing.

Adapted from Still & Hodgins (2003).[16]

of a preventive measure is carrying an object or a pouch filled with objects prescribed by a medicine man to ward off the evil of a witch. Do not remove medicine pouches from clients.

The various types of traditional practitioners among the Navajo are shown in Box 13-1.

Male healthcare providers are generally limited in the care they provide to women, especially during their menses. This practice is very common among elderly women. Provide a same-gender physical therapist whenever possible for conditions requiring intimate contact.

CASE STUDY SCENARIO

*M*rs. Spottedsnake, age 46 years, lives alone in her rural trailer home approximately 1.5 miles from the reservation-based health education center. She has been divorced for 12 years and is sharing her home with her 31-year-old daughter and three grandsons, ages 13, 11, and 6 years. Mrs. Spottedsnake is employed by a local reservation-owned casino, where she frequently lifts 30-pound bags of coins. Her net annual income is $14,050, and the casino does not provide health insurance. Mrs. Spottedsnake does not own a car and sometimes depends on community transit service for transportation; however, access is inconsistent.

Mrs. Spottedsnake has been under skilled physical therapy care for the past 2 weeks for chronic lumbar pain associated with disc herniation, status post 15 years. She is receiving care at the health education center. The nearest Indian Health Service hospital is many miles away in Aberdeen, South Dakota. Mrs. Spottedsnake has experienced some relief of symptoms with physical therapy interventions, but the physician feels that she should pursue surgical options in the near future. Upon questioning by the physical therapist, Mrs. Spottedsnake agrees that she would like to first obtain services from a traditional medicine man, but the nearest healer is located in the southwest region of the United States.

1. Describe the structure of the Indian Health Service, the system coordinating Mrs. Spottedsnake's healthcare services.

2. Identify three barriers Mrs. Spottedsnake must overcome to obtain healthcare.

3. How does Mrs. Spottedsnake's income compare with that of other ethnic groups?

4. Mrs. Spottedsnake has actively expressed interest in accessing a traditional healer. If you were unsure as to a patient's level of traditional beliefs regarding spirituality or use of native healers, describe a clinical strategy that might be useful in accessing such information.

5. Identify three factors that might be related to Mrs. Spottedsnake's level of acculturation into dominant society.

6. Describe three characteristics of communication that might affect Mrs. Spottedsnake's verbal and nonverbal interaction with non-Native healthcare professionals.

7. Mrs. Spottedsnake is divorced and is the head of her household. Compare gender role expectations for American Indians with those of non-Indian women.

8. Discuss five core spiritual beliefs that may influence Mrs. Spottedsnake's view of health.

9. Discuss the benefits of having Mrs. Spottedsnake consult the traditional medicine man.

10. Identify some potential negative outcomes of having Mrs. Spottedsnake consult the traditional medicine man.

11. Describe the role rehabilitation professionals might play in decreasing the impact of chronic health conditions on American Indian patients.

REFERENCES

1. US Bureau of the Census. American Factfinder. Available at: http://factfinder.census.gov/servlet/QTTable?_bm=y&-geo_id=D&-qr_name=DEC_2000_SF1_U_DP1&-ds_name=D&-_lang=en. Accessed May 29, 2004.

2. Indian Health Service. Diabetes among young American Indians. Available at: http://www.ihs.gov/facilitiesservices/areaoffices/billings/stats/population.asp. Accessed December 20, 2003.

3. Kramer BJ. Cross-cultural medicine—a decade later: Health and aging of urban American Indians. *West J Med*. 1992;157:281–285.

4. Hodge FS, Fredericks L. American Indian and Alaska Native populations in the United States: An overview. In: Huff RM, Kline MV, eds. *Promoting Health in Multicultural Populations: A Handbook for Practitioners*. Thousand Oaks, Calif: Sage; 1999:269–289.

5. Young IS, Kim EC. *American Mosaic: Selected Readings on American Multicultural Heritage*. Englewood Cliffs, NJ: Prentice-Hall; 1993.

6. Indian Health Services. Area offices and facilities. Available at: http://www.ihs.gov/FacilitiesServices/ AreaOffices/AreaOffices_index.asp. Accessed May 29, 2004.

7. Stubben JD. Working with and conducting research among American Indian families. *Am Behav Sci*. 2001;44:1466–1481.

8. Yeo G. Ethnogeriatrics: Cross-cultural care of older adults. *Generations.* 1997:72–77.

9. Brant CC. Native ethics and rules of behaviour. *Can J Psychiatr.* 1990;35:534–539.

10. US Bureau of the Census. American Indian education. Available at: http://www.census.gov/population/www/pop-profile/amerind.html. Accessed May 29, 2004.

11. Smedley BD, Stith AY, Nelson AR. *Unequal Treatment: Confronting Racial and Ethnic Disparities in Health Care.* Washington, DC: National Academies Press; 2003.

12. Jandt FE. Nonverbal communication. In: *Intercultural Communication: An Introduction.* 2nd ed. Thousand Oaks, Calif: Sage; 1998:97–119.

13. Cochran TM. Rehabilitation and American Indian elders. In: *Cultural Diversity.* Alexandria, Va: American Physical Therapy Association; 2003. Section on Geriatrics monograph series:1–12.

14. Jandt FE. Dimensions of culture. In: *Intercultural Communication: An Introduction.* 2nd ed. Thousand Oaks, Calif: Sage; 1998:213–233.

15. Hepburn K, Reed R. Ethical and clinical issues with Native American elders. *Clin Geriatr Med.* 1995;11:97–111.

16. Still O, Hodgins D. Navajo Indians. In: Purnell L, Paulanka B, eds. *Transcultural Health Care: A Culturally Competent Approach.* 2nd ed. Philadelphia, Pa: FA Davis; 2003:279–284.

17. Garwick A, Auger S. What do providers need to know about American Indian culture? Recommendations from urban Indian family caregivers. *Fam Syst Health.* 2000;18:177–189.

18. Morgan CO, Guy E, Lee B, Cellini H R. Rehabilitation services for American Indians: The Navajo experience. *J Rehabil.* 1986;23:25–31.

19. Earle KA. Working with the Haudenosaunee: What social workers should know. *New Soc Work.* 1996;8:27–28.

20. Marshall C, Johnson S. Cultural and environmental factors in the delivery of rehabilitation services to American Indians. In: Leavitt RL, ed. *Cross-Cultural Rehabilitation: An International Perspective.* Philadelphia, Pa: WB Saunders; 1999:247–258.

21. US Bureau of the Census. American Indian population. Available at: http://www.census.gov/population/www/pop-profile/amerind.html. Accessed May 29, 2004.

22. Grandbois GH, Schadt D. Indian identification and alienation in an urban community. *Psychol Rep.* 1994;74:211–216.

23. Hodge FS, Fredericks L, Kipnis P. Urban-rural contrasts, patient and smoking patterns in northern California American Indian clinics. *Cancer.* 1996;78:1623–1628.

24. Cochran TM, Jensen GM. Building community with American Indians: Balancing wisdom and vulnerability. *Gerinotes.* 2000;7:17–19.

25. Red Horse J. Clinical strategies for American Indian families in crisis. *Urban Soc Change Rev.* 1982;15:17–19.

26. Wolsey DH, Cheek JE. Epidemiologic patterns of morbidity and mortality. In: Galloway JM, Goldberg BW,

Alpert JS, eds. *Primary Care of Native American Patients: Diagnosis, Therapy and Epidemiology.* Boston, Mass: Butterworth-Heinemann; 1999:7–16.

27. Will JC, Strauss KF, Mendlein JM.. Diabetes mellitus and Navajo Indians: Findings from the Navajo health and nutrition survey. *J Nutr.* 1997;127(suppl 10):2106S-2113S.

28. Nelson RG, Gohdes DM, Everhart JE. Lower extremity amputations in NIDDM: 12–year follow-up study in Pima Indians. *Diabetes Care.* 1988;11:8–16.

29. Newman JM, Marfin AA, Eggers PW, Helgerson SD. End-stage renal disease among American Indians. *Am J Public Health.* 1990;80:318–319.

30. Elmer KB, George RM. HAIR-AN syndrome: A multi-system challenge. *Am Fam Physician.* 2001;63:2385–2390.

31. Kurzrock R, Cohen PR. Cutaneous paraneoplastic syndromes in solid tumors. *Am J Med.* 1995;99:662–671.

32. Nanney LB, Ellis DL, Levine J, King LE. Epidermal growth factor receptors in idiopathic and virally induced skin disease. *Am J Pathol.* 1992;140:915–925.

33. Matsuoka LY, Wortsman J, Gavin JR. Spectrum of endocrine abnormalities associated with acanthosis nigricans. *Am J Med.* 1987;83:719–725.

34. Matsuoka LY, Wortsman J, Goldman J. Acanthosis nigricans. *Clin Dermatol.* 1993;11:21–25.

35. Hud JA Jr, Cohen JB, Wagner JM, Cruz PD. Prevalence and significance of ancanthosis nigricans in an adult obese population. *Arch Dermatol.* 1992;128:941–944.

36. Bar RS, Harrison LC, Muggeo M, Gorden P, Kahn CR, Roth J. Regulation of insulin receptors in normal and abnormal physiology in humans. *Adv Intern Med.* 1979;24:23–52.

37. Indian Health Service. Trends in Indian health 1998–1999. Available at: http://www.his.gov/PublicInfo/Publications/trends98/trends98.asp. Accessed January 15, 2003.

38. Grieco EM, Cassidy RC. Overview of race and Hispanic origin. Census 2000 brief. Available at: http://www census.gov/prod/2001pubs/c2kbr01–1.pdf. Accessed July 22, 2003.

39. Demographic and Dental Statistics Section. Regional differences in Indian health 2000–2001. Available at: http://www.IndianHealthService.gov/NonMedical Programs/IndianHealthService_Stats/files/Regional_ Differences_Charts2.pdf. Accessed March 16, 2003.

40. Indian Health Service. *Indian Health Focus: Women, 1998–99.* Washington, DC: Author; 1999.

41. Bagheri MM, Burd L, Martsolf JT, Klug MG. Fetal alcohol syndrome: Maternal and neonatal characteristics. *J Perinat Med.* 1998;26:263–269.

42. Kaskutas LA. Understanding drinking during pregnancy among urban American Indians and African Americans: Health messages, risk beliefs, and how we measure consumption. *Alcohol Clin Exp Res.* 2000;24:1241–1250.

43. Chao HM. Alcohol and the mystique of flushing. *Alcohol Clin Exp Res.* 1995;19:104–109.

44. Cruz M. Alcohol and solvent abuse. In: Galloway JM, Goldberg BW, Alpert JS, eds. *Primary Care of Native*

American Patients: Diagnosis, Therapy and Epidemiology. Boston, Mass: Butterworth-Heinemann; 1999:263–268.

45. Grossman DC, Putsch RW, Inui TS. The meaning of death to adolescents in an American Indian community. *Fam Med.* 1993;25:593–597.

46. Cooper W, Boyce T, Wright P, Griffin M. Do childhood vaccines have non-specific effects on mortality? *Bull WHO.* 2003;81:11–34.

47. Iyasu S, Randall LL, Welty TK, et al. Risk factors for sudden infant death syndrome among Northern Plains Indians. *JAMA.* 2002; 288:2717–2723.

48. Indian Health Service. *Trends in Indian Health 1994.* Rockville, Md: US Department of Health and Human Services, Public Health Service, Indian Health Service, Office of Planning, Education, and Legislation, and Division of Program Statistics; 1994.

49. Indian Health Service. *Indian Health Focus: Elders, 1998–99.* Washington, DC: Author; 1999. Indian Health Service. (2004).

50. Grossman DC, Baldwin LM, Casey S, Nixon B, Hollow W, Hart LG. Disparities in infant family health among American Indians and Alaska Natives in US metropolitan areas. *Pediatrics.* 2002;109:627–633.

51. Teufel NI. Nutritional problems. In: Galloway JM, Goldberg BW, Alpert JS, eds. *Primary Care of Native American Patients: Diagnosis, Therapy and Epidemiology.* Boston, Mass: Butterworth-Heinemann; 1999:283–292.

52. Solomon CG, Manson JE. Obesity and mortality: A review of the epidemiologic data. *Am J Clin Nutr.* 1997;66(suppl):1044–1050.

53. White LL, Ballew C, Gilbert TJ. Weight, body image, and weight control practices of Navajo Indians: Findings from the Navajo Health and Nutrition Survey. *J Nutr.* 1997;127(suppl 10):2094–2098.

54. Byers T. Nutrition and cancer among American Indians and Alaska Natives. *Cancer.* 1996;78:1612–1616.

55. Teufel NI, Ritenbaugh CK. Development of a primary prevention program: Insight gained in the Zuni diabetes prevention program. *Clin Pediatr.* 1998;37:131–142.

56. Liu LL, Slap GB, Kinsman SB, Khalid N. Pregnancy among American Indian adolescents: Reactions and prenatal care. *J Adolesc Health.* 1994;15:336–341.

57. Horn B. Cultural beliefs and teenage pregnancy. *Nurse Pract.* 1983;8:35–39.

58. Chewning B, Douglas J, Kokotailo PK, LaCourt J, Clair DS, Wilson D. Protective factors associated with American Indian adolescents' safer sexual patterns. *Matern Child Health J.* 2001;5:273–280.

59. Cesario SK. Care of the Native American woman: Strategies for practice, education, and research. *J Obstet Gynecol Neonatal Nurs.* 2001;30:13–19.

60. Galloway JM, Goldberg BW, Alpert JS. *Primary Care of American Patients: Diagnosis, Therapy, and Epidemiology.* Boston, Mass: Butterworth-Heinemann; 1999.

61. Herring RD, Meggert SS. The use of humor as a counselor strategy with Native American Indian children. *Elem Sch Guid Couns.* 1994;29:67–77.

62. Napoli M. Holistic health care for native women: An integrated model. *Am J Public Health.* 2002;92:1573–1575.

63. Avery C. Native American medicine: Traditional healing. *JAMA.* 1991;265:2271–2273.

64. Andrews M, Boyle J. Religion, culture, and nursing. In: Andrews M, Boyle J, eds. *Transcultural Concepts in Nursing Care.* 3rd ed. Philadelphia, Pa: Lippincott; 1999:378–443.

65. Locust CS. *American Indian Concepts Concerning Health and Unwellness.* Tucson: University of Arizona, Native American Research and Training Center; 1985. Monograph series:2–19

66. Maugan TA. The spiritual history. *Arch Fam Med.* 1996; 5:11–16.

67. Hollow WB. Traditional Indian medicine. In: Galloway JM, Goldberg BW, Alpert JS, eds. *Primary Care of Native American Patients: Diagnosis, Therapy and Epidemiology.* Boston, Mass: Butterworth-Heinemann; 1999:31–38.

68. Indian Health Service. *A Roundtable Conference on the Traditional Cultural Advocacy Program.* Washington, DC: U.S. Department of Health and Human Services, Indian Health Service; 1993.

69. Hufflinger KW, Tanner D. The peyote way: Implications for cultural care theory. *J Transcult Nurs.* 1994;5:5–11.

70. Morse J, Young D, Swartz L. Cree Indian healing practices and Western health care: A comparative analysis. *Soc Sci Med.* 1991;32:1361–1366.

71. Thompson J, McKay S, Roundhead D. Depression in a Native Canadian in NW Ontario: Sadness, grief or spiritual illness. *Can Ment Health.* 1988;2:5–8.

72. Smedley BD, Stith AY, Nelson AR. Committee on Understanding and Eliminating Racial and Ethnic Disparities in Health Care. Unequal treatment: Confronting racial and ethnic disparities in health care. Available at: http://www.nap.edu/books/030908265X/html/. Accessed May 21, 2003.

73. Roubideaux Y. Perspectives on American Indian health. *Am J Public Health.* 2002;92:1401–1403.

74. American Psychiatric Association. *Diagnostic and Statistical Manual of Mental Disorders.* 4th ed. Washington, DC: Author; 1994.

75. O'Nell TD. Psychiatric investigations among American Indians and Alaska Natives: A critical review. *Cult Med Psychiatr.* 1989;13:51–87.

76. Putsch RW. Ghost illness: A cross-cultural experience with the expression of a non-Western tradition in clinical practice. *Am Indian Alaska Native Ment Health Res.* 1988;2:6–26.

77. Kraus LE, Stoddard S, Gilmartin D. *Chartbook on Disability in the US 1996: An InfoUse Report.* Washington, DC: National Institute on Disability and Rehabilitation Research; 1996:19–20.

Chapter 14

Cultural Considerations for Middle Eastern Cultures

- Elizabeth Dean, PT, PhD
- Surreya Mahomed, PT, DEd
- Aisha Omar Maulana, MPH

Nadyah Al-Mohannah is 37 years of age and the mother of four children. She emigrated as a teenager from the Middle East to the United States. She is a devout Muslim. Nadyah requires care for low back pain, which is complicated by obesity, diabetes, and high blood pressure. Her back problem can be considered secondary to her other serious life-threatening conditions.

This chapter focuses primarily on the culture of people who are Muslims and describes differences and similarities among Middle Eastern, Arabic, and Islamic cultures. In managing a patient of such a cultural heritage, the clinician needs to establish the patient's cultural identity with respect to being Arabic, Muslim, or originating from the Middle East, or some combination thereof. In addition, this chapter considers the individual who has immigrated to the West. The needs of Westerners who have converted to Islam are also distinct. To understand the role of culture on physical therapy in this context, the 12 domains of the Purnell Model for Cultural Competence[1] are used as a guide. This knowledge and an awareness of cultural differences will facilitate the physical therapist's capacity to build rapport and trust with the patient, to access the relevant information for the history, to conduct the physical examination, and to implement treatment. The intercultural competence of the physical therapist will increase the likelihood of the Muslim patient's adherence to the therapeutic recommendations and home program, and a successful long-term treatment outcome.

Overview of Heritage

The Middle East is a geographic region that includes the following countries: Bahrain, Egypt, Iran, Iraq, Israel, Jordan, Kuwait, Lebanon, Libya, Oman, Qatar, Saudi Arabia, Syria, Turkey (Asian region), United Arab Emirates, and Yemen. Many of the people of the Middle East are of Arabic descent. *Arabic* refers to the ethnic heritage defined by the customs, language, foods, and traditions of the people originating from the Arabian

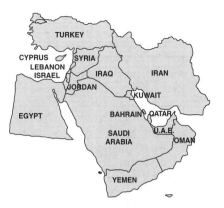

FIGURE 14.1 Map of the Middle East.

Peninsula, which includes Saudi Arabia (geographically the largest Muslim country) and the countries of the Arabian Gulf, namely Bahrain, Kuwait, Oman, Qatar, United Arab Emirates, and Yemen. Countries worldwide that are primarily Muslim—that is, whose people who adhere to the Islamic faith—are shown in Figure 14-1. Arabic and Islamic influences have extended to the countries of North Africa, collectively termed Maghreb, which includes Algeria, Comoros, Djibouti, Libya, Mauritania, Morocco, Somalia, Sudan, and Tunisia. Indonesia, however, an Asian country, has the largest Muslim population of any country in the world.[2,3]

Muslims adhere to the doctrines of the holy books, the Qur'an and the Haddiths. People who are Arabic can be of other faiths; likewise, Muslims can be of any ethnic origin and live in any part of the world, including the United States. Islam is the fastest-growing religion in the United States. At the current rate, Muslims in the United States will outnumber Jews by 2010, making Islam the nation's second largest religion.[4] One-quarter of the world's population is Muslim. Only 20% of the world's Muslims are Arabs.[5]

Over 100 million more Muslims live on the Indian subcontinent than live in all the Arab countries combined.[6] Israel has Arabic (Palestinian) and Muslim segments of the population along with significant segments of the population who are of the Jewish and Christian faiths. Thus, given their diversity, the healthcare needs of people who are Muslim can vary widely.[7]

The geopolitics and economic development of the Middle East reflect the discovery and drilling of oil over the past 70 years. Prior to that time, the people of this region lived relatively simple nomadic lives. Despite the oil-based wealth of some countries in this region, there are vast economic and developmental disparities across the Middle East.

Sociopolitical factors prevalent in the Middle East historically reflect tribal traditions of years gone by. The change from a nomadic lifestyle to one with modern conveniences has been rapid. The wealth from oil has afforded people from the oil-rich countries of the Middle East educational and travel opportunities. Those living in rural areas tend to be poorer with less access to educational and work opportunities.

Political structures and religion are linked in Islamic countries to varying degrees, with the stricter Islamic countries being headed by religious leaders. The head of state of the smaller Middle Eastern countries is often an *emir*, with a huge extended royal family, whose members tend to hold government posts. Power and influence in Islamic countries are often determined by the hierarchical status of the family within a given country. In many Islamic countries, women do not have the right to vote.

Communication

Although Arabic is the primary language spoken in Arabic countries (with the notable exception of Iran, where Farsi is spoken), each country has a unique dialect. The dialects are usually understandable among the residents of different countries and regions of the Middle East. The range of dialects, however, may be challenging for an Arabic interpreter. Arabic dialects are steeped in contextual meaning where often there is no direct translation, and meaning can be lost. Conversation is verbally and physically expressive. Gesticulation is common during speech and physical touching is integral to the conversation among those of the same gender if they are acquainted. As trust and rapport build between two people of the same sex, physical touching increases.

All social behavior in Islamic cultures is guided by the teachings of the Qur'an. In these cultures, men and women tend not to socialize together outside the family. Publicly, men greet each other in a more physical manner than in the West by hugging, and men can be seen walking together holding hands. There is also more physical contact between women publicly, including walking arm in arm. Interpersonal spatial distances are smaller compared with the West.

Strict Muslim men do not touch women other than their wives or other women in the family. Similarly, strict Muslim women will not touch men. This extends to a handshake, as it is believed to be disrespectful to the opposite sex and to the woman's family. If a Western man inadvertently extends his hand to a Muslim woman, she may either ignore the gesture or cover her hand.

Men and women avoid direct eye contact with each other when conversing. According to Qur'anic teaching, both men and women are to lower their eyes when speaking to the opposite sex. When speaking to a member of the same sex, however, personal spatial distance is close and direct eye contact can be maintained (Fig. 14-2).

Appointment times may be viewed as more flexible, with a tendency toward being late for scheduled meetings, although professional meetings are usually attended more punctually. Casual and formal meetings between Muslims begin with a traditional exchange of inquiries about the health and well-being of each person and his or her family. This is one example of the relative importance of the relational versus task orientation of people from the Middle East.

Inherent to Islamic belief is that Allah or God has ultimate control over one's life. This is illustrated in the use of the term *Inshallah* after many statements to signify "if God wills." Thus, much in life is attributed to God's will rather than to the individual.

Reflective Exercise

• A male physical therapist belongs to a Christian religion. How might he conduct himself when setting up an appointment for and when interviewing and treating a female patient who is Muslim? • What if the patient were male?

Family Roles and Organization

The Middle Eastern cultures are highly social and familial in orientation, and familial piety is central to their way of life. The family structure for most Muslims is patriarchal and based on the extended family (Fig. 14-3).[8] The family is the central structure, with a clear differentiation between the roles of men and women. Religious dictates require that men financially support their wives and children and provide equally for them. Traditionally, men's roles focus on activities outside the home and women's roles focus on activities within the home, including the care of the children.

Multiple generations continue to live in the same household, with deference given to older family members. Vast changes have occurred in Middle Eastern cultures with the discovery of oil

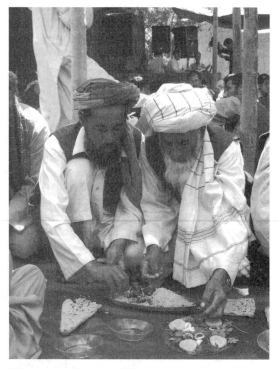

FIGURE 14.2 Men in the Middle East sharing a meal in close proximity. (Photo courtesy of Dan McLean.)

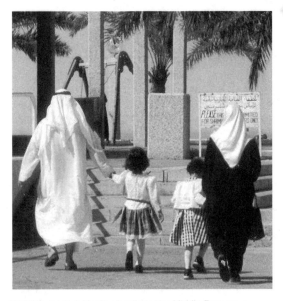

FIGURE 14.3 A Muslim family in the Middle East. (Photo courtesy of Elizabeth Dean.)

and economic growth, resulting in changed family dynamics and concern for the integrity of the nuclear and extended family structures and values. These changes cross two or three generations. Thus, as with most cultures, there is friction between parents and their children, and clashes between older, more traditional ways and more contemporary lifestyles.

Teenagers remain at home until they marry, which is usually in their young adulthood. A large proportion of men and women marry. Although less practiced today, polygamy persists. Divorce is permissible; however, divorced women have limited opportunities for remarriage. The rate of divorce is increasing. Unmarried women and couples without children are thought to live relatively unfulfilled lives based on Islamic doctrine, in which family is central. Unwed mothers are concealed by the family and may be sent out of the country to have their children born and put up for adoption.

Although present in Islamic countries, homosexuality is not overt because it is considered aberrant. Some cultures turn a blind eye, whereas in others it is criminally punishable to the point of death. Because of this, homosexuality is stigmatizing for the individual and the family.[3,9]

Reflective Exercise

• What cultural adjustments to the West might an Islamic teenager (male or female) and his or her parents need to make? • How might this impact family relationships? • What if the male were gay or the female lesbian?

Workforce Issues

Education is highly valued and viewed as a means toward an autonomous professional or business career, particularly for men in the Middle East, Arab, and Islamic cultures. Commonly, families have businesses that have been run by the family for generations. Although women have primary responsibilities with family and children, attending university has become increasingly acceptable for them (Fig. 14-4). In moderate Islamic countries, an increasing number of women are earning professional credentials as preparation for entry to the workforce. Today, a high proportion of women are enrolled in universities in the Middle East and a growing number of women are assuming nontraditional professions (Fig. 14-5). People from the Middle East who immigrate to Western countries tend to be well educated and pursue professional and business careers.[10]

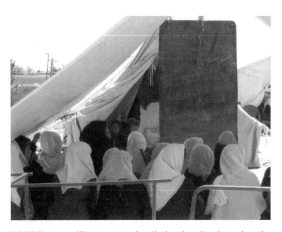

FIGURE 14.4 Women pursuing their education in a class in Afghanistan. (Photo courtesy of Elizabeth Dean.)

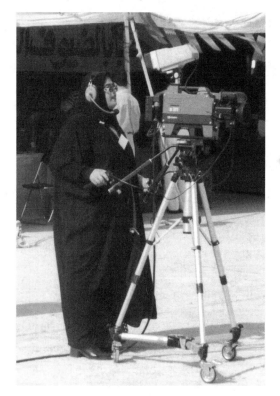

FIGURE 14.5 A woman who is Muslim in a nontraditional role in the workplace. (Photo courtesy of Elizabeth Dean.)

The wealthier Arabic and Islamic countries have large numbers of immigrants from neighboring countries who seek employment opportunities. Thus, labor, unskilled, and blue-collar jobs such as maids and drivers are filled by immigrants. White-collar and professional occupations are typically filled by the economically privileged indigenous population as well as educated expatriates.

With increased migration of people from around the world, physical therapy education programs need to include course content on cultural competence so that healthcare providers can treat patients effectively without jeopardizing internationally accepted professional standards and ethics. Physical therapy programs in the Middle East and the West may benefit from the inclusion of Islamic content and perspectives on health.

Physical therapy is a profession whose advances tend to reflect Western attitudes, beliefs, and values. As a profession that advocates largely noninvasive interventions, physical therapy exploits education and exercise, its primary "drugs," in the management of a wide range of conditions. Education is predicated on the value of perceived control. Muslims ascribe ultimate control to God and little to themselves.

Reflective Exercise

• Physical therapy education programs worldwide are modeled largely after Western programs, which have become the internationally recognized standard. How might such programs at home and in Islamic countries be modified to enhance the cultural relevance and sensitivity of their academic and clinical instruction without compromising internationally recognized practice standards?

Biocultural Ecology

The Middle Eastern countries have been influenced by migration from the Indian subculture and Africa. The Islamic world is vast and ranges to the north, south, east, and west; this contributes to a wide range of physical features, including eye color and shape, shape of the nose, hair color and texture, bone structure, and skin tones. Many people in Iran have fair skin and red hair. Distinctions made between Muslims based on these features vary from country to country. Thus, the appearance of the people ranges across the diversity of attributes common to the people of Egypt, India, and Africa.

In the oil-rich Middle Eastern countries, the leading causes of nonaccidental morbidity and mortality reflect the "diseases of civilization" that are epidemic in Western industrialized countries.[11-13] These conditions include heart disease, smoking-related lung disease, hypertension and stroke, diabetes, and cancer. The poorer Middle Eastern countries are afflicted with poor maternal and child health, poor nutrition, and infectious and parasitic diseases and illnesses. Compared with the West, the Middle East has higher rates of tuberculosis, hepatitis, typhoid fever, and dysentery. Outbreaks of cholera and hepatitis occur sporadically. Other conditions common in this region include sickle cell anemia and thalassemia. Congenital disorders are common due to marriage of close relatives, including first cousins, and women bearing children up until menopause.

The Middle East has been a region of political instability for many years. This is not without cost to the health of the people. Several countries have suffered internal strife, and others have been subjected to outside invasion, such as the state of Kuwait in the early 1990s. The long-term physical and psychosocial effects of the Gulf War on the residents of Kuwait are gradually becoming apparent. Chronic tension in Israel is taking its toll on the health of younger generations, who have never known peace.

Reflective Exercise

• Assuming you do not come from an Islamic culture, consider the relationship between socioeconomic status and lifestyle in your own culture. What similarities and differences do you observe between your culture and Middle Eastern and Islamic cultures?

Reflective Exercise

• Consider the impact of chronic political unrest and the threat of invasion on an individual's health. How might you investigate this potential impact on a patient's current complaint?

High-Risk Behaviors

With wealth in the Middle Eastern countries has come tobacco, fast food with poor nutritional quality, motorized vehicles, and inactivity and sedentary living. Although smoking is prohibited in the Islamic faith,[14] tobacco smoking continues to be socially sanctioned throughout the Middle East, and its prevalence there is among the highest in the world. Tobacco control and public awareness of health risks are in their infancy. The smoking of *sheesha* pipes is a long-standing social

tradition when men congregate in the evenings; however, the prevalence of *sheesha* pipe and cigarette smoking by women is believed to be increasing. Egypt and Syria are Islamic countries where women can be seen smoking *sheesha* pipes in cafes. Statistics on the smoking habits of women are more difficult to record because women's activities are home based and more private.

Reflective Exercise

• The American Physical Therapy Association has a strong position statement on smoking and smoking cessation. How would you reconcile the social acceptance of smoking by many individuals from the Middle East with your professional and ethical responsibility to inform patients of its undesirability and health hazards?

Alcohol and recreational drugs are also forbidden under Islamic law. Alcohol, however, is legally accessible in a few Muslim countries. Use of illegal drugs often leads to harsh punishment, including the death sentence in more fundamentalist countries such as Saudi Arabia. With respect to nutrition, the Qur'an dictates moderation in food consumption.

Social change has lagged behind technological change, particularly in the wealthy Arab countries. Wealth has led to the ownership not only of multiple vehicles per household, but also of fast, luxury vehicles, which has resulted in road accidents being a primary cause of death in the oil-rich countries. Community centers offering exercise programs do not exist, yet gyms and health clubs are becoming more common, particularly in the wealthier Islamic countries.

Vehicular accidents are a leading cause of death due to driving at high speeds, low rates of seatbelt and helmet use, and unpredictable driving habits. The incidence of HIV infection and AIDS is increasing in Islamic countries just as it is everywhere else in the world. Islam, like other religions, has been an important form of social control, particularly regarding sexuality issues. However, the taboos in this area have created a challenge to the development of public awareness campaigns and open discussion about this important social health concern.

Reflective Exercise

• Qur'anic teachings are consistent with the promotion of good health (see the Amman Declaration published by the WHO in 1989[15]). How might this knowledge be helpful to the Western physical therapist in planning and implementing a wellness or treatment program for a Muslim?

Nutrition

In many Middle Eastern countries, food is plentiful. However, in poor rural areas of Islamic countries such as Afghanistan, Iran, Iraq, and those in northern Africa, nutritional problems and even starvation can be seen. Avoidance of excess and allowing one meal to digest before beginning the next are traditionally valued in Islamic cultures.[15] With wealth in the oil-rich countries, obesity associated with hypertension and diabetes has become epidemic. A shift from the indigenous, simple diet of a nomadic people to food choices associated with wealth and affluence includes increases in animal saturated fats, sugar, refined foods, and meats and a reduction in fiber. These food choices, which are becoming culturally engrained, are irrefutably associated with the "diseases of civilization," namely heart disease, smoking-related lung disease, high blood pressure and stroke, diabetes, obesity, and cancers[11-13] (Fig. 14-6).

Western fast food chains are thriving in the Middle East. Strict Muslims do not eat pork, and animals for food need to be slaughtered in a ritualistic manner, *halal*. In traditional settings, eating utensils are not used and food is eaten with the right hand, which is not used for toileting. A Muslim family would consider it impolite not to have excess food on hand when entertaining visitors.

Reflective Exercise

• How would the increased social desirability and acceptability of both excess food and rich food choices impact your therapeutic relationship with a patient who is Muslim in the domain of health education?

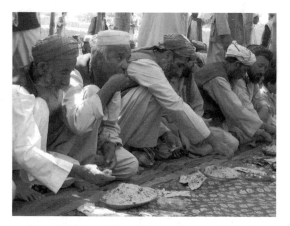

FIGURE 14.6 A Middle Eastern meal. (Photo courtesy of Dan McLean.)

Reflective Exercise

• Describe some ways you might consider promoting healthier eating practices in conjunction with an exercise program for a Muslim family.

Pregnancy and Childbearing Practices

Because the family is highly valued, so is fertility. Women who are unable to bear children are at risk of being divorced. Infertility can be treated legitimately in Islamic countries through artificial insemination and *in vitro* fertilization. Child adoption is rare. Although not discussed openly, birth control appears to be practiced, given the smaller family sizes compared with previous decades. Abortion is not permitted unless the mother's health is endangered.

Pregnancy and childbearing practices have become Westernized, and most children in the wealthier Middle Eastern countries are born in a hospital. In the rural and poorer regions, however, many children are born at home, with a high risk of infant mortality. Based on regional customs, following the birth of the child, the mother and child usually stay with the grandmother for a month before the mother returns home and assumes her spousal and household responsibilities. In terms of postpartum support, Muslim women receive considerable physical and emotional support from their families.

Reflective Exercise

• As a physical therapist, how could you use the cultural support system established for a Muslim woman by her family after the birth of her child, with respect to designing and implementing a reconditioning program for her?

Death Rituals

The Islamic perspective on health and illness incorporates the notion of receiving illness and death with patience, meditation, and prayers. Illness, suffering, and dying are viewed as a part of life and a test from Allah.[16] Muslims consider an illness atonement for one's sins and a means of knowing God;[17,18] death is a part of a journey to meet God.[19-21] Nevertheless, seeking care and treatment when one is ill is encouraged.[16]

For a Muslim, death is the transition from an earthly to a higher form of existence.[22] The daily prayers become more important during times of suffering. Patients are encouraged by their families to continue to pray as long as possible.[22] The conscious, dying patient may wish to face Mecca, the holy city in Saudi Arabia. Family and friends will recite passages from the Qur'an and pray for the patient's welfare in the life to come.[22] If no family members are available, the local Muslim community can provide religious comfort to the patient.

After death, the body should not be cut or harmed because it belongs to God.[23] Unless required by law, a postmortem examination is not performed.[21] The family may wish to perform after-death care of the body.[23] There are rituals for washing the body, cutting the hair of the deceased, shrouding the body, giving condolences, visiting the grave, and mourning.[24,25] The mourning period lasts several days for friends and relatives, and longer—up to several months—for closer family members, particularly a wife mourning the loss of her husband. Women traditionally wear black throughout the mourning period.

Reflective Exercise

• What role do you believe a physical therapist might have in providing supportive care to a Muslim patient who is dying?

Spirituality

Islam is a religion that pervades daily life and is based on the teachings and writings of the prophet Muhammad.[26,27] Muslims believe there is one God, Allah, and Muhammad is His prophet. The Qur'an, written in Arabic, consists of the messages from God given to Muhammad. Muslims celebrate Friday as their holy day. After the noon prayer, they usually gather as a family for picnics or outings. There are two primary schools of Islam, Sunnis and Shiites. Sunnis make up 85% of the Muslim population worldwide. The Shiites and Sunnis differ on many issues related to doctrine and practice. Iran is currently the only country that is predominantly Shiite.

There are five pillars of faith in Islam:[28]

1. The profession of faith. There is no God but Allah, and Muhammad is His messenger.
2. Prayer five times daily at specified times. The shortest prayer is 5 minutes before sunrise, and the longest prayer is in the evening, an hour after sunset, and is 20 minutes long. The daily prayers are conducted with the individual facing the holy city of Mecca. Prayer is the ceremonial recitation of prescribed words in Arabic accompanied by different body positions from standing to kneeling, to kneel-sitting, to prone kneeling with the head to the floor (prostrating in humility and adoration of the Creator). Individuals stop working during the day to pray privately in their offices or to go to a local mosque (Figs. 14-7 and 14-8). Mosques are prevalent so that people, mostly men, do not have to travel far. Women tend to pray at home or privately. To enter the mosque, the house of prayer, shoes must be removed and the feet washed. When women enter mosques, their heads and arms must be covered. Regardless of whether an individual prays at the mosque or elsewhere, prayer for a

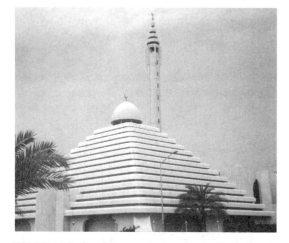

FIGURE 14.7 A contemporary mosque that calls Muslims to pray five times a day. (Photo courtesy of Dan McLean.)

Muslim requires facing Mecca, the holy city in Saudi Arabia where the *Hajj*, or pilgrimage, takes place. A Muslim can pray anywhere. A street worker or fisherman, for example, may be unable to reach a mosque, so he may pray at the side of the road or on the boat. Although a non-Arab who has converted to Islam may not understand the rote recitations from the Qur'an, it is believed that the recitation is understood by God, and this is what matters.

3. Fasting during the month of Ramadan. The timing of Ramadan is based on the lunar calendar, and Ramadan begins 10 days earlier each successive year. During Ramadan, eating, drinking fluids (including water), smoking, and sexual intercourse are prohibited from dawn to dusk. During this month, Muslims focus on obedience to God, self-sacrifice, gratitude to God, compassion for the needy, and rest.[29] Lactating or menstruating women, sick people, and travelers are exempt from fasting.[29] Instead these individuals fast at another time during the year or give alms to the poor. Additional prayers are not obligatory during Ramadan; rather, 20 passages from the Qur'an are recited repeatedly throughout the month.

4. Giving alms to the poor, *Zakat*. The prescribed amount is 2.5% of a person's wealth each year.

5. *Hajj*, a pilgrimage to Mecca during one's lifetime. This pilgrimage is made 70 days after Ramadan. Although not all Muslims are able to experience *Hajj*, everyone is encouraged to do so.

Reflective Exercise

• You are treating a Muslim patient in an outpatient clinic. You learn that Ramadan begins next week. What factors will you consider for the continuation of treatment during this month?

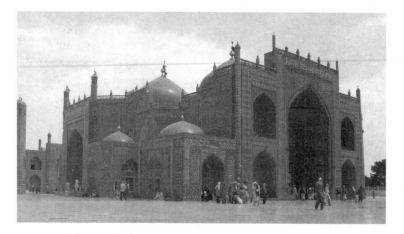

FIGURE 14.8 Elaborate mosque with great significance. (Photo courtesy of Dan McLean.)

The Islamic tradition requiring women to veil is practiced to divert the attention of men. This tradition is instituted before puberty. The decision for a woman to cover when in public is usually one made by the family, her husband, and herself. Some women do not wear a scarf, or *hijab*. Others wear the *hijab* in addition to having their outer clothing covered in public with a black *abbaya*. The *abbaya* covers the woman from head to foot, including the head and hair. Some women extend the covering to conceal the face and eyes with mesh fabric (the *burqa*) and wear gloves.

Reflective Exercise

• What are some questions that would be useful to include in the assessment and evaluation of someone of Arabic descent who is a Muslim regarding their religious beliefs and customs? • Why did you select these questions?

Healthcare Practices

Until several decades ago, when the people of the Middle Eastern countries practiced more nomadic lifestyles, they engaged in more daily physical activity and ate a basic but healthy diet. Healthcare was the responsibility of traditional healers and bonesetters. These healers continue to practice. Although Western-based medical care has become prevalent, particularly in the urban areas, traditional practices are still used. Passive treatments such as drugs and surgery and treatment with thermal and electrotherapy modalities are often perceived as having greater efficacy than noninvasive interventions. Some patients may feel that they have not been adequately treated unless some form of modality has been applied, drugs prescribed, or surgery scheduled. In Arabic and Islamic cultures, wellness and health promotion are not commonly understood or valued concepts.[30] Also, the effect of stress on health and psychosocial interventions are less prevalent concepts (Fig. 14-9).

People of Arabic descent usually express pain more freely than Westerners.[31] Most regard pain as unpleasant and something to be controlled

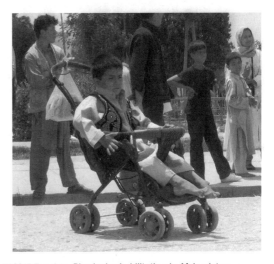

FIGURE 14.9 Physical rehabilitation in Afghanistan. (Photo courtesy of Dan McLean.)

externally. They may expect, for example, immediate postoperative relief of pain to be provided. Expressive, emotional, and vocal responses to pain, however, are usually reserved for the immediate family in situations such as childbirth and other potentially painful conditions. Additionally, pain may be expressed more freely in the presence of family as opposed to healthcare professionals. Thus, complete pain assessments are essential.

Attitudes toward blood transfusions and organ donation and transplantation vary not only on a personal basis but also from country to country in the Middle East and across the Arab and Islamic worlds.[32] Blood is donated most often by the expatriate population of Middle Eastern countries. Blood transfusions are usually accepted by Muslims. With respect to organ transplantation, the body is viewed as sacred and belonging to God, so that significant tampering with it is forbidden. However, with changing views, transplantation is becoming more accepted.

Reflective Exercise

• What questions would you need to ask a Muslim patient being treated postoperatively in a hospital in order to provide culturally sensitive and appropriate treatment?

Barriers to healthcare in North America experienced by Arabs and Muslims are frequently related to communication and expectations. A physical examination in Arabic and Islamic countries may involve little clothing removal or physical contact between the healthcare provider and patient. With gender segregation practices in Islamic countries, men and women may prefer same-gender healthcare practitioners. Being treated in the conventional open areas of physical therapy clinics in the presence of both sexes may be uncomfortable for both Muslim men and women. In addition, Muslims vary in their level of comfort with being treated by a healthcare practitioner of the opposite gender and disrobing for that individual. Some Muslims, women and men, will require a same-gender clinician. For a woman, disrobing in an open private practice treatment area or hospital outpatient department may be a concern. Some Muslim women require total privacy with the assurance of no possibility of being viewed by a man, even inadvertently.

Reflective Exercise

• A Muslim patient is referred to you for management of a neck injury from a car accident. How might you need to modify management for a male patient versus a woman?

With more relaxed attitudes toward appointment times throughout the Middle East, patients who are immigrants may be unaware of the tightly scheduled appointment slots in the West and may miss or run late with appointments. Thus, if time is a factor, the physical therapist must carefully explain the importance of punctuality. In their home countries, some Muslims and Arabs may be accustomed to exerting power and influence for themselves or family members to be put ahead on a waiting list and be seen immediately by the practitioner. One's socioeconomic status, which is often linked to one's family's status and ranking in society, provides one with certain rights and privileges in Middle Eastern countries. Waiting in a queue when one comes from a high-ranking family is not common in the Middle East. Explain the custom of waiting in line in the United States.

Treatment times may need to be scheduled

around prayer times and exclude Friday, the holy day. In Islamic countries, the weekend is Thursday and Friday, with Saturday and Sunday being regular weekdays. Attending a clinic for treatment may be less feasible for a Muslim during Ramadan because of fasting requirements (both food and water) and extra time for prayer and family. Also, because social gatherings may go throughout the night, Muslims may be short of sleep during Ramadan.

Self-responsibility as a means of effecting changes in health behavior is a strategy increasingly used in the West and advocated in Islamic countries. The World Health Organization has published the Amman Declaration on Health Promotion.[15] This declaration reflects a consensus of some 50 Islamic scholars on health-related issues and Qur'anic teaching. The declaration's recommendations promote illness and disease prevention based on the Islamic premise that your body is a gift from God for which you are responsible. Thus, an effective education strategy for Muslim patients is to focus on how following certain health recommendations will enable the individual to better serve God and the family.

Reflective Exercise

• How can the doctrines of Islam be used to promote good health? • What are some challenges of the doctrines of Islam to health promotion and to the practice of contemporary physical therapy?

Islamic countries are associated with a higher power distance between certain echelons of society, including health professionals. Thus, professionals tend to have a high position of power ascribed to them. In this case, patients expect to play a minor role in deciding what they have and what should be done, which are viewed as the doctor's responsibilities. Given the more relaxed way of life in Middle Eastern countries, however, the patient may not feel obliged to follow the physical therapist's instructions at home if he or she does not agree with them.

Exercising in public (for example, walking and running) may be an inappropriate option, particularly for women. Strategies need to be worked out that are culturally sensitive and acceptable for each patient. Health education and recommendations for the home program need to be tailored to the values as well as the needs of the patient; otherwise the recommendations will not be followed.

In Islamic countries, public exercise facilities are designed and used by boys and men. Boys and men also swim in the ocean. Women may accompany their children to the beach and, at most, sit in the water in their *abayas*. In some countries, women may be seen together for daily walks. Those who are accustomed to wearing the *hijab* and *abaya* will wear these while walking publicly.

Reflective Exercise

• You need to prescribe an exercise program for a patient who is Muslim. What factors would you take into consideration for a female patient versus a male patient?

The family of a hospitalized person is expected to be at the bedside. Many visitors and friends come to show their concern because visiting the sick is considered a good deed. Traditionally, the family provides spiritual care and support. Because the Qur'an encourages direct supplication for healing, the family may recite or read from the Qur'an.[29] However, if the patient is from another Islamic country, the family and friends can serve an important role in communicating with the patient. A large family and many friends in the patient's room can make provision of care difficult.

Reflective Exercise

• The Intensive Care Unit has made special provision for an Islamic patient to be in a private room in order to accommodate several relatives at the bedside. You need to mobilize the patient; however, the room is very crowded. How will you proceed?

As with other cultures, the attitudes, beliefs, and values of an individual in an Islamic culture have a major impact on that individual's health, wellness, and reactions to being unwell. There are wide differences in Arabic and Islamic countries regarding the degree to which traditional healers such as bonesetters practice, and the degree of Westernization in medical practice.

Healthcare Practitioners

Despite discussion of the Arabization of medical education in Arab countries in recent years, medical practice throughout the Middle East is largely based on a Western model. The proposition that an individual can control his or her health and influence ill health may not be shared by those Muslims who attribute what happens in life strictly to the will of Allah.

The Bedouin people of Middle Eastern countries tend to live in rural areas and to be less educated than other indigenous peoples. Also, they use traditional healers and bonesetters more often. An understanding of traditional healing may identify means by which contemporary physical therapy may fuse with traditional practices to make it more acceptable to certain patients without jeopardizing standards of practice and ethics.

Physical therapy is a developing profession in many Middle Eastern countries. Schools of physical therapy exist in Egypt, Iran, Kuwait, Saudi Arabia, and the United Arab Emirates. Physical therapists practice largely on referrals from physicians. In addition to this limitation to practice, the profession of physical therapy and its capacity to prevent, cure, and treat physical dysfunction both medically and surgically are apparently not as widely understood by the medical community in Middle Eastern countries as in many Western countries in which physical therapists have direct access to patients. Physical therapists are perceived as having lower status than physicians.

Reflective Exercise

• Establishing a Muslim patient's expectations of the provision of physical therapy is an important initial step in being able to treat this individual effectively. How would you establish a patient's expectations?

Healthcare professionals are of both genders, with the exception of nurses, who are primarily women in the Middle East. Given gender segregation, which varies from one Islamic country to the next depending on the level of orthodoxy, men tend to treat men, and women tend to treat women. One exception is in critical care. However, considerable variation exists, even among hospitals within a single Islamic country.

Reflective Exercise

• You are a female physical therapist. Your next patient is from Iran and requests a male therapist. How would you respond to his request?

Conclusion

The physical therapist needs to consider multiple cultural factors when treating a person who is Muslim, either in the West or when working abroad. Depending on the country and the socioeconomic status of the individual in the native country, literacy and language will vary. An interpreter may be needed, as well as translations of health education materials and home programs. In addition to conventional components, the assessment should include an overview of the patient's attitudes, beliefs, and values regarding his or her health and about the nature of the current problem, its remediation, and views of physical therapy. The assessment must identify cultural factors in the individual's history and background that will facilitate treatment and those that may be challenges. The physical therapist needs to establish compatibility with respect to the gender of the Muslim patient he or she is treating, an appropriate interpersonal distance, and a degree of eye contact and touching that the patient is comfortable with. The patient's expectations need to be identified, and the physical therapist needs to clearly define what her or his expectations are. To minimize miscommunication regarding scheduled appointments, the physical therapist may need to explain the scheduling system and the risk of missing an appointment or having a shortened treatment if the patient fails to arrive promptly. Interpersonal factors that build trust and rapport are integral to ensure that home programs and recommendations are followed, and to guarantee the overall success of the physical therapy treatment.

Reflective Exercise

• You are relocating your private practice to a neighborhood in a major North American city with a large Middle Eastern population. What factors might you need to consider in terms of designing the physical space to accommodate the needs of your Muslim patients? • What clinical considerations will your staff need to consider to provide culturally sensitive and congruent care?

CASE STUDY SCENARIO

Nadyah Al-Mohannah, a Muslim of Arabic descent, was born in the Middle East. She is 37 years old and the mother of four children ranging in age from 3 to 15 years. She immigrated to the United States after high school to study, and she earned a university degree before she married. She met her husband, also from the Middle East, in the United States, where they continue to live as citizens. Nadyah and her family are devout Muslims. She prays regularly, observes Ramadan, and wears a *hijab* outside the home.

Nadyah has been overweight since adolescence and has gained more weight after the birth of each child. Her weight is now 160 pounds. Her husband has been making remarks about her weight gain, which is a concern to her. Given her height, her body mass index is 34 (the ideal range is 20 to 25). She was diagnosed with high blood pressure at the time of the birth of her first child. She has been inconsistent in taking the "water pills." Her blood pressure at a recent medical checkup was 158/105 mm Hg. Her heart rate was 95 bpm.

Five years ago, Nadyah was diagnosed with type II diabetes. She was not surprised because her mother and aunt have long histories of type II diabetes. In her home country, Nadyah's relatives go to the hospital daily for insulin injections. Currently, Nadyah's physician is attempting to control her diabetes with hypoglycemic medications but believes she will require insulin if her blood sugar is not controlled within the next couple of months.

Nadyah was referred to you recently because she strained her back after lifting her youngest child. This problem began gradually some years ago. She has become particularly concerned about her health because she and her husband would like another child. The combination of excessive weight and inactive lifestyle increases the probability of symptoms related to chronic degenerative conditions, which will reduce her quality of life. With optimal nutrition, weight control, and regular exercise, she could lose weight, become normotensive, and reverse her diabetes, as well as eliminate or reduce her back complaints. Without effecting a lifestyle correction, this patient will have a markedly increased risk of heart disease, stroke, and cancer. Further, in the presence of obesity with its associated problems, Nadyah's risk of complications from minor illnesses or from routine medical procedures or surgery is significantly increased. Her back pain can be thought of as a secondary concern that interferes with the primary objective of her developing an active lifestyle and reducing the risk of succumbing to one or more diseases of civilization.

Prior to the formal part of the assessment, you take time to interact with Nadyah on a personal level. You learn about her family and that she is a Muslim. You learn that she prays regularly and that she and her family observe Ramadan. You also learn that Ramadan begins in six weeks, and that she and her family will return to the Middle East during this time. On further questioning you learn that Nadyah is particularly distressed because her back is preventing her from positioning herself to pray. There is also concern about her ability to sit during the long flight.

You observe her comfort with eye contact and interpersonal distance. You ask questions to learn about her level of comfort with being treated by you, her comfort with the open physical space in the clinic, and her need for use of the private examination room. In addition to the conventional assessment for her back complaint and vital signs, you establish that Nadyah is highly motivated to make some changes in her lifestyle so that she can safely have another child.

In the assessment and evaluation, you specify that she is well educated and that she has good English literacy skills—speaking, understanding, and reading. Further, her preferred learning style is verbal and experiential as opposed to written. With follow-up questioning, you confirm that she understands the relationship between the lifestyle of the mother and the health of her unborn child. Because of this, you review with her health education publications from the American Physical Therapy Association, the American Diabetes Association, and the U.S. Surgeon General.

To connect with her value system, you inquire about the health status, weight, and activity levels of her children and husband. You learn that the children tend to be heavier than they should be (according to Western standards), spending several hours every day using the computer and watching television. Additionally, they like to go to fast food restaurants. You discuss with Nadyah how she might best implement a healthy lifestyle within the context of her personal religious beliefs, traditions, and customs.

(continued)

Case Study Scenario Continued

Only one child, a son, participates actively in school sports. You learn that her daughters wear scarves and have been less actively involved with exercise and sports. Although you can provide exercise recommendations for Nadyah's children, including the girls, Nadyah herself is not keen to exercise as a family with her children, particularly in the presence of men.

1. What are the potential barriers to Nadyah's achieving an optimal level of health?

2. How might you help convert the apparent barriers into challenges?

3. What facilitators of optimal health are present and how might you incorporate them effectively into the physical therapy program?

4. How might you explain the importance of exercise and good nutrition and help Nadyah consider lifestyle changes while respecting her culture and values?

5. What modifications in her program might be needed during Ramadan?

6. How would you structure health education materials for Nadyah's specific needs given her cultural heritage and traditional beliefs?

7. List the short-term and long-term goals you would recommend for Nadyah. How might you ensure that they are culturally appropriate and acceptable to her?

REFERENCES

1. Purnell LD, Paulanka BJ, eds. *Transcultural Health Care: A Culturally Competent Approach*. Philadelphia, Pa: FA Davis; 2003.

2. CIA. Factbook: Indonesia. Available at: http://www.cia.gov/cia/publications/factbook/geos/id.html#Intro. Accessed May 27, 2004.

3. Kulwicki A. (2003). People of Arab heritage. In: Purnell L, Paulanka B, eds. *Transcultural Health Care: A Culturally Competent Approach.* 2nd ed. Philadelphia, Pa: FA Davis; 2003:90–106.

4. Power P, Joseph N, Rhodes S. The New Islam. *Newsweek.* March 16, 1998;131:34–37.

5. McKennis A. Caring for the Islamic patient. *J Assoc Oper Room Nurs.* 1999;69:1187–1196.

6. Blank J. The Muslim mainstream. *US News World Rep.* July 20, 1998;125:22–25.

7. Lawrence P, Rormus C. Culturally sensitive care of the Muslim patient. *J Transcult Nurs.* 2001;12:228–233.

8. Daneshpour M. Muslim families and family therapy *J Marital Fam Ther.* 1998;24:355–390.

9. Hafizi O, Lipson J. People of Iranian heritage. In: Purnell L, Paulanka B, eds. *Transcultural Health Care: A Culturally Competent Approach.* 2nd ed. Philadelphia, Pa: FA Davis; 2003:177–194.

10. Zogby J. *Arab America Today: A Demographic Profile of Arab Americans.* Washington, DC: Arab American Institute; 1990.

11. World Health Organization. Annual health report, 1999. Available at: http://www.google.com/u/who?q=annual+report+1999&sa=Go&sitesearch=who.int&domains=who.int. Accessed December 14, 2003.

12. World Health Organization. Annual health report, 2000. Available at: http://www.google.com/u/who?q=annual+report+2000&sa=Go&sitesearch=who.int&domains=who.int. Accessed December 14, 2003.

13. World Health Organization. Annual health report, 2001. Available at: http://www.who.int/whr/en/. Accessed December 14, 2003.

14. World Health Organization. Islamic ruling on smoking. Available at: http://www.google.com/u/who?q=Islamic+Ruling+on+Smoking&sa=Go&sitesearch=who.int&domains=who.int. Accessed December 14, 2003.

15. World Health Organization. Amman Declaration on Health Promotion. Available at: http://www.emro.who.int/Publications/HealthEdReligion/AmmanDeclaration/Chapter2.htm. Accessed December 14, 2003.

16. Rassool GH. The crescent and Islam: Healing, nursing and the spiritual dimension. Some considerations towards an understanding of the Islamic perspectives on caring. *J Adv Nurs.* 2000;32:1476–1484.

17. Al-Ghazzali M. *The Mysteries of Fasting.* Lahore, Pakistan: Ashraf Press; 1968.

18. Al-Ghazzali M. *The Mysteries of Purity.* Lahore, Pakistan: Ashraf Press; 1970.

19. Athar S. *Islamic Perspectives in Medicine. A Survey of Islamic Medicine: Achievements and Contemporary Issues.* Indianapolis, Ind: American Trust; 1993.

20. Athar S. *Information for Health Care Providers When Dealing with a Muslim Patient.* Chicago, Ill: Islamic Medical Association of North America; 1998.

21. Athar S. Information for health care providers when dealing with a Muslim patient. Available at: http://www.islam-usa.com. Accessed December 2, 2003.

22. Sheikh A. Death and dying—A Muslim perspective. *J R Soc Med.* 1998;91:138–140.

23. Green J. Death with dignity: Islam. *Nurs Times.* 1989;85:56–57.

24. As-Sayyid S. *FIQH us-SUNNAH. Funerals and Dhikr. IV.* Jaddah, Saudi Arabia: International Islamic Publishing House; 1991.

25. Bin Abdul-Aziz al-Musnad M. *Fatwa Islamiyah. Islamic Verdicts from the Noble Scholars: Shayk Abdul-Aziz bin Abullah bin Baz; Shaykh Muhammad bin Salih Al-Uthaimin and Shaykh Abdulla bin Abdur-Rahman Al-Jibreen along with the Permanent Committee and Decisions of the Fiqh Council. Darussalam.* Riyadh, Saudi Arabia: Global Leaders in Islamic Books; 2002.

26. Abdalati H. *Islam in Focus.* Indianapolis, Ind: American Trust; 1975.

27. Farah CE. *Islam.* 6th ed. New York, NY: Barron's; 2000.

28. Ahmed A. *Discovering Islam: Making Sense of Muslim History and Society.* Boston, Mass: Routledge Kegan Paul; 1988.

29. Ali N. Providing culturally sensitive care to Egyptians with cancer. *Cancer Pract.* 1996;4:212–215

30. Kulwicki A, Miller J, Schim S. Collaborative partnership for culture care: Enhancing health services for the Arab community. *J Transcult Nurs.* 2000;11:31–39.

31. Reizian A, Meleis A. Arab-Americans' perception of and responses to pain. *Crit Care Nurs.* 1986;6:30–37.

32. Ali Albar M. *Contemporary Topics in Islamic Medicine.* Jeddah, Saudi Arabia: Saudi Publishing & Distributing House; 1995.

chapter 5

Cultural Considerations for Jewish Clients

● Ronnie Leavitt, PhD, MPH, PT

M rs. Bertha Epstein, age 67 years, practices Orthodox Judaism and is very active in her synagogue. She lives in Brooklyn, New York, with her husband of 47 years. Her children and grandchildren live within walking distance of her home. Recently her long-standing osteoarthritis has been giving her so much pain that she cannot comfortably complete her community responsibilities and personal activities of daily living. A visit to the physician is scheduled for next week. Passover is next month.

This chapter provides an overview of Jewish principles and laws as they relate to life's daily practices and health-related decisions. As a physical therapist concerned with cultural competence, one needs a basic understanding of how individuals define their Jewishness; and if they are religious, how does religion influence their worldview and daily practices as well as their interaction with the healthcare system? Generally speaking, the more orthodox Jewish people are in their religious outlook, the more literal and faithful they are in interpreting the word of God, as put forth in the Hebrew Bible (*Torah*), the *Talmud* (the oral tradition), and the consultation of Jewish scholars and rabbis. In any case, the physical therapist will need to respect and adhere to the religious practices of the client and family in order to be culturally competent.

Overview/Heritage

As with all cultural groups identified in this book, it is impossible to speak about a group with one voice because the group members vary according to the primary and secondary characteristics of culture (see Chapter 1). For some, Judaism is a religion. For many, however, being Jewish is a personal and group identity having more to do with culture, ethnicity, and a secular lifestyle than with religion. It may be a "way of life." Part of understanding modern Jewish identity is knowledge of the different Jewish subcultures. Judaism, as a religion, has three main branches: Orthodox, Conservative, and Reform. Within each of these, further intracultural diversity is prominent. There is also a strong secular movement within Judaism, that is, Jews who identify as being Jewish but do not practice an organized religion. If the physical therapist is unfamiliar with the Jewish religion, he or she may benefit from first reading the section on spirituality in this chapter to obtain an overview of the three major branches of Judaism.

Also relevant, especially with regard to the incidence and prevalence of diseases and cultural habits, is one's identity as an Ashkenazi Jew or Sephardic Jew. During the Middle Ages two geographically based communities of European Judaism developed: the Sephardic and the Ashkenazic. Today, Ashkenazi Jews make up 82% of the world's Jewish population.[1] About 90–95% of American Jews are Ashkenazic,[2] with ancestors primarily from Germany, Eastern Europe, and Russia; the smaller group of Sephardic Jews are mostly from Spain, North Africa, the Middle East, and the Mediterranean area.[3]

To understand Jewish identity, one must realize that Jewish people are very sensitive to anti-Semitism. In maintaining their cultural identity and resisting assimilation, the Jewish people incurred the hostility of the Babylonians (Judaism was founded by Abraham in the pre-Babylonian city of Ur), the Greeks, and the Romans. The destruction of Jewish Jerusalem in 70 A.D. by the Romans led to the Diaspora of hundreds of thousand of Jews, primarily throughout the Mediterranean world, but also to northern Europe, the Middle East, and even Africa and India. These fragmented communities of Jews continued to resist cultural assimilation. This contributed to the expulsion of Jews from countries such as Spain, Portugal, and Italy or to their confinement to ghettos in countries such as Germany, Poland, and Russia. The most egregious example of anti-Semitism was the Holocaust of World War II, where more than 6 million Jews and others from discriminated groups were exterminated. Some in contemporary society may assimilate into the mainstream culture without being signaled out as part of a historically persecuted minority. For others, it is nothing short of an imperative to maintain a strong Jewish identity.

The desire to return to a "Biblical homeland" and to escape anti-Semitism has contributed to the expansion of the Zionist movement. This secular political movement, calling for the resettlement of the dispersed Jewish world population, began in earnest with the destruction of the Ottoman Empire following World War I and led to the founding of the Jewish state of Israel in 1948 (Fig. 15-1). Most Jewish people have a strong connection to Israel, although there is considerable disagreement concerning Israeli politics. By definition, the word *Israel* refers to all Jews throughout the world.

Residence

People of Jewish heritage are a "minority" group within the United States, making up approximately 2% of the population. Thus, some American physical therapists have little knowledge of, or interaction with, people who identify as Jewish. In 1990 there were approximately 17.8 million Jews in the world, with 5.7 million in the United States, 3.5 million in Israel, 3.5 million in Europe, and 2.3 million in the Americas excluding the United States.[4]

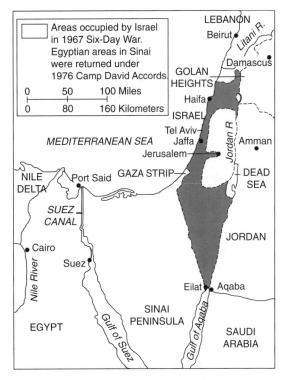

FIGURE 15.1 Map of Israel.

The 2000–2001 National Jewish Population Survey, sponsored by the United Jewish Communities,[5] the umbrella agency representing over 500 North American Jewish federations and communities, is by far the largest and most comprehensive ever conducted of North American Jews. Jews are concentrated in the Northeast (43%), with the West and South each having 22% and the Midwest having the smallest share, with 13%. Physical therapists are more likely to work with Jewish people in large cities such as New York, Los Angeles, or Chicago. However, there are pockets of Jews, including ultra-Orthodox Jews, in smaller cities and rural areas.

Eighty-five percent of adult Jews were born in the United States. The largest number of recent Jewish immigrants came from the former Soviet Union (44%), and they tend to settle on either the East or West Coast. Ten percent of Jewish immigrants come from Israel. For new Jewish immigrants, as with any new immigrant population, the degree of acculturation and the cultural way of life in the country of origin are significant considerations.

Reflective Exercise

• What is your level of familiarity with people of Jewish heritage? • Are you aware of any stereotypes when identifying Jewish people? • Do you know any Jewish immigrants who have come to the United States? • To what degree have they acculturated? • How do you respond when you hear Jewish people talk about the Holocaust? • What are your feelings when you hear about Israel in the news?

Education and Occupations

Education has always been an emphasized and respected value in Judaism. More than half, 55%, of Jews have a bachelor's degree, compared with 28% of the general population, and 24% have a graduate degree. The majority of employed Jews, 59%, work in management, business, and professional positions. Historically, Jews were barred from owning land or lending money. The median household income is slightly above the median income of all U.S. households ($50,000 compared

with $42,000). One-fifth (19%) of all Jewish households are low income, defined as $25,000 or less per year, compared with 29% of all U.S. households.[6]

Education is the most important variable with respect to health status. Of special significance is the fact that higher levels of education are associated with increased genetic counseling and screening.[2,7]

Jewish values reflect a love of family and the community. Spiritual and moral qualities are taught by example in the home. The synagogue is the most important Jewish institution outside of the family and is a cultural center as well as a place of worship.[2] Although the American value orientation toward individualism is strong among Jews, there is also a high value for collectivism when it comes to members of the Jewish family and community. A person's health and well-being are a concern to the community as a whole. The value of joyfulness, *simcha,* helps one to maintain a positive outlook toward life.

The Jewish people reflect a love for tradition. Jewish religious customs and health-related behaviors have always been intertwined. The Jewish religion and culture directly influence lifestyle behaviors that affect health. Examples include the practice of circumcision for a boy, a ritual bath for a woman, and death and funeral practices. Participating in a *minyan* (prayer group) is reported to increase one's sense of personal identity and self-esteem and to provide psychological support for someone in crisis.[8]

Reflective Exercise

• Have you observed the presence of Jewish values or traditions among your clients? • What values and traditions do you hold dear in your religion?

Communications

Dominant Language and Dialects

American Jews primarily speak English. Hebrew, part of the Semitic language family, is the official language of Israel, and it is the language used most often in religious rituals and prayers.

Hebrew uses a unique alphabet and is written from right to left; books are read from left to right as well. Yiddish is a Judeo-German dialect used by many first-generation Jews. Today, there is a resurgence of efforts to maintain the Yiddish heritage. Many Yiddish words have become common in the American English language, including *kvetch* (to complain a lot), *tush, tushie,* or *tuchus* (backside, buttocks), and *nosh* (to snack). Common Hebrew expressions include *l'chaim* (to life), *shalom* (peace), and *mazel tov* (congratulations), to name a few. There is more than one way to pronounce and spell many Jewish words. For example, the word to describe the period from sundown on Friday to sundown on Saturday may be *Shabbat* or *Shabbos.*

Cultural Communication Practices

Communication practices for Jewish people, to a large extent, depend on their personal style and American upbringing. There are no prohibitions against speaking freely and openly. Style tends to be informal and lively. Humor, as among other cultural groups, may be a way to alleviate a sense of pain and alienation. However, jokes that reinforce negative stereotypes or refer to the Holocaust are typically considered to be in poor taste.

Among the ultra-Orthodox, touching between a man and woman who are not married is not allowed. If a female physical therapist extends her hand for a handshake, an ultra-Orthodox male will not respond. As for temporality, most Jews balance remembering the past, enjoying the present, and planning for the future, as evidenced by their high regard for education. Punctuality is the norm for appointments and in business arrangements, but time commitments are more relaxed in social settings.

Reflective Exercise

• Do you notice a difference between your style of communication and that of your Jewish clients?
• Do your Jewish clients speak more directly and more quickly than the style to which you are accustomed? • Are you comfortable with these differences?

Family Roles and Organization

Head of Household and Gender Roles

In many respects, family roles and organization have been affected by Jewish law. Historically, Judaism developed in a patriarchal society, and the husband was viewed as the dominant figure. According to the *Talmud,* Jewish husbands are required to provide food, clothing, medical care for the family, and conjugal relations. They are prohibited from "beating their wives, forcing them to have sex, or restricting their free movement"[1] (p. 236).

Women are recognized for their role in the household; traditionally, they have generally run the home and are responsible for raising the children. The Jewish mother, a main theme in Jewish folklore and the media, is a source of strength. In modern times, particularly in the Conservative and Reform movements, men and women are generally considered equal partners. Certain restrictive rules remain for women in the Orthodox community. For example, in the Orthodox community, women are not allowed on the *bima* (the stage from which religious services emanate and the *Torah* is housed), and only men may become a *mohel,* the person who performs a circumcision on a newborn male child.[9] The Conservative and Reform movements will count women in a *minyan* (the quorum required to conduct a prayer service) and will ordain women as rabbis.

Reflective Exercise

• What is your opinion about the roles of men and women in religious life? • If you have been to a religious event at different synagogues, what differences do you observe between them?

Marriage is considered a sacred covenant, and a couple is expected to build a Jewish home, a place of serenity devoted to the performance of good deeds. The importance of a loving family and home is a cardinal principle of Judaism. Divorce is allowed.[10] "Mixed" marriages among people of different Jewish ideologies and between Jews and people of other religious faiths are common. The rate of intermarriage is of great concern to Jewish leaders both for "religious" reasons and for fear of a "vanishing Jewish population."

Developmental Tasks and Child Rearing Practices
Judaism values children as a blessing from God. Procreation is a "commandment" and adoption is considered equal to procreation: "Be fruitful and multiply" (Genesis 1:28). One of the fundamental tenets of Judaism is that every child is created pure. Also, each child is to be treated equally, including children with disabilities. The blessing of parenthood should be shared with the entire community, and the community shares in the responsibility of raising a child.[10]

Today, Jews are having fewer children, with a fertility rate of 1.8 children, than are needed to maintain the population (2.1). Fifty-two percent of Jewish women ages 30–34 have not had any children, compared with 27% of all American women. The median age of the Jewish population has risen from 37 to 41 years (compared with 35 for the total U.S. population), and over half are age 45 years or older. There are considerably more Jewish elders over 65 years than in the general population (19% vs. 12%) and 9% of the Jewish population are over 75 (vs. 6% of the total U.S. population). Children 17 years and younger make up 19% of the Jewish population, compared with 21% a decade ago and 26% for the general U.S. population.

Conservative and Reform Jews respect the rights of parents to use contraception and to determine how many children they should have.[10] For the Orthodox, contraception may be allowed if one has already fulfilled the commandment of procreation. Sterilization is forbidden for the Orthodox, except in cases where the paramount principle of saving a life comes into play.[11] Generally, due to the sanctity of life, abortion is supported in cases where the life or health of the mother is in danger; this takes precedence over protecting the fetus,[10] and a woman is forbidden to give her life in exchange for the life of her fetus.[12]

Emotional health is as important as physical health. The permissibility of abortion, when genetic disease or malformations are probable, is difficult to judge because abortion is permitted only if the mother is affected.[10] Concerning all matters of reproduction, for some Jews the memory of the Holocaust, the rate of intermarriage, and the low birth rate are reminders of the need to promote procreation.

Rituals and prayers are required for a Jewish child to be brought into the covenant (community) of the Jewish people. In a ceremony widely observed among all Jews, boys are circumcised by a ritual circumciser, a *mohel*, trained in both the medical procedure and the details of Jewish law, in a celebratory gathering known as a *bris* (or *berit*). If a *mohel* is not available, a Jewish physician can perform the circumcision, along with a rabbi in attendance. In the Reform movement, girls also have a *berit* service, sometimes in the form of a naming ceremony.

Children are frequently named for someone who has died. Each child is given a Hebrew name that is used when they are older and called to the *Torah*.[9,10] The *Bar* or *Bat Mitzvah* ceremony (for boys 13 years old and girls $12\frac{1}{2}$ or 13 years old, depending on which branch of Judaism one belongs to) is a major rite of passage for children that marks the beginning of adult religious responsibility. Jewish education can continue through high school in confirmation classes for Reform Jews.[10]

Reflective Exercise

• Have you ever been to a bris or a Bar or Bat Mitzvah ceremony? • What did it symbolize to you?
• Do you have similar traditions in your religion?

Jews traditionally affix a *mezuzah* to the upper part of the right doorpost of a Jewish home or in each room. The *mezuzah* is a small parchment scroll, inserted into a tubular case, on which are passages from the *Torah* and the *Shema Yisrael*, a blessing that speaks to the love of God[10] (Fig. 15-2). When one is entering a home, the *mezuzah* serves to remind one how to act in a home; upon leaving the home, one is reminded of the high level of behavior expected wherever one goes.[13]

The practice of *tzedakah*, or doing righteous acts, is one of the main attributes of Jewish living that is learned from observing actions in the

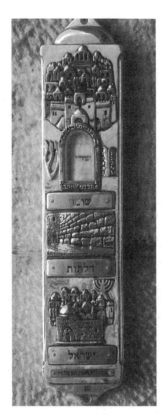

FIGURE 15.2 A *mezzuzah*, which is traditionally mounted on the doorpost of a home.

home and at the synagogue. Often the word *tzedakah* is translated to mean charity, but the Hebrew root of *tzedakah* means justice and righteousness. Fulfilling the act of *tzedakah* allows one to be responsible toward humankind. Because every human being is created in God's image and is entitled to have his or her needs met, if one cannot meet those needs, it is the responsibility of members of the community to help the person do so.

Jewish family life is characterized by honoring one's father and mother. Honoring one's parents, the fifth of the Ten Commandments, is a transition between the first four, which are human obligations toward God, and the next five, which are human obligations toward other human beings. This is to be done joyously and will be rewarded both in this life and in the world to come. The Orthodox, especially, would consider studying the *Torah* and doing good deeds as ideal ways to honor one's parents.[9]

Roles of the Aged and the Extended Family

The Jewish ideal regarding the treatment of the elderly, including grandparents, demonstrates deference, honor, and respect. The elderly are considered worthy of special charity and treatment according to many medieval Jewish ethical and *halachic* (rabbinic interpretations of Jewish literature) works; families have the responsibility for supporting their elders. If this is not possible, it is the role of the larger Jewish community. The first Jewish home for the aged in the United States was founded in 1855. Now almost every large Jewish community has one. In response to the increase in the older population, both in absolute numbers and as a percentage of the total population, Jewish community centers, social agencies, and synagogues are increasing the money and amount of programming devoted to the elderly.[9]

A physical therapist, especially one doing home visits, may encounter the Jewish value of welcoming a stranger into one's home. Practicing hospitality toward a guest is a tradition rooted in biblical times. An invitation to a meal would not be uncommon.[9]

Reflective Exercise

• If you have visited a Jewish home, did you observe the display of any unique religious symbols? • What have you noticed about the style of child rearing or family dynamics of Jewish people compared with non-Jews? • In what ways are the structure and practices of the extended family similar to and different from your family's?

Alternative Lifestyles

In today's American society, gender roles are increasingly blurred and alternative households continue to evolve as a result of such factors as the increasing divorce rate and the elective decision to become a single parent or to couple with someone of the same sex. Both men and women are generally expected to serve as role models to their children and give service to the community.

Biocultural Ecology

Skin Color and Biological Variations
Jewish people are generally Caucasian, although there are some black Jews, most notably the Falasha, originally from Ethiopia. Sephardic Jews tend to have darker skin and hair coloring. Increasingly, children adopted by Jewish people may be Asian, black, or of mixed race.

Hereditary and Genetic Conditions
There is a growing body of knowledge concerning which groups have a greater inherited susceptibility to particular diseases. Ashkenazi Jews have a genetic link to Tay-Sachs, Niemann-Pick, and Canavan's diseases, which are progressive, fatal childhood diseases. Familial dysautonomia, torsion dystonia, and cystic fibrosis are also genetically linked disorders more common to Ashkenazi Jews.[14] The most common genetic disease affecting Ashkenazi Jews is Gaucher's disease, a lipid storage disorder that results in weakening of the bones due to infarctions, anemia, and platelet deficiencies. About 10% of Ashkenazi Jews are carriers of this disease.[1]

Jewish people of Eastern European decent (i.e., Ashkenazi Jews) also have an increasing predisposition to the breast cancer 1 gene mutation (BRCA1). This group has a 0.9% carrier rate for this single mutation, which is at least three times higher than the estimated carrier rate for all BRCA1 mutations combined in the general U.S. population. This mutation, isolated in 1994, increases the risk of breast and ovarian cancer. For those who inherit the mutated gene, there is up to a 90% lifetime chance of developing breast cancer and up to an 84% chance of developing ovarian cancer. In the U.S. general population, inherited BRCA1 is estimated to account for 4% of breast and 12% of ovarian cancers.[14]

In contrast, some genetic variations have a protective effect against diseases, and it has recently been discovered that Jewish people have a genetic mutation called ADH2*2 that protects against alcoholism. It is estimated that 20% of Jewish people have this variation, which is associated with drinking less frequently, consuming less alcohol overall, or causing an unpleasant reaction to liquor.[15]

Carrier screening and prenatal tests are increasingly available for some of these diseases. Ashkenazi Jews have high levels of participation in research relating to the acceptance rate of genetic counseling. It is possible that these high rates are associated with Jewish cultural and theological beliefs, an obligation to learn about one's health to benefit oneself and others, or a higher educational level.[7] Issues associated with this knowledge include the appropriateness and effectiveness of genetic counseling and screening to reduce morbidity and mortality rates, genetic therapy, and the possibility that increased release of information may lead to discrimination in health insurance and employment.

Medical conditions seen with greater-than-expected frequency among Jews include inflammatory bowel diseases such as ulcerative colitis, Crohn's disease, and colorectal cancer.[1] Jewish females have a low incidence of uterine and cervical cancers.[2]

Variations in Drug Metabolism
The drug clozapine, used to treat schizophrenia, has a higher rate of side effects among Ashkenazi Jews. This is apparently associated with a specific genetic haplotype that causes agranulocytosis.[1]

Reflective Exercise

• How do you think you would feel regarding genetic testing if you believed you might be at greater risk for a particular gene? • What are the advantages of genetic testing? • What are the disadvantages of genetic testing?

Nutrition

Meaning of Foods and Common Foods
Food and eating are important to people of Jewish ancestry. Traditional Jewish foods are typically associated with religious celebrations and are a unifying component of ethnic identity. Foods commonly associated with Jewish living are chicken soup (sometimes referred to as "Jewish penicillin"), bagels and lox (smoked salmon), *knaidle* (matzah meal dumplings served in soup at Passover or on the Sabbath), chopped

liver, *kugel* (noodle pudding), gefilte fish (ground freshwater fish served in oblong pieces with horseradish), blintzes (crepes filled with fruit or cheese), and more.

Rituals and Limitations

Jewish dietary regulations are defined according to Jewish laws of *kashrut*. When one maintains specific dietary practices with regard to food and utensils, one is considered *kosher*. Certain foods are restricted, and any food or utensil that is not *kosher* is *treif*. For example, one may not eat pork because the animal from which it comes does not chew its cud, or shellfish or nonscaled fish (shrimp, lobster, and shark) because they do not have fins or scales. Foods that are permitted, such as chicken or beef, are to be slaughtered in a way that minimizes the animal's pain; blood is then drained from the meat. Meat (*fleishik*) and dairy (*milchik*) foods are separated in preparation, serving, and eating. Foods that are neither are *pareve*, or neutral, and may be eaten with milk or meat.

Most important is that these dietary commandments come from God, and therefore following them makes one holy. In today's world, variations in the degree of adherence to all kosher rules exist, but it is safe to assume that Orthodox people are kosher and some individuals from the other Jewish groups are as well. Alcohol is used in many traditional rituals and is regarded as a legitimate pleasure of life. Asking about specific dietary restrictions and habits is wise.[9,16] It is essential for a healthcare facility serving people of the Jewish faith to observe the laws of *kashrut* for their clients' meals. This may be done through the facility's own dietary services or by contracting with a kosher caterer.

Reflective Exercise

• Have you eaten food associated with Jewish culture? • What foods do you or your family eat that are associated with your cultural heritage? • How does eating these foods make you feel? • What do they symbolize to you? • What foods do you eat regularly that may have originally been associated with a different cultural or ethnic group?

Death Rituals

Jewish tradition encourages a realistic acceptance of the inevitability of death and respect for the dead. The *mitzvot* ("commandments") related to death are meant to prescribe conduct and practices at the bedside of a dying person in preparation of the body for burial, at the funeral, and at the house of mourning. Judaism teaches the sacredness of grief, sympathy, and memory, but one is not expected to become obsessed with grief. Responsibility toward the deceased involves burial as soon as possible, usually within a day or two. A delay is acceptable only if time is required to gather the immediate family or if the Jewish Sabbath or a Jewish holiday is about to commence.[10]

Because a basic principle of Judaism is the preservation of human life, and Jewish sources command one to cure another, active euthanasia is classified as murder. Nevertheless, when a cure is not possible, it is generally permissible to let nature run its course.[16]

For the Orthodox, specific rituals are proscribed. A body is not to be left alone from the moment of death until burial. The body is dressed for burial in a simple white burial shroud. A man is traditionally buried with his prayer shawl.[9] Jewish law forbids embalming and cremation, although some Reform rabbis will officiate at funerals involving either practice. The body is generally placed in a plain wooden coffin. Viewing the body is discouraged, and a closed coffin is present at the funeral service. All people, the poor and the rich, the weak and the great, are to be treated with equal depth of compassion during the rituals associated with death and mourning.

Funeral services may occur in a synagogue, funeral parlor, or cemetery chapel. They are generally brief, with psalms recited, a eulogy given, and a memorial prayer offered known as the mourner's *kaddish*. At the cemetery, there are additional prayers. Once the coffin is lowered, handfuls (or shovelfuls) of dirt are placed over the coffin by close friends and relatives. People wear modest, generally dark clothing, and Orthodox and Conservative men (and some women) cover their heads with a skullcap (*kippot* or *yalmuke*).

Following the service, people return to the home for a traditional meal prepared by family friends—often dairy—including hard-boiled eggs, which symbolize the circle of life.

Bereavement Practices

The burial is followed by a weeklong mourning and consolation period, where friends and family members visit at the home of either the deceased or another family member. This is known as "sitting *shiva*." In the house, mirrors will be covered, mourners will not shave or bathe more than is necessary for hygiene, and they will sit on boxes or low benches. It is customary to bring food as a gift so that mourners do not need to concern themselves with the mundane necessities of life. In general, one can expect to stay anywhere from a few minutes to several hours, depending on the relationship with the mourners. The traditional mourning period and recitation of the *kaddish* prayer in memory of the loved one will vary depending on one's degree of religiosity and the level of intensity and obligation following the death.

Planting living trees or making a charitable donation in honor of the deceased some time after the funeral is customary. In Jewish tradition, the number 18 represents life: Donations featuring the number 18 or multiples of 18 are especially meaningful. Floral arrangements are not appropriate.[10,17]

Reflective Exercise

• What are your personal and religious beliefs about death and end-of-life decision making? • Can you compare your own religious practices following the death of a loved one with those for people of the Jewish faith? • Have you ever made a shiva call?
• What do you think are the advantages and disadvantages of death-related traditions?

Spirituality

Dominant Religion and Use of Prayer

Religiosity refers to religious attendance, practice, or activity. Spirituality is more difficult to define. It may be a uniquely individual inner quality that facilitates connectedness with the self, others,

and nature, or it may involve one's acknowledgment of and relationship with a Supreme Being.[18] People affiliated with different streams of Judaism will likely have differing definitions of how these concepts apply to themselves and will have a wide range of religious practices. Some Jews go to synagogue daily, and some may never go and still celebrate some of the holidays. Many Reform and Conservative Jews consider themselves to be strongly affiliated, and they may practice their own form of Judaism with a strong commitment in a consistent manner. Orthodox Jews may not accept these practices as "legitimate."

As a religion, Judaism is the oldest monotheistic faith, with a belief in one God who entered into a covenant with Abraham and his descendants. The writings of Judaism, or the Hebrew Bible, include the five books of Moses, the *Torah*, which was handed down from God at Mt. Sinai. Christians refer to this part of the Bible as the Old Testament. The heart of Judaism is found in the words "Hear O Israel, the Lord is our God, the Lord is One" (Deuteronomy 6:4).

A Jewish house of worship is referred to as a synagogue, *shul*, or temple (Fig. 15-3). Each synagogue will have *Torahs*, handwritten parchment scrolls of Hebrew writings, in the "holy ark" under an "eternal light." The rabbi is the spiritual leader of a congregation.

Religious life is based on the commandments that are found in the *Torah* and additional Jewish literature, including the *Mishnah* and the *Talmud*. Moses Maimonides, a twelfth-century sage,

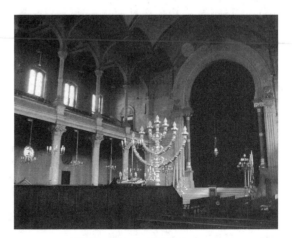

FIGURE 15.3 A Jewish synagogue.

wrote the *Mishnah,* or code of Jewish law, which is a compendium of what Jews should and should not do with regard to all aspects of living. The *Mishnah* is also the primary source on medical matters; Maimonides was a physician as well. The *Talmud* is the oral tradition based on the rabbinic commentary of the *Mishnah.* The rabbinic interpretation of Jewish law is known as the *halacha.* This body of jurisprudence, often cited by rabbis and scholars, is used to develop the principles and practices of contemporary Jewish life.[3,16]

The three major branches of Judaism developed during the eighteenth century when Jews were emancipated from the Jewish ghettos. Historically, ghettos were walled-off and gated sections of a city to which Jews were restricted. The word *ghetto* originated in Venice, Italy, circa 1516, and was used to describe a neighborhood on the site of the city's foundry.[19] Jews had new options with regard to how to define themselves. To a great extent, these groups represent the accommodation of, or rejection of, modernity to varying degrees. Orthodox Jews, accounting for approximately 7% of Jews in the United States, are the most traditional and most serious with regard to practicing the time-honored rules of observance and piety. They believe that God passed the whole *Torah* to Moses at Mt. Sinai and that it remains intact and unchanged. They keep the Sabbath, follow a strict kosher diet, and dress conservatively. There is a strong belief among them in the virtue of modesty; women, in an attempt to make themselves less desirable to men, cover their arms and legs; married women may wear a *sheitel,* or wig, to cover the head. A man will not touch a woman who is not his wife. Orthodox men wear a *kippot* (also known as a *yalmuke*), a small, circular head covering, at all times. Orthodox Jews celebrate more holidays and do so with a greater degree of strictness. The Orthodox Jew tends to be more insular.

Hasidic, or Chasidic, Jews are a subgroup of the Orthodox Jews, sometimes referred to as "ultra-orthodox." The Lubavitch, who have their headquarters in New York, are the most well known. Hasidic Jews are often identified by their clothing: The men wear eighteenth- and nineteenth-century black coats and hats and may have long, curled sideburns, and the women dress modestly (Fig. 15-4). When working

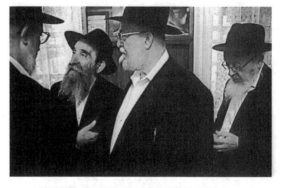

FIGURE 15.4 Dress of Orthodox Jewish men.

with Orthodox Jews, the physical therapist may encounter beliefs and behaviors that must be taken into consideration if one is to be culturally competent.

The Reform movement grew from the admired ideals of democracy and secular ideas taking root in North America with the arrival of an increasing number of Jews from Europe. Although Reform Jews, about 42% of all Jews and growing, believe that the *Torah* is a valuable cultural and philosophical body of work, it is not considered by them to be a divine revelation that occurred at one time; rather, it has developed over centuries. Their emphasis on adaptation to modern society is based on ethical and moral teachings and an understanding that each individual is free to decide what to believe.[3]

Conservative Judaism, representing about 38% of Jews in the United States, developed as a middle-ground alternative to the Orthodox and Reform traditions. While Conservative Jews believe that sacred Jewish writings did come from God, they acknowledge a human component. Conservative Judaism considers the *Talmud* to be authoritative yet adaptable to each generation in order to blend tradition and change. The Reconstructionist movement, comprising about 1% of American Jews, grew out of the Conservative movement and a need to "reconstruct" Judaism to fit contemporary traditions while maintaining the intentions of the past.[20] Jewish identification is generally noted through one's belonging to an Orthodox, Conservative, or Reform synagogue. Additionally, because Jewish identity is an amalgam of religion and cultural factors, there is a strong secular movement within Judaism—that is, Jews who identify as Jewish but do not practice organized religion.

Reflective Exercise

• If you know any Jewish people, to what branch of Judaism do they belong? • Do you know anyone who is an Orthodox Jew? • How does this affect your relationship with him or her? • Have you ever discussed religious beliefs and practices with your friends or patients? • What are your feelings about sharing your own religious beliefs or learning about other people's beliefs?

Authentic Jewish living, no matter with what branch of Judaism one identifies with, involves the following of *mitzvot*. Although *mitzvah* is translated from the *Torah* as "commandment," it has a broader meaning signifying both ethical and ritual "signs of the covenant, affirmed and reaffirmed throughout the ages at various turning points in which Jewish existence stood in the balance"[10] (p. 105). The performance of *mitzvot*, sometimes referred to as good deeds, is a "means of enriching one's personal and family life and contributing to the perpetuation of Judaism"[10] (p. 98). Although the original source of *mitzvot* is the *Torah*, the *Talmud* is where the *mitzvot* are specified and enumerated. There are a total of 613 *mitzvot*—248 positive ones, corresponding to the bones of the human body, and 365 negative ones, equal to the number of days in a solar year.[9] Orthodox Jews may perceive *mitzvot* truly as a commandment from God, while a Conservative or Reform Jew may consider doing *mitzvot* a part of one's tradition.

Religious Holidays

The celebration of *Shabbat* and holidays is a core element of Judaism and the Jewish home. Many home-centered rituals, such as reciting a prayer while lighting candles, sipping wine, or cutting a *challah* (a type of bread), evidence this, especially for Orthodox Jews. *Shabbat* is for rest and spiritual reawakening, a day to participate in special home and synagogue activities. Orthodox Jews observe the *mitzvot* that are permitted or forbidden on *Shabbat*. Other observant Jews celebrate

Shabbat to varying degrees in a variety of ways. *Shabbat* begins at sundown on Friday evening and ends after sunset on Saturday evening. The *havdalah* ceremony, separating the holy from the ordinary, ends the *Shabbat*. The major prohibitions associated with *Shabbat* relate to work and traveling. "Work" is defined not only as making a living, but as an action that is expected to bring about a change in a particular condition. Thus, observant Jews are not allowed to do such things as turn electric appliances or lights on or off.

Jews who observe the *Shabbat* must be home before sundown on Friday. This is a potential conflict at some places of employment. An observant Jew may be willing to work on a Sunday. One can take part in activities on *Shabbat* that are otherwise prohibited, such as using the telephone to call a physician or driving a car to get to the hospital, if the life of an individual is at stake. Likewise, certain activities performed by a physical therapist at a hospital or during a home visit, if medically necessary, are permitted. However, once at the hospital, an Orthodox Jew would not be able to drive home, use money to purchase meals, or push the buttons on an elevator to go to another floor.

The dates for Jewish holidays vary because they are based on the lunar calendar. An extra month is periodically added to account for the lunar year being 11 days shorter than the solar year.[1] Most Jewish holidays celebrate events in Jewish history. All holidays begin on the eve before the day of the holiday and end at sundown after the holiday. The "High Holy Days," which commence the Jewish year, occur around the early fall. *Rosh Hashana* celebrates the creation of the world and is considered the "New Year." *Yom Kippur*, the "Day of Atonement" and a day of fasting, falls 10 days later.[13] *Sukkot*, which signifies the end of the harvest and commemorates the 40 years of wandering by the Jews in the desert on their way to the "Promised Land," is also celebrated in the fall.

Hanukkah, a popular and joyous holiday, symbolizes the successful revolt of the Jewish revolutionaries against Syrian anti-Semitic oppression in 167 B.C. According to Jewish tradition, oil that should have lasted one day burned for eight days. To commemorate this "miracle," Jewish people light candles in a *menorah* for eight nights.

Although a minor holiday within the Jewish calendar because it falls near Christmas, which is widely celebrated in a predominantly Christian country, *Hanukkah* has come to be associated with the tradition of gift giving.

Passover, or *Pesach*, is in the spring, close to Easter. It commemorates the miracle of the exodus from Egypt and the beginning of Jewish nationhood. This is the most celebrated Jewish holiday around the world, when Jews, even if they are not strongly affiliated, join together with family and friends to have a *Seder*. A *Seder* involves reading from the *Hagaddah*, a text that tells the story of the exodus, and also includes many ritual foods and practices. An employer or organizer of professional activities needs to be sensitive to the requirements of *Shabbat* and Jewish holidays.

Reflective Exercise

• What religious holidays do you observe, and how do they impact your life? • How would your life be different if you observed the Sabbath? • Do you value the observance of Shabbat or religious holidays? • How do you think Jewish people might feel as a result of the fact that many American holidays are based on Christianity? • How would you feel if your holidays were not taken into account in your school or place of employment?

Healthcare Practices

Focus of Healthcare

The sanctity of life is a core tenet of Judaism, and health maintenance is a human responsibility. The prominent values of justice, charity, and kindness demonstrate a concern for the health and well-being of all people in the world. Religiosity influences the response to signs and symptoms of illness through rituals associated with disease and disease prevention, and health promotion and wellness. In particular, religious observances involving social, moral, and dietary prescriptions tend to increase communal activities and social support functions that promote health and aid in adaptation to stress-related diseases and trauma.[18]

Responsibility for Healthcare

The relationship between (a) Judaism and Jewish culture and (b) patterns of illness and the creation of health belief systems and related behaviors is well documented. For Jews, there has been a strong religious or cultural concern for health throughout history. One also has a responsibility to properly care for the body and not destroy it. Illegal drugs, permanent tattooing, and suicide are forbidden. Matters of hygiene, diet, exercise, and sleep are subjects involving religious obligations.[16]

In earlier times, and among the most traditional Jews, the link between God the creator and health and disease was a direct one. The idea was that sin is the cause of disease, and blood is the causal agent—hence the notion of bloodletting. In modern times, this notion is challenged by contemporary germ theory.

A rich tradition of cure and prevention using a combination of the empirical, the religious, and the magical is based on the Bible. With rare exceptions, contemporary Jews embrace the developments of medicine and would consider it sinful to forgo life-saving medical ministrations. Today the Jewish obligation to heal is demonstrated by the relatively large proportion of Jewish physicians and hospitals, all of which are open to people of any background. In fact, it is a *mitzvah* for a physician to heal and for the sick to seek medical treatment.[11]

God is still recognized as the ultimate healer, and praying to God is a part of treatment. Visiting people who are sick and being helpful to them is considered a *mitzvah* as well.

Traditional and Folk Practices

Belief in the evil eye, one of the oldest and most common folk illnesses, persists among some Jews, especially older immigrants. In Yiddish, *kayn aynhoreh* is the expression uttered by Jews after a compliment or expression of luck is made to prevent the casting of an evil spell on someone else's health. The speaker may spit three times after reciting the words.[21]

Folk practices, such as using the *mezuzot* to ward off disease, although not common, may still have a place in the lives of the more traditional.[16] A "Jerusalem amulet" may be hung in the home to protect the family from the evil eye and other

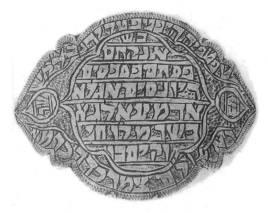

FIGURE 15.5 A Jerusalem amulet.

dangers, to heal pain and end suffering, or as a talisman for success and good luck[21] (Fig. 15-5). Other traditional practices to ward off the evil eye are having a red ribbon woven into clothes or attached to a crib (Eastern European Jews) or wearing a blue ribbon or bead (Sephardic Jews).[21]

Cultural Responses to Pain

Zborowski's[22] seminal study on pain concluded that Italian and Jewish people tend to complain about pain more frequently and with more emotion than the "old American Yankee," who tends to be more stoic, and the Irish, who tend to ignore the pain. Additionally, Jewish people worry more about the long-term implications of pain and do not want to use medications for fear that they would mask a more serious problem.

Reflective Exercise

• In what ways do your religious beliefs influence your health beliefs and behaviors? • Can you think of any health-related practices in your family that have been passed from generation to generation? • Have you ever considered the meaning and implications of pain to your clients from different ethnic groups?

Blood Transfusions and Organ Donation

Traditional Judaism respects the dead and at one time would consider death to occur only after cessation of both breath and heartbeat. In modern times, most Jewish people, even the Orthodox, accept the common medical practice of defining death as the state when one is brain dead.

Autopsies traditionally are not allowed because they constitute destruction and desecration of God's property. Modern interpretation allows for an autopsy because it may be considered a way to benefit medical science and thus, potentially, another life. With respect to organ donation, rabbinic authorities have permitted the use of organs for the life or health of other living humans, reasoning that this does not desecrate, but rather honors, the dead person. One may actually be duty bound to overlook traditional religious law in favor of the obligation to save a life.[16]

Receiving blood and blood products is usually not a problem for Jews, regardless of their degree of religiosity. However, some are reluctant to receive blood for fear of contracting HIV/AIDS.

Healthcare Practitioners

There is a long tradition of Jewish people becoming healthcare practitioners. Generally speaking, an Orthodox Jewish patient might be more comfortable with a physical therapist of the same gender if a long-term patient-practitioner relationship is expected to develop. Issues of touching and modesty would be alleviated. However, during an acute medical crisis, someone of either gender can give medical care.

Reflective Exercise

• How do you feel about going to see a healthcare provider who is of a background similar to yours?
• Do you mind going to see someone who has a lifestyle very different from yours?

Conclusion

People of Jewish heritage represent a wide array of beliefs and behaviors, both religious and cultural. When working with Jewish people, the physical therapist must respect and incorporate these ideas and practices in order to be culturally competent. It is impossible to know everything about a group or individual; thus, the best practice is to learn as much as possible, to ask your patient the appropriate questions, and to develop your culture-related skills.

Mrs. Epstein has visited her primary care physician, and they have agreed that a female physical therapist (PT) will visit her at her home for an evaluation and intervention. The PT (Jane) arrives on Wednesday afternoon and is immediately offered coffee and *rugella* (a homemade pastry). Thinking that this would be a good way to open her initial interview with Mrs. Epstein, she accepts the offer. Jane observes that Mrs. Epstein walks slowly through the kitchen and leans on appliances and counters when possible. During their conversation, Mrs. Epstein, who has an accent, uses several words with which Jane is unfamiliar, although she thinks she understands the gist of their meaning. For example, Mrs. Epstein, who is moaning while walking about and complaining about the pain in her legs, is talking about her need to begin preparation for *Pesach*. Many relatives will be visiting her, including some cousins from Israel, and she must prepare many dishes for the *Seder*: *choroses*, gefilte fish, *matzoh* ball soup, brisket, and more. This is her favorite holiday, and she looks forward to it every year, but how can she do it all with so much pain and weakness? She gets so tired. Also, Mrs. Epstein explains that the entire kitchen must be cleaned out and all the food that is not specially "*kosher* for Passover" must be taken to the basement. This is extremely important. Mrs. Epstein has been considering asking people at her local *shul* for some assistance in preparing for the holiday. Several years ago, Mrs. Epstein was part of the Caring Community Committee and she helped her neighbor during the "High Holidays."

Upon physical examination, Jane finds general weakness in the lower extremities; limitations of range of motion consistent with moderately severe osteoarthritis of the hips and knees, right greater than left; and some swelling of the ankles. Mrs. Epstein notes that her physician has given her some new medications and says she might consider a total hip procedure on the right if the pain limits her preferred lifestyle. She does not use any assistive devices, although she reports more frequent rest periods and reduced capability of doing all she wants.

Jane has recently moved to New York City from Iowa. She is working for a home care agency in Brooklyn, and they said that they needed a female therapist to see this patient. Many of the patients she expects to see are Orthodox Jews, and she admits that she has never knowingly worked with this population before. Jane has been thinking a lot about her own personal biases since coming to such a large city with people of so many backgrounds. Jane wants to become culturally competent. She knows that Mrs. Epstein will require considerable patient education with regard to energy conservation, an exercise program to increase strength and functional activities, and maintenance or recovery of range of motion. Jane has some ideas about assistive devices that may be helpful.

1. What cultural differences are evident in this scenario?

2. What potential challenges or cultural barriers might Jane face?

3. Describe how Mrs. Epstein may feel. Identify her values and beliefs that may affect the physical therapy care program.

4. How might Jane negotiate the interaction in a culturally competent manner?

5. How might Jane negotiate the interaction in a culturally incompetent manner?

6. Is the timing of Jane's scheduled visits to the home an important consideration?

7. Do you believe Mrs. Epstein's children should be involved in the PT program? Why or why not?

8. How might both Jane and Mrs. Epstein benefit from the encounter?

REFERENCES

1. Selekman J. People of Jewish heritage. In: Purnell L, Paulanka B, eds. *Transcultural Health Care: A Culturally Competent Approach.* 2nd ed. Philadelphia, Pa: FA Davis; 2003:234–249.

2. Jacobs L, Giarelli, E. Jewish culture, health belief systems, and genetic risk for cancer. *Nurs Forum.* 2001;36:12–17.

3. Infoplease. Judaism. Available at: http://www.infoplease.com/ipa/A0001462.html. Accessed April 25, 2003.

4. Infoplease. Jews. Available at: http://www.infoplease.com/ce6/society/A0826266.html. Accessed April 28, 2003.

5. Taking the pulse of Jewish opinion. *Am Jew Comm J.* 2003;3.

6. National Jewish Population Survey 2000–2001. Jewish virtual library. Available at: http://www.us-israel.org/jsource/US-Israel/ujcpop.html. Accessed April 25, 2003.

7. Culver J, Burke W, Yasui Y, Durfy S, Press N. Participation in breast cancer genetic counseling: The influence of educational level, ethnic background, and risk perception. *J Genet Couns.* 2001;10:215–231.

8. Scheidlinger S. The minyan as a psychological support system. *Psychoanal Rev.* 1997;84:41–52.

9. Binder Kadden B, Kadden B. *Teaching Mitzvot: Concepts, Values, and Activities.* Denver, Colo: A.R.E.; 1996.

10. Maslin S. *Gates of Mitzvah: A Guide to the Jewish Life Cycle.* New York, NY: Central Conference of American Rabbis; 1979.

11. Lewittes M. *Principles and Development of Jewish Law.* New York, NY: Bloch; 1987.

12. The American scene: Roe reaches 30. *Hadassah Mag.* 2003; (suppl).

13. Telushkin J. *Jewish Literacy.* New York, NY: William Morrow; 1991.

14. Cahan A, Bock G. Specific BrCa1 gene mutation identified in Ashkenazi Jewish population. Available at: www.wehealnewyork.org/advances/ashkenazi.html. Accessed April 28, 2003.

15. Hasin D, Aharonovich E, Liu X, et al. Alcohol dependence symptoms and alcohol dehydrogenase-2 polymorphism: Israeli Ashkenazis, Sephardics, and recent Russian immigrants. *Alcoholism: Clinical and Experimental Research.* 2002;26:1315–1321.

16. Numbers R, Amundsen D. *Caring and Curing: Health and Medicine in the Western Religious Traditions.* New York, NY: Macmillan; 1986.

17. Funeral customs and etiquette. Available at http://www.nvo.com/finalplans/nss-folder/htmlcode/funeralcustoms-andetiquette.html. Accessed April 25, 2003.

18. Musgrave C, Allen C, Allen G. Spirituality and health for women of color. *Am J Public Health.* 2002;92:557–560.

19. Pearson K. Ghetto: Etymology. Available at: http://www.tcnj.edu/Dictionary /ghetto/htm. Accessed June 16, 2003.

20. Infoplease. Branches of Judaism. Available at: http://www.infoplease.com/spot/judaism1.html. Accessed April 25, 2003.

21. Spector R. *Cultural Diversity in Health and Illness.* Stamford, Conn: Appleton & Lange; 1996.

22. Zborowski M. Cultural components in responses to pain. *J Soc Issues.* 1952;8:16–30.

Highlighting the Culture of Various
Physical Therapy Populations

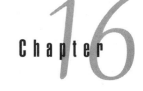

Chapter 16

Disability across Cultures

● Ronnie Leavitt, PhD, MPH, PT

● Ronnie Leavitt, PhD, MPH, PT

Vignette

Julio Gonzalez, age 25 years, recently emigrated from Mexico. He was in a motor vehicle accident 4 weeks ago and suffered a complete spinal cord injury at T8. He is now undergoing physical and occupational therapy at a rehabilitation hospital. Julio has many visitors, and the staff find this distracting. The visitors are family and extended family, and they are constantly assisting Julio rather than encouraging his independence. Julio is uncomfortable with the rehab staff assisting him with his personal care, and prefers that his family do this. Not all of the family members speak English, and when they are present, all communication is in Spanish. Julio appears to be depressed and unmotivated, and states that he does not want to experience the stigma of being disabled. Julio and his family have very limited resources.

This chapter addresses disability from a cross-cultural perspective using the Purnell Model for Cultural Competence to facilitate understanding of people with disabilities from selected cultures. Additionally, it addresses attitudes toward people with disabilities within a cultural context, the macro- (society and community) and micro- (individual and family) level responses to disability, and culturally congruent strategies that can be implemented by physical therapists. In essence, this chapter is an introduction to the emerging field of disability studies, a specialty area that focuses on sociocultural perspectives rather than focusing only on biomedical factors to appreciate the lives of people with disabilities. Disability

studies, which is a relatively new field with limited research, is fast becoming recognized as a key body of knowledge for rehabilitation professionals. Disabilities exist in all societies; yet how much does the physical therapist understand about the meaning of disability? How does one ever understand the lived experiences of people with disabilities?

Metaparadigm Concepts

Global Society and Disability
Patterns of health and disease determinants and their consequences are changing from what they

were in previous decades. The major health problems in the world are shifting from acute infectious diseases and perinatal problems to chronic degenerative conditions and injuries resulting from violence, warfare, and traffic accidents.[1] This process, known as the epidemiological transition resulting from an increase in longevity worldwide, is leading to greater rates of disability. At the same time, there is a major paradigm shift occurring in social institutions, communications, advanced technology, and world cultures that will affect how disability is defined, encountered, and interpreted.[2]

In reality, the concept of disability is not a cultural universal. That is, disability as Westerners know it is not a concept found in all cultures. Sometimes people with disabilities are expected to follow the same life cycle as everyone else in their dominant cultural group. As Ingstad and Whyte[3] state, "In many cultures, one cannot be 'disabled' for the simple reason that 'disability' as a recognized category does not exist. There are blind people and lame people and 'slow' people, but 'the disabled' as a general term does not translate easily into many languages . . . the concepts of disability, handicap, and rehabilitation emerged in particular historical circumstances in Europe"[3] (p. 7). If disability does exist as a recognized category, variations in meaning exist across cultures. The significance of a disability for the individual and his or her family depends on each society's values. Also varying among cultures and societies are attitudes toward people with disabilities; concepts of rehabilitation; the sociocultural, biological, and economic implications of disability; and policies affecting people with disabilities (Fig. 16-1).

Reflective Exercise

- What attributes about people do you value highly?
- Do you see an association between these values and your attitudes toward people with disabilities?

People with disabilities have always been part of human society, although documentation of their life experiences is limited. In Iraq a skeleton of an elderly Neanderthal with a withered arm and blindness in one eye has been found.

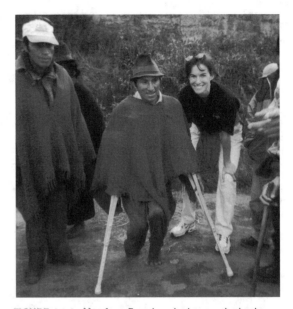

FIGURE 16.1 Man from Ecuador who has cerebral palsy. Despite hip, knee, and plantarflexion contractures, he walks a half-mile and back to his job, where he farms in a field. Prior to receiving a pair of crutches, he managed with a stick for support.

The grave site, covered with flowers, gives an indication that he was a valued member of society. Ancient art and early legends from Greece, Rome, India, China, and the Americas show evidence of the existence of people with disabilities.[4,5]

Prevailing attitudes toward people with disabilities in earlier times point to a mixed picture. For example, the Old Testament commanded, "Thou shall not curse the deaf nor put a stumbling block before the blind, nor maketh the blind to wander out of the path" (Leviticus 19:14) while also warning, "if you do not follow His commands and decrees . . . all these curses will come upon you and overtake you: the Lord will afflict you with madness, blindness, and confusion of mind" (Deuteronomy 28:15, 28–29).[4]

Other sources lead us to believe that people with disabilities were often held in high esteem. For example, a number of tribal groups in East Africa and the Southern Pacific were known to treat children with obvious impairments with great kindness and full acceptance.[5] Conversely, it is known that people with disabilities have been subject to discrimination, ranging from minor embarrassment to neglect. Although it is exceptionally rare, a small number of groups, such as the Kuna Indians of Panama and the Cofan Indians in Ecuador, have practiced infanticide, usually by abandoning an infant after birth (Larry Purnell, personal communication, December 1, 2003). Additional reports of killing deformed babies include practices of the Masai in Africa, the poisoning of children with polio on the Ivory Coast, and country-specific holocausts such as Nazi Germany, where people without disabilities were killed as well.[4–6] Outright killing of older children or adults because of disability is almost unheard of. In general, through the pre-industrialized era, even when they were perceived as "misfits," people with disabilities were generally maintained in a life-supporting environment (including institutions) and marginally integrated into society.[4,7]

The subculture of disability may be more or less significant. For example, for people with hearing impairments, deafness may be one's major identifying factor. Therefore, deafness is not viewed as a limitation but rather as a biological characteristic that has given rise to a specific culture and the slogan of "deaf pride" among the deaf (and, similarly, "disability pride" among disabled athletes)[5,6] (Fig. 16-2). In the United States, a disability subculture is typically associated with a disability rights movement or patient advocacy group. In contrast, much of the world does not share the concepts associated with the subculture of disability; here the disability rights movement is absent or in the early stages of development, which may influence the interaction between the physical therapist and the patient. For example, patients may not understand their rights or capabilities to pursue life's options unless they are guided by an advocate or role model (Fig. 16-3).

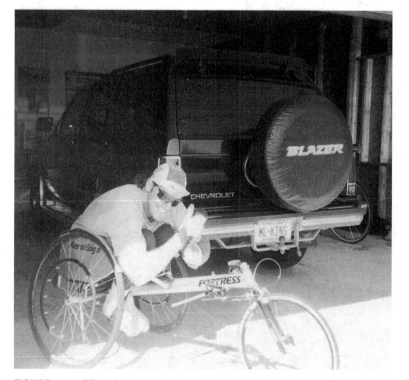

FIGURE 16.2 Wheelchair sports represent a subculture within the subculture of disability. Mike King has paraplegia secondary to traumatic spinal cord injury and has participated in wheelchair racing internationally.

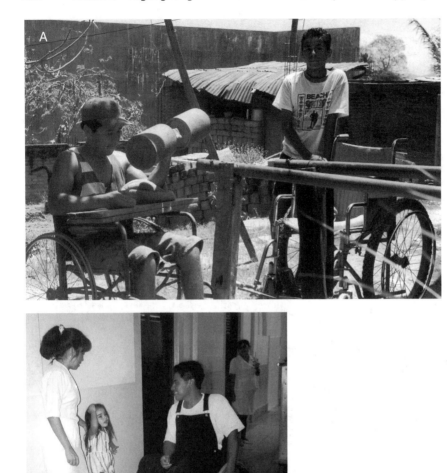

FIGURE 16.3 Osso is young Mexican man who has paraplegia secondary to traumatic spinal cord injury. Not only has he constructed a rehabilitation gym in his backyard (*A*), but he has pioneered a support group in his rural province for people with disabilities (*B*).

Reflective Exercise

• What is your understanding of disability? • What do you think of when you think of someone with a disability? • How has your understanding of disability changed over time? • What has caused the change?

During the industrial era, European American societies began to think of people with disabili-

ties as sick, helpless, and needing to be taken care of. Although social Darwinism and the eugenics movement gained momentum during the 1800s, this period is best characterized as fostering an institutional service model that continued to call for the segregation and marginalization of people with disabilities. Patients were presumed to be unable to function in their own best interest and were expected to take on the "sick role," being freed from normal social roles and responsibilities. Medical advances and the development of interventions have led to a biomedical model with little emphasis on the sociocultural context of the patient. In this model, healthcare providers are presumed to be the experts and are likely to view the patient as a compilation of body parts and systems, with little attention directed to the whole. The intention was benevolence.

Reflective Exercise

• Do you personally have a friend or family member with a disability? • How does your attitude toward the friend or family member differ from your attitude toward your patients?

Hanks and Hanks[8] hypothesized that the degree to which a society is willing or able to bear the costs of caring for people with disabilities depends on several interrelated materialistic and cultural factors. Some of these determinants are listed in Box 16-1. These differences, although influenced by sociocultural practices, primarily reflect the wide economic gap between the two groups.

In modern times, there continues to be a range of variation with regard to how people with disabilities are treated in society. On the one hand, people with disabilities have continually experienced a greater stigma, more pervasive prejudice, and more discrimination than any other group, including being subjected to forced sterilization and institutionalization.[9] Yet, as we move into a new millennium, at least in the industrialized nations, the biomedical model of care is generally being replaced with family-, community-, and consumer-based models that are more oriented toward human rights. Career opportunities for the disabled are growing as well (Fig. 16-4).

Beliefs about the meaning of disability in a particular culture are one component of a society's general belief system about health and sickness, and they have meaning in terms of what form of rehabilitation will be developed in a society. The cultural interpretation of disability depends on how a society attaches value and meaning to a particular type of disability. The interventionist, patient, and family may each have a different perspective.

BOX 16.1

Determinants of Societies Able to Care for Those with Disabilities

(a) The relative socioeconomic status of the society, which includes such factors as the number and type of productive units.

(b) The need for labor, the amount of economic surplus, and its mode of distribution.

(c) The social structure of the society, including whether or not the society is egalitarian or hierarchical, how it defines achievement, and how it values age and gender.

(d) The cultural definition of the meaning of the disability: Does the symptom of the disability require magical, religious, medical, legal, or other measures?

(e) The position of the society in relation to the rest of the world. Although there are significant differences in health status and healthcare systems, including rehabilitation, among contemporary societies, the differences are most extreme between the more and less developed societies.

Source: Hanks and Hanks (1948).[8]

Reflective Exercise

• Is there such a thing as "normal"? • Can you imagine that someone with a disability might choose not to change or eliminate his or her disability if given a choice?

Methodological limitations on research regarding attitudes toward disability exist. In the less developed world, data collection on people with disabilities is still in the early stage of development. As recently as 1987, the largest nation in the world, the People's Republic of China (PRC) did its first nationwide count of *canji*, adults and children with disabilities, in the National Sample Survey of Disabled Persons.[10] According to Kohrman,[10] especially in developing nations, the interplay of the global "disability movement" and nation-state development encourages the

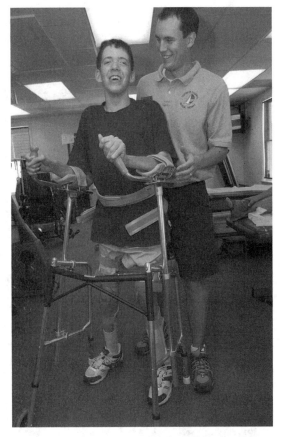

FIGURE 16.4 Career opportunities for individuals with disability are growing. Sumner Spence is pursuing a college education and a degree in business. (Photo courtesy of Daniel Cook.)

collection of biostatistical data. Often, statistics can foster attention or mold attitudes toward the issue of disability.

Leavitt[11] noted that general healthcare and rehabilitation for people with disabilities have historically been very low priorities throughout the world for several reasons. First, the cost-benefit ratio of providing rehabilitation to people with disabilities has always been considered poor compared with other health programs. Second, traditionally the potential achievement of a person with a disability has been underestimated. Third, a history of negative attitudes toward persons with disabilities exists. In many societies, people with disabilities have historically been seen as deviant from the norm and have been attributed with a social stigma or "attitude that is deeply discrediting . . . a failing, a shortcoming, a handicap"[12] (p. 3). Fourth, when discrimination limits participation by people with disabilities in various social roles, they become even more invisible. Fifth, there is an apparent absence of urgency. Rehabilitation is associated with disease and illness that is, for the most part, neither acute, communicable, nor "exciting." The general public will not be at risk, nor will its opposition be mobilized, if rehabilitation services are not delivered to the populations in need. Sixth, on an individual level, mainstream biomedical practitioners tend to reflect a value orientation that stresses one's mastery of disease and taking personal credit for recovery.

In cases in which an individual has a disability, often very little dramatic improvement can occur; in some instances, further loss of function is anticipated. Although a wide array of simple and complex technologies are available, the provision of these services does not ensure dramatic results. Thus, many caregivers find rehabilitation frustrating and often not worthwhile. Finally, individuals with disabilities are a disadvantaged minority and, accordingly, have had little political influence when lobbying for the opportunity to affect public policy (Fig. 16-5).

Reflective Exercise

• Do you see variations among cultures in how some people with disabilities identify with disability? • Do you personally, or does your employment, facilitate the development of a disability-related subculture or advocacy group?

Reflective Exercise

• What evidence do you see in the health professions of the value orientation of mastery over the disease and taking personal credit for recovery? • Do you sense frustration within the health professions when cures are unattainable and further loss of function is expected?

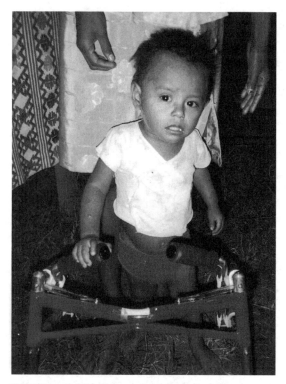

FIGURE 16.5 This Mexican child with a disability is likely part of a disadvantaged minority with little promise of political influence.

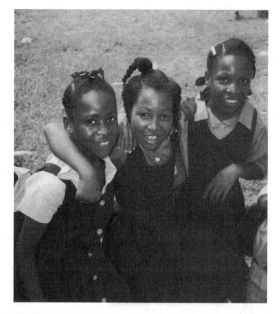

FIGURE 16.6 Camilla is a young Jamaican girl who has cerebral palsy. Without assistive devices or a wheelchair, she is dependent on her girlfriends to transport her to and from school.

Community and Disability

The idea of triangulation of data sources is important, especially in cross-cultural research and when the researcher is less familiar with the gestalt of the community. This may be impractical in some instances. For example, as cited by Brown[13] in a study by the Ethiopian National Children's Commission, community leaders felt that the community was sympathetic and ready to assist children with disabilities. However, the families had negative attitudes, such as feeling ashamed of the child. One does not know the opinion of the families. Similarly yet conversely, Leavitt[14] based her research on children with disabilities in Jamaica on interviews with family members but did not interview key community leaders or government officials. In this case, the families were, for the most part, loving and accepting, and believed it was the community and government leaders who were not facilitating the integration of children with disabilities into Jamaican society—for example, by failing to provide assistive devices or wheelchairs to school children (Fig. 16-6).

Can one assume that there is a direct link between what people say about their attitudes and beliefs and what they actually do? Assessing attitudes through participant observation is often how judgments are made. In the developing world, there are ample reports of pervasive negative attitudes toward people with disabilities. In India, for example, Pinto and Sahur[15] report that people with disabilities remain highly marginalized. In some villages they are shunned or abused, especially when the disability is thought to be the result of parental sin or God's displeasure. In the cities, there may be increased exposure to people with leprosy, amputations, or visual impairments because it is not uncommon for people with disabilities in India to be beggars. Typically, they have experienced limited social opportunities and civil rights.

Attitudes toward people with disabilities are formed in the home—for example, with the disappointment or even rejection of a child born with a congenital anomaly—and then perpetuated in society as the child enters school. Attitudes toward people with disabilities are generally more positive with increased age and experience and for women. Personality characteristics such as self-esteem and role identity are relevant as well.[16,17]

In contrast, Ingstad[18] has argued that the overwhelming reactions of negativity and rejection are "myths." They are in conflict with the fact that most families try their best to care for their loved one with a disability. Furthermore, she argues that these myths undermine efforts by people trying to foster a disability rights movement and serve as an excuse for governments not to address the issues of prejudice and discrimination in education and employment.

Reflective Exercise

• How and why do you think your ideas about disability have developed? • How are people with disabilities portrayed in the media in American society? • In other societies? • What language have you heard in the media and among peers regarding people with disabilities?

Reflective Exercise

• How has your understanding of disability changed over time? • What has caused the change? • Does your profession support progressive societal changes with regard to how people with disabilities are perceived and treated?

The Family, the Individual, and Disability

Although intercultural and intracultural variations exist, three major categories of social beliefs seem to exist cross-culturally and tend to predict how well a person with a disability will fare in a particular community. These categories are designated valued and disvalued attributes, causality, and anticipated role. If the society values physical strength and beauty, as defined by that particular culture, then people who do not display these attributes will be considered less likable, less worthy, and more disabled. If the society favors intellectual capability, then being physically limited by a wheelchair might be seen as less significant.

Core values held by most Asian cultures, as well as some other cultural groups, emphasize collectivism, where family and the group are placed above the individual. Children must remain loyal because of the sacrifices their parents have made. Children are expected to provide financial, emotional, and practical support for their parents, especially when self-care becomes a concern.

Associated with disvalued attributes is stigma. Although there is not complete consensus, people with disabilities are generally considered to have the disvalued attribute of an observable deviation from the norm, which typically results in their being branded with stigmata, that is, "marks" or "blemishes." The stigmata are used to assign a negative value to the deviant person.[12] The construction of individual and societal models of stigmatization of people with disabilities seems to be intimately connected to beliefs concerning causation of disabilities, typically those that are supernatural in origin. As Goffman states,[12] "A disability is often considered evidence of God's displeasure of one's own or one's family's past behavior . . . a stigmatized individual is presumed to be not quite human, and often a sign of danger" (p. 5). Stigma associated with disability may increase the family's fear of exposure to criticism and disgrace for themselves and their ancestors.[19]

Ingstad and Whyte[3] note that in Botswana, Uganda, Nicaragua, Sarawak, and other countries, people with disabilities are accepted not on the basis of their physical or mental condition, but on their likelihood of conforming to the defining characteristics of full personhood in the particular society. These characteristics are based on sociability, kinship identity, the ability to marry and have children, and the ability to contribute to the household economy. If one cannot partake in these obligations, it is up to the family to make it possible. Thus, personhood in some developing countries depends more on social identity and the fulfillment of family obligations than on individual ability.[18]

An individual with a disability, or the individual's family member, is likely to seek some form of intervention in an attempt to "cure" or minimize the effect of the disability. Beliefs might impact the patient's decision regarding what medicines to use, what foods to eat, or what exercises to do. Behaviors vary substantially among cultures and can be quite different from those held by European Americans. Depending on the individual's sociocultural background, services may be provided by a "Western"-style healthcare professional, by a "traditional"/indigenous healer, or by a lay person or family member. Examples of traditional healers include, but are not limited to, curanderos (Mexican American), espiritistas (Puerto Rican), santerios (Cuban), vodoo priests (Haitian), diviners (Southeast Asian American), singers (Native American), and the more generalized herbalists and astrologers. Each has his or her own repertoire of skills and rituals. In reality, the practical issues of availability, cost, and severity of an episode may account for the choice of practitioner.[20]

Still, room for optimism exists. A new paradigm based on self-determination, self-representation, and human rights is emerging. The United Nations Year *of* Disabled Persons (as opposed to *for*) in 1981 marked a turning point on the international scene with regard to the perception of people with disabilities. Originally, the action plan called for increased institution size and more training of professionals. However, as people with disabilities became more involved themselves, a new model emphasizing cooperation and partnership evolved. The theme of the year became "full participation and equality." The Decade of Disabled Persons (1983–1992) was built on the promotion of equalization of opportunities and rights for people with disabilities.[21] "Undoubtedly, the major achievement of the decade was the increased public awareness of disability issues among policy makers, planners, politicians, service providers, parents, and disabled persons themselves."[22] Antidiscrimination legislation has since been enacted to varying degrees throughout the world. In the United States, the Americans with Disabilities Act (ADA) of 1990 declares that people with disabilities have a right to pursue "equality of opportunity, full participation, independent living, and economic self-sufficiency"[21] (p. 159).

Reflective Exercise

• Do you support the ADA? Do you have experience with the costs and benefits of the ADA? • Can a person with a physical disability be a physical therapist? • Does the kind of disability matter? • What kind of disability would prevent a person from becoming a physical therapist?

What role do physical therapists have in advancing this newer way of approaching the presence of people with disabilities in society? As the world, and likely one's place of employment, becomes increasingly multicultural, the need for cross-cultural research investigating the attitudes, beliefs, and behaviors relevant to disability and rehabilitation will become both pragmatic and morally vital. Physical therapists have the opportunity to support and advocate for children with disabilities (Fig. 16-7).

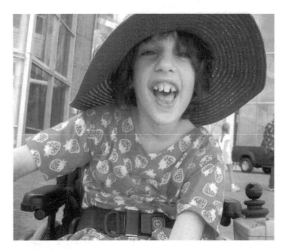

FIGURE 16.7 Physical therapists have the opportunity to support, encourage, and advocate for children with disabilities to help them pursue their goals and dreams. Selina attends a school in Baltimore for children who are gifted in science and math, and she wants to be an astronaut. (Photo courtesy of John Lee.)

Reflective Exercise

• When working with people with disabilities, do you remember to consider the client's ideals, values, and behaviors that might relate to his or her cultural or socioeconomic status? • Do you consider how one's disability status can affect his or her identity?

In today's times, psychological research on attitudes toward illness and disability is often focused on a particular disorder such as AIDS, Parkinson's disease, or cardiovascular diseases. Regarding people with disabilities, the Attitudes Toward Disabled Persons Scale by H. E. Yukor and J. R. Block is commonly used for research.[23]

Reflective Exercise

• Do your views toward a person with a disability vary depending on factors having to do with a particular diagnosis? • Time and mode of onset? • Degree of disability? • Perceived likelihood of catching the disability? • Whether the person has an alternative belief system to yours? • What effect do these views have on your relationship?

Communication

One way to assess attitudes cross-culturally is through the language that is used to describe something. Even in the European American societies, there is disagreement over the most appropriate terminology to use. Some argue that "person with a disability" is the preferred term because it places emphasis on the person first and the disability second. However, within the disability subculture, some argue that the phrase "person with a disability" is illogical. To those who follow the World Health Organization's definitions of impairment, disability, and handicap, it would be appropriate to say "person with a sensory, cognitive, or motor impairment"; disability occurs only when one encounters an inhospitable environment. Thus, it is not that the person is disabled[24] but that the environment is limiting the person's ability to function.

Reflective Exercise

• Are you comfortable communicating with someone with a disability? Do you make accommodations? • Do you interact in a distancing or paternalistic manner or as an equal partner in the rehabilitation experience?

The traditional terms for disability used in China are *canfei,* meaning "handicapped and useless"; *canji,* meaning "handicap and illness"; and *canji ren,* meaning "handicapped and sick people." The term *gong neng zhang ai zhe,* meaning "individuals with disabilities," is rarely used.[19] In Bantu, terms related to physical disability relate to sorcery or reincarnation.[25] The language used internationally among multiple societies and cultures is beyond the scope of this chapter. However, the physical therapist must keep current on society's view of politically correct language when referring to people with any of an array of possible disabilities.

Reflective Exercise

• What terms do you use when referring to a person with a disability? • Have the terms changed over time? • Why or why not?

Family Roles and Organization

The role people can play as adults and how much they can contribute to the household is important to consider. The material conditions of a community are bound to affect belief systems and decisions regarding disability and adult roles, especially in poor communities. If there is fear of economic cost to the family and no economic gain, a negative attitude is more likely to result.

Some people with disabilities may find work outside the home (Fig. 16-8), but more commonly people with disabilities contribute by watching children, doing housework, or helping with farm work. Some may be assigned tasks that others do not want. For example, Groce[5] sites a study from Ecuador where rural families who were introduced to iodized salt for the purpose of

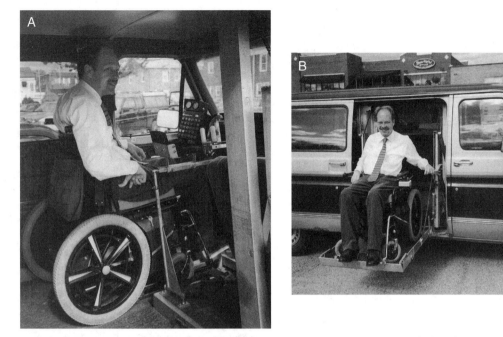

FIGURE 16.8   (*A, B*) Jesse Charles has quadriplegia secondary to a complete traumatic spinal cord injury. He gets to and from his office job in his custom-equipped van and returns home each day to his wife and child.

eliminating iodine deficiency syndrome (mild mental retardation and hearing loss) were concerned that there would be no one to collect firewood, draw water, or herd animals.

In some societies, people with disabilities have been, and still are, expected to contribute to the family income through their role as beggars. In some cases, begging is clearly associated with disgrace. On the other hand, in a rural Mexican community, Gwaltney[26] described elderly persons who became blind as a result of onchocerciasis. They beg for a living but are treated with respect. The blind villagers derive a sense of approved and purposeful participation in the life of their pueblo, and the community has made cultural accommodations.

Workforce Issues

Do healthcare professionals demonstrate more positive attitudes toward disabilities than do the general public? As reported in Aiken,[16] the attitudes of healthcare professionals are similar to those of the general public: They report being more accepting of people with asthma, diabetes, heart disease, or arthritis and less accepting of people with AIDS, mental retardation, psychiatric illness, or cerebral palsy. Basnett[27] also notes that medical professionals are similar to the general population with regard to people with disabilities, and that the dearth of research in this area is likely related to the low priority accorded to disability. Basnett, a physician with a cervical spinal cord injury, argues that in Western societies "health professionals are not just mirrors of society, taking an individualistic interpretation and accentuating it, but are also active promoters of a paradigm that strengthens their own role. This makes understanding disability in terms of social control and oppression much more difficult for individuals trained in that environment"[27] (p. 452). Susan Roush,[28] a physical therapist, suggests that physical therapists are similar to other healthcare professionals, although she believes that they have a unique background and perspective as well as a special responsibility to change their own attitudes and those of others. One possible line of inquiry is to look more formally at the attitudes of physical therapists toward people with disabilities and to apply the results to more-structured training programs in order to produce more positive attitudes and behaviors.

Reflective Exercise

• How have your attitudes toward people with disabilities changed since you went to physical therapy school? • Since you began practicing among people with disabilities? • Do you believe that professionals' attitudes toward people with disabilities are different from those of the general public? • Does your personal response to people with disabilities enhance their likelihood of successful adaptation to the disability?

A second example of needed research is addressing the lack of cultural competence when it comes to measuring functional activities. Scales to assess patient status and intervention efficacy have generally been standardized for the European American culture and lifestyle; however, in the United States, people of non-European American heritage are at greater risk for disability and experience greater secondary complications and mortality rates associated with disability. Merely translating an assessment tool into another language is insufficient.

Research on the Denver Developmental Screening Test (DDST), a commonly used pediatric instrument, has demonstrated that some developmental skills emerge at significantly different ages for Alaska Native children compared with white middle-class children in the United States.[29] Similarly, Gannoti[30] found differences between the normative group and a population of children living in Puerto Rico using the Pediatric Evaluation Disability Inventory (PEDI). Gannoti noted several social customs affecting the age at which developmental skills were expected to occur. For example, young children in Puerto Rico, in contrast to European American

children in the United States, typically use a bottle at night until 6 or 7 years of age and may not be expected to use a fork for fear of injury. Are the DDST and PEDI appropriate tests to use to evaluate children's development if the expected developmental age is different for the child's cultural group?

For adults, Duncan, as reported by Leavitt,[20] has validated a new Stroke Impact Scale for 14 culturally and linguistically diverse European groups. However, it has not been tested on people from South and Central America, Asia, or the Caribbean, the areas from which most immigrants to the United States come. Typically used functional tests do not take into account activities such as eating with chopsticks or hands, or moving in and out of the squat position. These activities may be everyday requirements for people from Asia. Research in this area will help lead to cultural proficiency; that is, when cross-cultural research is held in high regard and is disseminated, new approaches are developed in response to perceived need.

Concerning employment opportunities, a Chinese client looking for a job was frightened about the idea of being "tested" by a government agency and never returned to the counselor's office.[31] Employers may not understand the fear of such intrusions and the problems of limited English proficiency. Thus, the employer may presume someone is not cooperative or not sufficiently involved and therefore not worthy of the job. Moreover, the process of self-directed decision making favored by American healthcare professionals is anathema to many Asians, who have a worldview that stresses respect for health professionals' knowledge, a collectivist responsibility for one's health and/or disability, and a belief that the condition was ordained by spirits or the gods, which means that it would be useless to try to deal with the government.[31]

Healthcare Practices

Responsibility for Health and Beliefs about Disability

The noted anthropologist Arthur Kleinman[32] sees the healthcare system as a special kind of cultural system that includes such elements as patterns of belief about the causes of illness, decisions about how to respond to specific episodes of sickness, and the actions taken to effect a change. The beliefs and behaviors exhibited by an individual are influenced by macrosocial and bioenvironmental factors. Specifically, Kleinman has developed the theory of an "explanatory model"(EM) to analyze this kind of cultural system."EMs are the notions about an episode of sickness and its treatment that are employed by all those engaged in the clinical process. The study of patient and family EMs tell us how they make sense of given episodes of illness, and how they choose and evaluate particular treatments"[32] (p. 105). To derive an EM, the physical therapist might ask the questions posed in Box 16–2 to elicit the client's (or family's) personal point of view regarding the disability and the role the therapist will take to facilitate rehabilitation.

Causality refers to the cultural explanations for why a disability occurs. Few societies have only one explanation, and there may be different explanations for different disabilities. The variation in the beliefs concerning cause is considerable. Furthermore, people often "hedge their bets," incorporating the notion of multicausality for one diagnosis. Typically, remarks might be prefaced with "I don't know, but maybe . . ." or "I believe . . ., but my mother [husband, neighbor, etc.] thinks . . ." "Natural" or "supernatural" possibilities exist. Groce[5] contends that this need to ascribe causality is related to one's ability to justify demands made on social support networks and community resources.

Natural causation is also an explanation used in other cultures, but some explanations are more "scientifically sound" than others. For example, in Jamaica, a "scientific" natural explanation could be "Fits damage the brain," "The doctor say long time it take to born . . . ," "The afterbirth is coming before . . . ," or "I had lots of clots . . ." However, some naturalistic belief systems are not supported by scientific reality. Again from Jamaica: "Like how I have the children fast and the food me eat . . ."or "Me had a problem with me big daughter . . . sent her to buy shoes and she run away with a guy and she never come back until long after the baby born. I was very worried"[14] (p. 115). In this case, the diagnosis was Down syndrome.

In many Asian cultures, naturalistic explanations often focus on the suspected failure of the mother to follow prescribed healthy practices during pregnancy and the postnatal period. For example, Chan[33] reports a mother being blamed for her son's epilepsy because she ate lamb, a forbidden food, during pregnancy. The Chinese expression for epilepsy, *yang dian feng*, translates as "shaking of the lamb." Excessive "cold wind" and shellfish have also been held responsible for disability.

Alternatively, an imbalance of elements, or humors, may be naturalistic causes of a disability. In much of the world, the belief exists that there needs to be a balance of complementary forces for one to be in harmony with nature—a balance of "hot" and "cold" (Hispanic), yin and yang (Chinese), *fret* and *cho* (Haitian), *am* and *dong* (Vietnamese), or *garm* and *sard* (Iranian), for example.[34-39]

Leavitt[14] interviewed family members who had children with a disability in a poor, rural area of Jamaica. A majority of the interviewees did not believe their child was stigmatized. In fact, most noted that their family and neighbors seemed to be quite fond of the child in question. When a subject reported hearing negative comments, it was generally believed to be an isolated incident. Nevertheless, it is likely that stigma may have been a factor in some of the households.

BOX 16.2

Kleinman's Explanatory Model for Disability

1. What do you call your problem?
2. What do you think caused your problem?
3. What do you think your sickness/disability does to you?
4. What are the chief problems your illness/disability has caused you?
5. What are the most important results you hope to get from your treatment?
6. What are the consequences that you most fear as a result of your disability?

Source: Kleinman (1980).[32]

People from the European American cultures typically ascribe disability to natural causes such as viruses and bacteria, environmental agents such as accidents and toxins, or genetic disorders. Nevertheless, people might unhesitatingly ask a mother of a child born with a disability if she drank, smoked, or used drugs during pregnancy. A man with paraplegia is often given more sympathy if the disability is a result of fighting for his country as opposed to driving while drunk.

Although there is evidence that attitudes toward people with disabilities are becoming more positive in the United States, there is limited theoretical research linking cultural variables with attitudes toward people with disabilities. One such study, "Attitudes toward Disabilities in a Multicultural Society,"[40] investigated differences in the attitudes of six cultural groups in Australia with regard to 20 diagnoses. Overall, people with disabilities were accepted most by the German community, followed by the Anglo, Italian, Chinese, Greek, and Arabic groups. Interestingly, the results did not show significant differences with regard to the concept of stigma hierarchy; in all communities, people with asthma, diabetes, heart disease, and arthritis were the most accepted, and people with AIDS, mental retardation, psychiatric illness, and cerebral palsy were the least accepted.

A few studies examining attitudes toward people with disabilities for specific cultural groups have been conducted. Greeks and Greek Americans were compared with regard to attitudes toward people with disabilities, and the analysis indicated that ethnicity accounted for 28% of the variance, with more positive attitudes found among Greek Americans.[41] Saetermoe, Scattone, and Dim[42] found that Asian American respondents were more likely to stigmatize people with disabilities than were their African American, Latin American, or European American counterparts. Furthermore, Asian-born participants demonstrated more negative attitudes than the U.S.-born participants, supporting the idea that acculturation decreases stigmatization. Iwakuma and Nussbaum[43] reported that Japanese subjects have a strong sense of shame for having a disability, and for the "pollution" of the disability spreading to family members. Japanese folklore associated with disability is illustrated by concepts involving death and decay. As for less industrialized societies, Somali immigrants in the United States reported that people with disabilities are treated as part of the family and community, like any other member would be.[44] Of interest is that Nepalese children's attitudes toward people with disabilities were found to be more positive toward people who are obese, as obesity is associated with wealth, power, and food availability; this preference departs from all Western findings.[45] For people from a European American individualistic culture, the conditions listed in Box 16-3 are more likely to be present and contribute to a subculture of disability.

Reflective Exercise

• Do you believe that you have a responsibility to change the attitudes of others with regard to people with disabilities? • Why or why not? • In what ways might you attempt to influence others' attitudes?

BOX 16.3

American Subculture of Disability

1. Medical treatment makes survival with disabilities common.
2. Culture-wide concepts of normality and disability exist.
3. Cultural values stress individualism and achievement, and people with disabilities are likely to strive for independence and autonomy.
4. Disability is an overriding determinant of status and identity.
5. People with disabilities have opportunities to meet and interact with one another.
6. People with disabilities have access to education and technology that facilitate their interaction with others.
7. People with disabilities have access to a modern infrastructure such as transportation and communication systems.

Source: Loveland (1999).[46]

Disability across Cultures

In most communities, having a disability makes one stand out from the group; for example, in Native American communities, being different and calling attention to oneself is particularly stressful.[36] Some Native American parents discourage their children from having any contact with people with disabilities or even touching assistive technology. Likewise, being labeled as deviant is associated with the notion of contagion. There is fear that a disability might be "caught" or that one could become "contaminated," and in Kenya a hut for a people with disabilities may be built far away from the others and the person's belongings forbidden to be touched.[5]

In Nepal, there are many more boys reported to have polio than girls. The assumption is that girls do not survive because they either are placed at greater risk by being less well nourished or not adequately immunized, or are not allotted resources to facilitate survival or recovery.[5]

In Korea, deviance often leads to isolation, possibly due to uneasiness associated with not knowing what to do. If people do help those with disabilities, there is a tendency to over compensate and be overprotective, resulting in infantilization of people with disabilities.[47] Kim-Rupnow[47] also reports that in Korea the mother may be held responsible for a child with a disability if she did something during pregnancy to create an imbalance of metaphysical forces, *myang*.

Magicoreligious Beliefs

In many cultures, religious beliefs are highly associated with a supernatural belief system. Divine intervention is implicit in the Old Testament when people with disabilities were not allowed to approach the altar, and in the New Testament when Christ, upon restoring sight to a blind man, is reported to have said, "Go and sin no more." The Buddhist and Hindu religions also suggest the effect of retribution, with a sin in a past life being responsible for one's present situation.[48]

In contrast to these beliefs are those in which a supernatural cause is ascribed to the disability. Not infrequently, supernatural belief systems are associated with witchcraft, spirits, or ancestors who are punishing the people with disabilities, or

in the case of a child, the parents, who engaged in "inappropriate" behavior.[5,14,15,47] These explanations, however, must be viewed with caution. It is quite possible that informants underreport their belief in supernatural causes. Alternatively, one can believe in the supernatural but not associate it with his or her personal situation.

In rural Jamaica, supernatural explanations often include mention of the *duppy*.[14] The *duppy*, meaning ghost or spirit, is frequently blamed for things that go wrong or are evil. *Duppies* can be visible or invisible, and they can work through people, animals, birds, and plants. *Duppies* live and play around the silk cotton tree and are especially fond of the night. They are thought to be unpredictable, sometimes helpful and sometimes harmful. "The *duppy* . . . well, because babies are small, people who pass off like to play with them. That's what caused the life of my last baby. . . . When you leave baby alone, the *duppies* play with him. The *duppies* want to give assistance"[14] (p. 116).

In Jamaica, the Kumina Queen, a religious leader who is the "adoptive mother" of a mentally retarded boy, says, "It's a kind of spiritual order . . . the mother leave him at night and when she coming back for it nobody there to look about the baby. Spirit come and fingle it [plays with it or caring for it] . . . me give the child sugar and water and the spirit no like that . . . the father says spirit feed him—him sick and vomit up some green things [the child vomits up the bad spirit food]"[14] (p. 117).

Additional examples from Jamaica involving God's role in a child's disability are "I just believe God make him and he make everyone of us to his own likeness"[14] (p. 117) and "Sickness is not our fault. God gave it to us. We have faith in God"[14] (p. 117). In contrast, a few people in the Jamaican study specifically stated that they did not believe God had any connection to their child's problems. "I don't believe that God make him sick like that. Me say is me the problem come from since me was young"[14] (p. 117) and "God don't make anyone sick. Sickness is from the devil"[14] (p. 117).

In India the belief in karma, or payment for past deeds, underlies the belief system.[15] Alternatively, according to popular beliefs in Mexico, God can select parents who will be particularly kind to and protective of "special" children.[49] In Botswana, the birth of a child with a disability can be seen as either a sign of God's trust in the parents' ability or a punishment for a past transgression.[50]

Most Hispanics/Latinos are Roman Catholic and rely heavily on Catholicism to support them during times of stress. Religious beliefs are closely tied to folk remedies. Physical therapists are generally familiar with beliefs such as the power of holy water to ward off evil or the necessity of bringing a sick elder to pray before the image of a saint. At the period of death and dying the recitation of the Rosary and last rites are representative behaviors. Additionally, the "hot/cold" paradigm is relevant. For example, blood is "hot" and is associated with strength, virility, and machismo. A person who is anemic needs to eat more "hot" foods such as organ meats, which are considered blood products.

People of Hispanic origin may also become sick (i.e., be punished) if they have sinned or violated a taboo, thereby causing the wrath of God or invoking some source of wickedness. Belief in the evil eye is not uncommon. Generally, the concept implies that an evil spell has been put on another, which causes the victim to fall ill. The motive is usually envy. Other folk beliefs associated with supernatural forces include the notion that a pregnant woman must be careful using a sharp object or the child may be born with a cleft palate; and if she is knitting clothes for the child, she cannot wind the yarn into a ball or the child will be born with the cord wrapped around his or her neck.[39]

People of Asian origin may also believe in supernatural causes, divine punishment, and the need to maintain harmony by balancing hot and cold forces of nature. In the highly acclaimed and very readable book *The Spirit Catches You and You Fall Down*, Anne Fadiman[51] describes the cultural conflict between a Hmong family whose daughter Lia has a seizure disorder and her American physicians. The Hmong people are a traditional group from Laos, many of whom have unwillingly immigrated to the United States as a result of the Vietnam War. The Hmong see illness as a spiritual matter linked to everything in the universe, while the medical community in the United States attributes it to a division between the body and spirit. The Hmong call Lia's illness *quag dab peg*—"the spirit catches you and you fall down"—that is, the soul is taken and you cannot get well until the soul is returned.

For the Hmong, traditional healing practices including animal sacrifice and special ceremonies involving such tools as a saber, gong, rattle, finger bells, and a "flying horse" are paramount, as is the role of the *txiv neeb*, an indigenous healing practitioner. Not only are these very different practices from those used in the United States, but many Hmong also believe that American doctors remove organs from their patients to eat or to sell as food, that they anesthetize patients to allow the soul to escape, and that they cut the "spirit-strings" from patients' wrists, thus disturbing their "life-souls."[51]

For the American Indian, supernatural causes may relate to spirit loss, spirit intrusion, spells, or witchcraft.[36] Thus, physical therapists must be holistic in their approach to interventions for them to be effective.

Leavitt[14] describes health behaviors associated with children with disabilities in rural Jamaica. Many Jamaican respondents believed in the possibility of a supernatural cause for the disabling problem and used a variety of traditional healing practices. The Jamaicans' belief in African forms of witchcraft and animism is relevant to their behavioral response to the presence of disability. *Obeah*, or the practice of witchcraft, is essentially a magical means whereby an individual may obtain his personal desires, eradicate ill health, procure good fortune in life and business . . . , evince retribution or revenge upon his enemies, and generally manipulate the spiritual forces . . . to obtain his will.[52] The *obeah* man or woman keeps his "things" in his *obi* place. These "things" are composed of blood, feathers, parrot's beak, grave dirt, rum, and eggshells, and his "bush" is a concoction of medicinal herbs. The *obeah* may sometimes cause a problem by "putting" the spirit sickness on a person, or the *obeah* may "work it off." Many people visit an *obeah*, even though it is forbidden by law. Strongly linked with the concept of *obeah* is the belief in *duppies*. Religion appears to be as important a factor in the caretaker's behavior with regard to treatment practices as it is in the caretaker's belief system, as shown in Box 16-4.

BOX 16.4

Examples of the Influence of Religion on Caretakers' Behaviors and Beliefs in Jamaica

- "Need great faith . . . Darvey [the child] no have faith."
- "I'm a Christian you know, and he weren't like this you know [the child had been functioning at a lower level]. I took him to the Throne of Grace, and I laid on him right here and I prayed on him day and night and I ask God to touch him because he used to run all over the place as though him mad . . . but I entreated him to God and I laid on down on him and I pray and I say God touch him. I kept on asking the Lord to touch him, and I can see for *sure* him better."
- The Kumina Queen: "You have to call to God before you do anything . . . me deal with God direct . . . me no deal with the *duppy* one [*obeah* man] . . . me speak seven different languages and speak in tongues . . . I can't make him [the child] talk, God has to give that."

Source: Leavitt (1992).[14]

BOX 16.5

Folk Tales Regarding the Prevention of Disabilities in Babies in Jamaica

- Place an opened pair of scissors or a horseshoe over the bedroom door where the baby sleeps to keep away evil spirits.
- *Duppies* are afraid of red; newborn babies should have a red ribbon tied around their left wrist and wear red clothes to ward off evil spirits.
- Do not let menstruating women hold a baby or it will get stomach cramps.
- If a pregnant woman has sex with a man other than the baby's father, the baby will be handicapped.
- When the baby's navel stump falls off, the mother must bury it outside under a young plant to ensure that the baby will grow strong and healthy.
- Do not cut a baby's hair before he can talk or he will have problems talking.

Source: Leavitt (1992).[14]

Folk and Traditional Practices

Associated with these healing practices are folk tales that relate to prevention of a disability rather than treatment of an existing disability. The examples listed in Box 16-5 were shared by a group of women who worked with a pregnant Peace Corps volunteer.[14]

Jamaican folk medicine practices can be as simple as the use of a bush tea for a cold, avocado to lower high blood pressure, and pawpaw to get rid of a boil, or as complex as the treatment by an *obeah* man employing many of the previously mentioned materials. Most "bushmen" are not *obeah* men but rather spiritualists who believe that herbs can strengthen the physical body and help to ward off ailments. Often the spiritualist believes in the necessity of supporting the healing herbs with religious ceremony, charms, fresh air, and sunlight, or foods such as cock soup or roasted animal testes. Examples of statements concerning the use of indigenous healing practices for the treatment of a child with a disability in rural Jamaica are listed in Box 16-6.

Reflective Exercise

- Do you ask your clients about complementary and alternative forms of medicines and treatments?
- How do you feel about these treatments? • Do you serve as a cultural broker between the world of biomedicine and community healers?

Barriers for People with Disabilities

In today's world, barriers to full participation in society in such areas as education, vocational rehabilitation, healthcare, and employment for people with disabilities continue to exist. For people who are also from ethnic minorities, the barriers are even greater than those for white, middle-class people with disabilities, supporting

BOX 16.6

Use of Indigenous Healing Practices for the Treatment of a Child with a Disability in Rural Jamaica

- "I use baths a whole lot of times, in the night, put wash pan of water over here, and put two sticks and cross them—let it stay overnight, and bathe him in the morning."
- "I put milk in the bath, and no talk with anyone until after the bath."
- "Dig a hole to the level of the waist. Bury him in it for one hour, remove him and stand him."
- "Me use grapefruit juice and brandy to wet his mole [brain]. It helps to keep his brain steady."
- "Yes, I wouldn't hide you that [going to a mother lady], cause I had to try all that because I see and get the vision and maybe it can be a different inferior spirit come along and hurt her."
- "The mother lady sent me to the bush doctor shop. Get some kind oil to use on her and bush to boil."

Source: Leavitt (1992).[14]

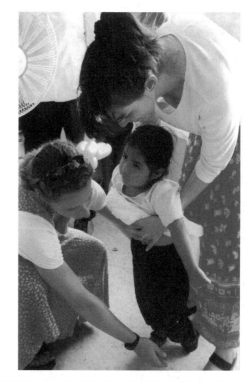

FIGURE 16.9 A child with a disability in Mexico faces more barriers to full participation in society than does a white, middle-class child.

the idea that some people are faced with a "double burden" (Fig. 16-9).

Linguistic and cultural barriers exist for people at all points in the life span. For example, Hampton,[31] who focused on Asian American people with disabilities, noted that medical expenditures for people with disabilities varied according to ethnicity. According to a study published in 1996 (with data from 1987), "Whereas white children spent $1,898 per child, African Americans spent $977 and Asian Americans $864. The presumption is that Asian Americans in fact do have a great need for services, but they are not being accessed secondary to lack of knowledge about healthcare services or lack of resources. Low utilization of available services has been reported specifically for Korean and Vietnamese populations."[31,53]

In 1990, Asian American students, constituting approximately 3% of the total school population, were thought to be underrepresented in special education (0.9%), suggesting that these students were either not being identified or not receiving the services to which they were entitled. Also, students were identified as not having the language support/modifications and services needed for successful completion of their individualized education plans' identified goals. Barriers identified by parents of Asian American students with disabilities were related to language, inappropriate referral and assessment practices, a lack of awareness about educational systems and processes (including their rights), and lack of cultural awareness by professionals.[31]

Older Asian Americans with disabilities are less likely to have Medicare, pensions, disability insurance or other benefits, or to participate in community-based health programs or live in nursing homes compared with their white counterparts.[20,31,53] Again, language barriers, lack of citizenship, limited access to insurance, and lack of advocacy skills are all potential burdens that can be added to the presence of disability or health problems.

Conclusion

The concept of intracultural diversity is supported by the wide variation in beliefs and behaviors with regard to disability and rehabilitation. It is easy to imagine how both a traditional people and the Western medical practitioner view the other as strange, ignorant, and stubborn. Conflict can easily arise. The clinician must acknowledge and accept, rather than ridicule, differing belief systems and behaviors associated with disability as long as they are not harmful to a person. Some folk remedies do include arsenic, lead, or opium, and these can be dangerous.

The future is likely to witness an increasing number of people with disabilities from a range of cultural groups. People with disabilities exist in every society along with specific sociocultural systems and explanatory models that account for beliefs about the disability and the cultural practices with regard to disability diagnosis and treatment. The social construction of disability is undoubtedly related in part to societal attitudes toward disability, the material realities of the environment, and the adaptive mechanisms that are available to the individual and family. In removing barriers, disability rights activists across nations are advancing toward theories of social justice, where disability is viewed as a form of human variation—a belief that bioethics groups and society should promote a collectivist mindset characterized by interdependence and human community rather than independence and personal autonomy, self-determination rather than self-sufficiency.

The newest paradigm, focusing on a client- or family-centered model, including community-based rehabilitation (CBR), independent living, and attention to the client's and family's sociocultural environment, has yet to be embraced by all. The process of change is slow, as evidenced by the many physical, political, societal, and personal obstacles people with disabilities face in their everyday lives. Nevertheless, society and the field of rehabilitation are moving in this direction.

Physical therapists must begin to appreciate the reality of disability for their clients. We have a role to play in advancing a modern approach to disability rights and the notion that cultural competence is as important as clinical competence. Embracing cultural diversity and developing the most appropriate service models and public policy to enhance the lives of all people with disabilities are moral imperatives for the physical therapy profession.

CASE STUDY SCENARIO

*D*wight Shattuck, a bright 4-year-old boy, has athetoid cerebral palsy. Although he is able to move along the floor by creeping, he is unable to sit independently or pull himself to a standing position. He is dependent in all self-care activities. He does not have any assistive devices and is carried everywhere by his mother or siblings. Dwight and his family—mother, age 30 years, and three siblings, ages 3, 9, and 14—came to Connecticut 5 months ago from Jamaica. They live in a small, run-down home within the Hartford city limits. Paula, his mother, works a few hours a week when her oldest child is home to care for Dwight. Dwight's father is "away for good," and Paula does not believe that Dwight's condition had anything to do with why the father left her and the children. As for her decision on where to move, Ms. Shattuck knew that a lot of Jamaican people live in Hartford, including some people she knew from home. She also knew that the United States had a good system for helping children with disabilities.

(continued)

When asked to describe the history of Dwight's illness, his mother said, "Dwight has brain damage; that's what the doctor tell me." Before seeing the doctor, she "didn't know what it was," but she suspected something was wrong since birth. "She told me something might be wrong with him . . . he take a long time before he was born, and the oxygen cut off from his brain and . . . she take him to Children's Hospital." Upon further prodding, his mother admitted that "he wasn't doing much like a child at 4 or 5 months. He just laying down . . . The fits took him when he was about 2."

Paula used to take Dwight to a community rehabilitation clinic when she lived in Jamaica. The worker there taught her some exercises and talked with her at her home. When asked about specific home remedies, Paula said, "Oh yes, I try some olive oil and so forth . . . olive oil and lotion." She also uses leaf of life and mint tea, but those are used for all the children if they are sick. Paula used to put Dwight in red clothes (dressing children in red clothes is believed to keep away evil spirits), but she no longer does. "I pray a lot for him, and neighbors pray for him too."

Regarding Ms. Shattuck's perception of whether Dwight is stigmatized, she said, "If you tell them (neighbors and friends) it brain damage, they just finish it and don't ask you no more questions." This, she feels, is much simpler that having "to explain everything" with the use of words such as cerebral palsy. When asked if others talk nastily about Dwight, she responded, "I don't know if they say it behind my back but not in front . . . [but] yes, some of them would . . . that he is handicapped and he's not going to walk." Nevertheless, Paula takes Dwight outside as she would take the other children, although this is becoming increasingly difficult because Dwight barely fits into the baby stroller.

Paula is most concerned about Dwight not yet sitting up or walking. She would like him to go to school, but she knows "nobody is going to look after him as I do it, understand him and have the patience." Does this make her angry? "No, not a bit . . . I know he's mine and I just have to make up my mind and stay with him until he's much better."

1. What explanatory model for Dwight's disability does the mother hold? How might this influence physical therapy interventions?

2. Does this family present with more characteristics of a collectivist culture or an individualist culture? How would this potentially affect the physical therapy interventions?

3. What traditional healthcare practices are present in this scenario? What more should the physical therapist know about them? How might they affect physical therapy interventions?

4. What barriers to physical therapy care exist in this scenario? How might the physical therapist assist in overcoming these barriers?

5. What evaluative tool might the physical therapist use? What considerations should the physical therapist make to ensure that the instrument is culturally appropriate?

6. What perceptions of disability are evidenced in this scenario? What influence might the physical therapist have on the perceptions of disability?

Adapted from Leavitt (1992).[14]

REFERENCES

1. Brundtland GH. The future of the world's health. In: Koop CE, Pearson C, Schwartz M, eds. *Critical Issues in Global Health.* San Francisco, Calif: Jossey-Bass; 2001:3–11.

2. Albrecht G, Selman K, Bury M. *Handbook of Disability Studies.* Thousand Oaks, Calif: Sage; 2001.

3. Ingstad B, Whyte SR. *Disability and Culture.* Berkeley: University of California Press; 1995.

4. Braddock D, Parish S. An institutional history of disability. In: Albrecht G, Selman K, Bury M, eds. *Handbook of Disability Studies.* Thousand Oaks, Calif: Sage; 2001:11–68.

5. Groce N. Health beliefs and behavior towards individuals with disability cross-culturally. In: Leavitt R, ed. *Cross-Cultural Rehabilitation: An International Perspective.* London, UK: WB Saunders; 1999:37–48.

6. Ravaud JF, Stiker HJ. Inclusion/exclusion: An analysis of historical and cultural meanings. In: Albrecht G, Selman K, Bury M, eds. *Handbook of Disability Studies.* Thousand Oaks, Calif: Sage; 2001:490–512.

7. Scheer J, Groce N. Impairment as a human constant: Cross-cultural and historical perspectives on variation. *J Soc Issues.* 1988;44:22–37.

8. Hanks J, Hanks L. The physically handicapped in certain non-occidental societies. *J Soc Sci.* 1948;4:11–20.

9. Smart J. *Disability, Society and the Individual.* Gaithersburg, Md: Aspen; 2001.

10. Kohrman M. Why am I not disabled? Making state subjects, making statistics in post-Mao China. *Med Anthropol Q.* 2003;17:5–24.

11. Leavitt R. *Cross-Cultural Rehabilitation: An International Perspective.* London, UK: WB Saunders; 1999.

12. Goffman E. *Stigma: Notes on the Management of Spoiled Identity.* Englewood Cliffs, NJ: Prentice-Hall; 1963.

13. Brown SC. Methodological paradigms that shape disability research. In: Albrecht G, Selman K, Bury M, eds. *Handbook of Disability Studies.* Thousand Oaks, Calif: Sage; 2001:145–170.

14. Leavitt R. *Disability and Rehabilitation in Rural Jamaica: An Ethnographic Study.* Associated University Presses; 1992.

15. Pinto P, Sahur N. *Working with People with Disabilities: An Indian Perspective.* Buffalo, NY: Center for International Rehabilitation Research Information and Exchange; 2001.

16. Aiken LR. *Attitudes and Related Psychosocial Constructs: Theories, Assessment, and Research.* Thousand Oaks, Calif: Sage; 2002.

17. Tervo R, Azuma S, Palmer G, Redinius P. Medical students' attitudes toward persons with disability: A comparative study. *Arch Phys Med Rehabil.* 2002;83:1537–1542.

18. Ingstad B. Disability in the developing world. In: Albrecht G, Selman K, Bury M, eds. *Handbook of Disability Studies.* Thousand Oaks, Calif: Sage; 2001:772–792.

19. Liu GZ. *Chinese Culture and Disability: Information for US Service Providers.* Buffalo, NY: Center for International Rehabilitation Research Information and Exchange; 2001.

20. Leavitt R. Developing cultural competence in a multicultural world. *PT Mag.* January, 2003:56–69.

21. McColl M, Bickenbach J. *Introduction to Disability.* London, UK: WB Saunders; 1998.

22. Boutris-Ghali, B. Message of the Secretary General: World programme of action opens way to full participation in society. In: *Disabled Persons Bulletin.* Vienna, Austria: United Nations Center for Social Development and Humanitarian Affairs; 1992. No. 2, Publication 64.

23. Antonek R, Livneh H. *The Measurement of Attitudes toward People with Disabilities: Methods, Psychometrics and Scales.* Springfield, Ill: Charles C Thomas; 1988.

24. Neufeldt A. "Appearances" of disability, discrimination and the transformation of rehabilitation service practices. In: Leavitt R, ed. *Cross-Cultural Rehabilitation: An International Perspective.* London, UK: WB Saunders; 1999:25–47.

25. Devlieger P. Physical "disability" in Bantu languages: Understanding the relativity of classification and meaning. *Int J Rehabil Res.* 1998;21:51–62.

26. Gwaltney J. *The Thrice Shy: Cultural Accommodation to Blindness and Other Disasters in a Mexican Community.* New York, NY: Columbia University Press; 1970.

27. Basnett I. Health care professionals and their attitudes toward and decisions affecting disabled people. In: Albrecht G, Selman K, Bury M, eds. *Handbook of Disability Studies.* Thousand Oaks, Calif: Sage; 2001:450–486.

28. Roush S. Shifting the paradigm of disability. *PT Mag.* June 1993:48–52.

29. Kerfield C, Guthrie M, Steward K. Evaluation of the Denver II as applied to Alaska Native children. *Pediatr Phys Ther.* 1997;9:23–31.

30. Gannoti M. *The Validity and Reliability of the Pediatric Evaluation of Disability for Children Living in Puerto Rico.* University of Connecticut; 1998. Dissertation abstract.

31. Hampton NZ. Asian Americans with disabilities: Access to education, health care, and rehabilitation services. In: *Asian Americans: Vulnerable Populations, Model Interventions, and Clarifying Agendas.* Boston, Mass: Jones and Bartlett; 2003.

32. Kleinman A. *Patients and Healers in the Context of Culture.* Berkeley: University of California Press; 1980.

33. Chan S. Families with Asian roots. In: *Developing Cross-Cultural Competence.* Baltimore, Md: Paul H Brookes; 1998:251–344.

34. Colin J, Paperwalla G. People of Haitian heritage [chapter on CD-ROM]. In: Purnell L, Paulanka B, eds. *Transcultural Health Care: A Culturally Competent Approach.* 2nd ed. Philadelphia, Pa: FA Davis; 2003.

35. Haifizi H, Lipson J. (2003). People of Iranian heritage. In: Purnell L, Paulanka B, eds. *Transcultural Health Care: A Culturally Competent Approach.* 2nd ed. Philadelphia, Pa: FA Davis; 2003:177–194.

36. Joe J, Malach R. Families with Native American roots. In: *Developing Cross-Cultural Competence.* Baltimore, Md: Paul H. Brookes; 1988.

37. Nowak T. People of Vietnamese heritage. In: Purnell L, Paulanka B, eds. *Transcultural Health Care: A Culturally Competent Approach.* 2nd ed. Philadelphia, Pa: FA Davis; 2003:327–345.

38. Zoucha R, Purnell L. People of Mexican heritage. In: Purnell L, Paulanka B, eds. *Transcultural Health Care: A Culturally Competent Approach.* 2nd ed. Philadelphia, Pa: FA Davis; 2003:264–279.

39. Zuniga M. Families with Latino roots. In *Developing Cross-Cultural Competence.* Baltimore, Md: Paul H. Brookes; 1998:209–250.

40. Westbrook M, Legge V, Pennay M. Attitudes towards disabilities in a multicultural society. *Soc Sci Med.* 1993;34:615–623.

41. Zaromatidis K, Papadaki A, Gilde A. A cross-cultural comparison of attitudes toward persons with disabilities: Greeks and Greek-Americans. *Psychol Rep Part II.* 1999;84:1189–1196.

42. Saetermoe C, Scattone D, Dim K. Ethnicity and the stigma of disabilities. *Psychol Health.* 2001;16:699–714.

43. Iwakuma M, Nussbaum F. Intercultural views of people with disabilities in Asia and Africa. In: Braithwaite D, ed. *Handbook of Communication and People with Disabilities:* *Research and Application.* Mahwah, NJ: Lawrence Erlbaum Associates; 1999.

44. Greeson C, McCarthy V, LeRoy B. A qualitative investigation of Somali immigrant perceptions of disability: Implications for genetic counseling. *J Genet Couns.* 2001;10:359–378.

45. Harper D. Children's attitudes toward physical disability in Nepal: A field study. *J Cross-Cult Psychol.* 1997;28:710–729.

46. Loveland C. The concept of culture. In: Leavitt R, ed. *Cross-Cultural Rehabilitation: An International Perspective.* London, UK: WB Saunders; 1999:15–24.

47. Kim-Rupnow WS. *An Introduction to Korean Culture for Rehabilitation Service Providers.* Buffalo, NY: Center for International Rehabilitation Research Information and Exchange; 2001.

48. Miles M. Some influences of religions on attitudes towards disabilities and people with disabilities. In: Leavitt R, ed. *Cross-Cultural Rehabilitation: An International Perspective.* London, UK: WB Saunders; 1999:49–58.

49. Madiros M. Conception of childhood disability among Mexican-American parents. *Med Anthropol.* 1989;12:55–68.

50. Ingstad B. Problems with community mobilization and participation in CBR. In: Leavitt R, ed. *Cross-Cultural Rehabilitation: An International Perspective.* London, UK: WB Saunders; 1999:207–216.

51. Fadiman A. *The Spirit Catches You and You Fall Down.* New York, NY: Farrar, Straus and Giroux; 1997.

52. Morrish I. *Obeah, Christ and Rastaman: Jamaica and Its Religion.* Cambridge, UK: James Clarke; 1982.

53. Ling W. *Cultural Diversity of Older Americans: An Overview of East Asian Cultures for Physical Therapists.* APTA, Section on Geriatrics; 2003.

Chapter 17

Veteran and Military Culture and Physical Therapy

● Stephanie Beaman, MPT, and Jill Black Lattanzi, PT, EdD*

*S*ergeant Walker is a 24-year-old female special operations communications specialist in the U.S. Army. She has recently returned home from Iraq after sustaining gunshot wounds to her right leg. After being placed in a military hospital for 1 week for acute treatment of her wounds, she has been honorably discharged and will be continuing her medical care at her local VA hospital. She has been experiencing 8/10 constant, burning pain in her right leg, despite taking multiple narcotic pain medications. This pain is interfering with her ability to sleep and her ability to walk short distances. Sergeant Walker has been referred to outpatient physical therapy for gait training, strengthening, range of motion (ROM), and modalities prn.

Introduction

People who have served in the military share a subculture. Their training and experiences give them commonalities that may cross dominant cultural lines. Indeed, active participation in the military subjects one to the culture of the military. Military culture includes specific values, customs, traditions, and philosophical principles that have combined to create a common framework for those in uniform. Military culture provides a common institutional and organizational ethos and influences standards of behavior, discipline, teamwork, loyalty, and selfless duty.[1]

Physical therapy professionals may interact with servicemen and women, and thereby inter-act with the military culture, in their professional practice. The military's health system is one of the largest in the world. Each branch of the military has its own network of healthcare facilities. The Army's network alone manages the care for 3 million beneficiaries spread across 600 hospitals and clinics worldwide.[2] Most reputable is Walter Reed Army Hospital, in Washington, DC. In addition to active military hospitals, the Veterans' Health Administration (VHA) serves the needs of U.S. military veterans and is the largest employer of physical therapy professionals. In fact, employment data for 2003 shows 982 physical therapists employed by the VHA. This is up from 677 in 1995.[3] This chapter is important because of the significance of military culture as well as the large number of physical therapy professionals who

*Special thanks to Peter Glover, DPT

will interact in professional practice with clients of a military culture.

Reflective Exercise

• Have you had physical therapy clients with a military background? • Have you ever considered working for the Veteran's Health Administration?

Overview / Heritage

The U.S. Military Culture

As one serviceman stated, irony exists in that the individual freedoms of the world's strongest democracy are defended by a military culture that functions like a strong dictatorship. The young serviceman was identifying the contrast between the values of civil society and those of military society in the United States. Civil society values individual freedom, autonomy, and self-expression, while military society downplays personal liberties and individualities and emphasizes duty, loyalty, self-sacrifice, and obedience to command. The values emphasized by the military are essential for success in combat and in the defense of U.S. civilian freedoms.

Reflective Exercise

• Do you believe that military culture is more of an individualistic culture or a collectivist culture? • Why? (You may wish to refer to Table 2-1.)

Military statutes and values are recognized and upheld by the laws of the United States and have been consistently supported by the Supreme Court. The culture of the U.S. military has its foundation in the Declaration of Independence, in the U.S. Constitution, and in more than 225 years of experience defending the freedoms of U.S. civilians.[1]

While U.S. military culture differs among branches of military service, commonalities of culture permeate all service branches and all levels of command. All military personnel, be they enlisted members or officers, experience a boot camp or basic training as a rite of passage for new initiates. Boot camp or basic training achieves the

transformation of civilians into service members through the indoctrination of military culture and ideology over individual civilian freedoms. By stripping recruits of their civilian clothes, shaving off their hair, forbidding them accustomed freedoms, taxing them physically, depriving them of sleep, and forcing them to depend on the team for survival, the military deindividualizes recruits and then reshapes and molds them such that military discipline and culture become second nature.[4,5] Thus, recruits emerge with a new worldview, one of "service before self," and a commitment to the potential ultimate sacrifice, that of their lives for the sake of their country's civilian freedoms.[6] The recruits also emerge with an understanding of the rules and procedures of military culture, an appreciation for military rituals and traditions, and an understanding of military discipline. Enlisted recruits are taught to follow; officer recruits are taught both to lead and to follow.

Reflective Exercise

• Compare military boot camp to physical therapy school. What similarities and differences do you see?

Military culture is protected, communicated, demonstrated, and upheld by the officers of the armed forces. The officers of all service branches turn military values into action, lead by example, and communicate the viewpoint of the military institution.[1,7] In addition, each service branch functions as a meritocracy, with advancement determined by merit. Service members advance from the bottom of the enlistment ranks or the bottom of the officer ranks, with few opportunities to enter laterally on either ladder. President Truman in 1948 reaffirmed the practice of military meritocracy in the face of U.S. civilian society racism when he wrote an executive order requiring "equality of treatment and opportunity for all persons in the armed services without regard to race, color, religion, or national origin."[8] Thus President Truman theoretically "opened the doors of the nation's greatest meritocracy to a large group of disenfranchised African Americans who found in the military opportunity for advancement that was closed to them in the society at large."[4] Table 17-1 depicts the rank order for the different military services. The physical therapist

TABLE 17.1

U.S. Military Hierarchy

RANK	ARMY/AIR FORCE/MARINE CORPS	NAVY/COAST GUARD
Commissioned Officers		
Special	Five-star general	Five-star admiral
O–7 to O–10	General (1–4 stars)	Admiral (1–4 stars)
O–6	Colonel	Captain
O–5	Lieutenant colonel	Commander
O–4	Major	Lieutenant commander
O–3	Captain	Lieutenant
O–2	1st lieutenant	Lieutenant junior grade
O–1	2nd lieutenant	Ensign
Warrant Officers		
WO 1–5	Warrant officers (Army/MC 1–5) (Air Force—none)	Warrant officers (Navy 1–4 only) (Coast Guard 2–4 only)
Enlisted Ranks		
E-9	Sergeant major (Army/MC) Chief master sergeant (AF)	Master chief petty officer
E-8	Master sergeant (Army/MC) Senior master sergeant (AF)	Senior chief petty officer
E-7	Sergeant 1st class (Army) Gunnery sergeant (MC) Master sergeant (AF)	Chief petty officer
E-6	Staff sergeant (Army/MC) Technical sergeant (AF)	Petty officer 1st class
E-5	Sergeant (Army/MC) Staff sergeant (AF)	Petty officer 2nd class
E-4	Corporal (Army/MC) Senior airman (AF)	Petty officer 3rd class
E-3	Private 1st class (Army) Lance corporal (MC) Airman 1st class (AF)	Seaman
E-2	Private E-2 (Army) Private 1st class (MC) Airman (AF)	Seaman apprentice
E-1	Private (Army/MC) Airman basic (AF)	Seaman recruit

Note: U.S. military ranking is divided into commissioned officers, warrant officers, and enlisted ranks. Commissioned officers are at the top of the military hierarchy and are confirmed at their ranks by the Senate. Servicemen with professional degrees are awarded commissioned officer status. Warrant officers are specialists in certain military capabilities and hold warrants from their service secretary. Enlisted-rank servicemen can be promoted to warrant officer status by successful completion of specialized technical training. Enlisted ranks range from the new recruits to servicemen with advanced training or skills.

working in settings where military personnel come for healthcare should be familiar with the ranks.

Reflective Exercise

• To what degree does the military culture value authority? • Autonomy? • Respect? • Equality? • How might these values affect the physical therapy interaction?

The military uniform bespeaks the military culture by signifying rank, identity, and hierarchy[9] (Fig. 17-1). Separating soldier from civilian, private from general, and pilot from seaman, the distribution, fitting, and wearing of uniforms signal a rite of passage in military training. New recruits learn conformity, obedience, and attention to detail from the many military regulations governing the wearing of the uniform.[10] Military uniforms denote a mindset as well as an image and represent an embodiment of military culture.

James Burk[11] identified four essential components of military culture common across all services: discipline, professional ethos, ceremony and etiquette, and cohesion and esprit de corps. Discipline requires obedience to orders without question and self-sacrifice for the good of the unit and the nation. Discipline is essential for success on the battlefield and distinguishes the U.S. military from an armed mob. The professional ethos of military culture encompasses the willingness to engage an armed opponent and the willingness to sacrifice oneself for the good of the nation, the mission, and comrades. Professional ethos is essential to meet the rigorous demands of armed combat and includes physical and moral courage and discipline. Ceremony and etiquette, the most visible aspect of military culture, includes salutes, uniforms, ribbons and medals, and the playing of "Taps" (Fig. 17-2). Burk[11] describes these as "institutional

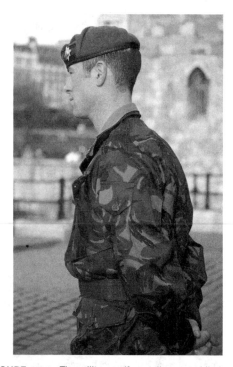

FIGURE 17.1 The military uniform tells us a soldier's rank, identity, and hierarchy.

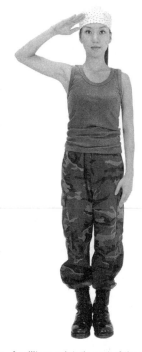

FIGURE 17.2 A military salute is part of the ceremony and etiquette of the military culture.

imperatives to acknowledge lawful authority, control or mask anxiety, affirm solidarity, and celebrate the unit or the individual" (pp. 451–452). These traditions create bonds and unity and contribute to military effectiveness. The bonds and unity or "cohesion and esprit de corps" constitute the fourth common cultural element described by Burk. "Cohesion is the shared sense of sacrifice and identity that binds service members to their comrades in arms"[11] (p. 452) and includes loyalty and unity, which results in the formation of strong bonds in the face of military hardships.

Individual Service Overview

With military culture as a common base, the individual services build elements of their own culture into the structure of military culture. Hence a serviceman or woman self-identifies as soldier, sailor, airman, marine, or coastguardsman. The delineation of service culture permits the military person to concentrate on the respective skills and doctrines necessary for specific missions on land, on sea, or in the air.[1]

The United States Army is the oldest of the service branches, with roots reaching to the colonial militiamen of the Revolutionary War. Formally established by the Continental Congress on 14 June 1775, the U.S. Army has faithfully trained men and women to be soldiers with an emphasis on land combat. Most recently, the Army changed its slogan from "Be All You Can Be" to "An Army of One" to place importance on unity amidst the diversity of individual soldiers (Fig. 17-3).[12] The United States Navy began as the Continental Navy and was founded 13 October 1775 by the Continental Congress. The Department of Navy was established 30 April 1798 and has grown to include four principal components: the Department of the Navy, with executive offices mostly in Washington, DC; the Operating Forces, which includes the Marine Corps; the Reserve Components; and the U.S. Coast Guard in times of war (the U.S. Coast Guard reports to the Department of Homeland Security in times of peace).[13]

The U.S. Marine Corps was also birthed in the time of the Revolutionary War, having been established on 10 November 1775, just 5 months after the Army and 1 month after the Navy. The Marines represent a smaller number of warriors

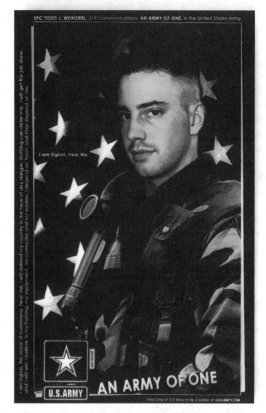

FIGURE 17.3 "An Army of One" is the U.S. Army's new slogan. (Photo courtesy of U.S. Army.)

and are described as "the aggressive tip of the military spear" and the "only forward-deployed force designed for expeditionary operations by air, land, or sea."[14] *Semper fidelis,* or *semper fi,* meaning "always faithful" in Latin, is the Marine Corps motto describing Marines' commitment to each other, to the organization, and to the country. The Corps core values are honor, courage, and commitment.[15]

The Unites States Air Force had its beginnings as a branch of the Army in the early 1900s, just after the Wright brothers' first flight at Kitty Hawk, North Carolina. In July 1909, the U.S. Army purchased the first plane from the Wright brothers. The U.S. Army Air Corps was formally organized under the Army in July 1926, and the National Defense Act of 1940 appropriated the necessary funds to purchase 6,000 airplanes. In June 1941, the U.S. Army Air Force was established and became a strong participant in World War II. On 18 September 1947, the U.S. Air Force was established as a service branch independent of the U.S. Army.[16]

Today, the four services work closely together and yet separately as they each train and prepare for diverse aspects of their mission to defend the United States of America. Improvements in technology and communications permit the different branches to advance in expertise and improve in cooperation with one another. All service members share the same goal, defending the freedoms of the people of the United States of America.

Reflective Exercise

• Within the U.S. armed services, what intercultural and intracultural similarities and differences exist?

The Veterans' Health Administration

The Veterans' Health Administration (VHA) is the nation's largest integrated healthcare system and is devoted to serving the needs of America's veterans by providing primary care, specialized care, and related medical and social support services[17] (Fig. 17-4). Founded in the early 1900s, it began as an inpatient, facility-based system. In 1995 the VHA underwent a major transformation in line with the nationwide shift in healthcare toward a more outpatient- and community-based focus. Since 1995, the VHA has eliminated more than 6,000 inpatient beds and provided in-

creased outpatient and home care services. The VHA also responded to a need to improve mental/behavioral health services by establishing more than 2,000 psychosocial residential rehabilitation beds.

By 1997, the VHA had instituted a practice of servicing clients via primary care teams. Primary care teams are designed to meet the complex needs of veterans through continuity of service and coordination with integrated health team members. Integrated primary care team members include a primary care provider and can include a triage nurse, other supportive nursing staff, a behavioral health provider, a social worker, a dietician, and a pharmacist.[18] There is an emerging model in the VHA that adds physical therapy as an integral member of the primary care team (Fig. 17-5). The system is known as the Primary Care Model for Physical Therapists and is discussed in further detail later in this chapter.

As of July 2002, the VHA operated approximately 163 hospitals, 850 ambulatory care and community-based clinics, 137 nursing homes, 43 domiciliaries that function as intermediate treatment and transitional living facilities for disabled veterans, 206 readjustment counseling centers, and 73 comprehensive home care programs.[19] The VHA also offers a number of specialty services, including treatment of spinal cord injury, rehabilitation of the blind, geriatrics, and treatment for traumatic head injury.

The number of enrollees in the VHA system increased from 2.9 million to 6.8 million during

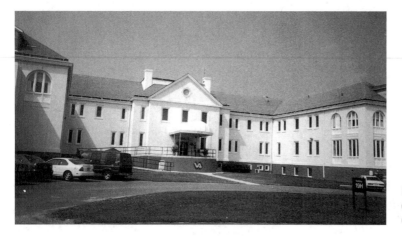

FIGURE 17.4 A VHA medical campus. (Photo courtesy of Peter Glover.)

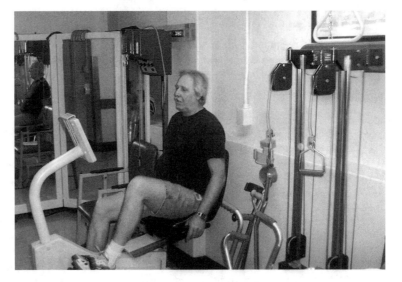

FIGURE 17.5 A military veteran undergoing rehab in a VHA hospital. (Photo courtesy of Peter Glover.)

the period from 1996 to 2002. This growth was largely due to a policy change in 1996. Traditionally, VHA enrollees were restricted to low-income veterans who had suffered injuries or illnesses related to their time of service. In 1996 Congress acted to allow almost all veterans care through the VHA system. This has posed great challenges to the system and healthcare personnel as they attempt to meet the healthcare needs of a much larger population.

Reflective Exercise

• Why might a physical therapist consider working for the Veterans' Health Administration (VHA)? • How might working for the VHA differ from working in another setting?

Communication

Dominant Language

The United States military conducts all communication in English, and yet physical therapists in veteran's hospitals report encountering patients whose primary language is something other than English. In World War II, many men from the Philippines enlisted in the U.S. military to assist in the defense of their country; therefore, some of the older veterans receiving medical care in the veteran's hospitals speak Filipino as their primary language.

The U.S. Census of 2000 indicates that 4.3% of the veteran population is of Latino/Hispanic origin.[20] The physical therapist in the military or veteran's system may readily encounter clients who communicate better in Spanish than in English.

Contextual Use

The contextual use of language in the U.S. military differs from that in U.S. civilian society. As discussed in Chapter 4, the dominant U.S. society communicates in a low-context manner, relying on explicit explanations and many words to communicate effectively. The U.S. military culture, steeped in traditions and codes of conduct, represents high-context communication. For example, the specifics of the uniform communicate rank and implicitly dictate behavior. The understood code of conduct dictates order and procedure without explicit explanations. In this way, the culture of the U.S. military more closely resembles the high-context communication patterns of Asian and Middle Eastern cultures. The physical therapist working within a military setting would be wise to study and learn the implicit patterns of communication present within this environment. In this way, he or she might avoid a cultural misunderstanding, offense, or faux pas.

Reflective Exercise

• Is military culture communication more high-context or low-context? • What implications might this have on physical therapy interactions? • What must the physical therapist do to avoid miscommunication?

Like all cultures and subcultures, military culture has invented its own jargon, using numerous terms with unique meanings and creating a status position for its members, adding to the insider/outsider hierarchy. One cannot be a member of a group without understanding and speaking the group's language. A physical therapist working in the VA system gives this account:

There was a veteran who had survived a failed suicide attempt. The veteran had jumped off an overpass and had shattered bones in both legs. The veteran was a member of the 173rd Airborne Brigade in Vietnam, a small airborne unit that had numerous casualties. When the veteran found out that I was to arrive as a new physical therapist and that I had been a member of the 82nd Airborne division, he said he would hold off on his physical therapy until I arrived. We hit it off immediately, and I learned during the physical therapy evaluation that the suicide attempt had been an attempt to end the "survivor guilt" this veteran had been experiencing since the Vietnam War. He also discussed why he felt he had survived his leap off the overpass. In his training as a paratrooper, he had done hundreds of parachute landing falls (PLFs), a technique used to decrease injuries when landing from a parachute jump. I was the only healthcare provider who had any idea what a PLF was, and what the 173rd Airborne Brigade was. He had mentioned these things to other providers, but they never questioned him about PLFs or his service as a paratrooper. I'm sure most of his providers didn't know the term, but also didn't bother to ask. Sometimes, just inquiring about the terms can help reassure a veteran that you are interested in him or her and genuinely care about his or her experiences. (Marilyn Rodgers, personal communication, August 21, 2003)

In this case, the therapist had been a member of the group and understood the language as well as the stresses and trials of military combat. In general, the physical therapist does not have to know or use the group's terms, but some understanding of them or a demonstrated interest in or asking about them may help in gaining rapport with military clients.

Reflective Exercise

• How might a physical therapist without military experience gain knowledge and understanding of military terms and expressions?

Greetings and Names

The U.S. military uses a formal pattern for greetings and names. Those in active military service should first be called by their rank followed by their last name. Physical therapists practicing within the military hospital system should follow the same practice. This pattern of address is not expected among nonactive veterans. Here the physical therapist should follow the same procedure for names as one would in civilian society, always being more formal, using title such as Mr., Mrs., Miss, Ms., or Dr. until told to do otherwise.

Reflective Exercise

• In the initial vignette, how should the therapist greet the client?

Time

The military uses military time, and the military physical therapist will need to do so as well. Military time uses a 24-hour time scale, with 0000 corresponding to midnight and 2300 corresponding to 11 P.M. There is no need for an A.M. or P.M. designation. Timeliness is valued within military culture, with events seen as occurring in a sequential rather than a circular manner. In this way, U.S. military culture is characterized by a monochronic perception of time. Appointments and events are expected to start on time.

Physical Touch

As with U.S. civilian culture, the physical therapist should always explain the procedure to the patient and ask specific permission to touch the patient before doing so. Professional, respectful touch is appropriate when the patient has given permission. This is especially important when working with a client who has been in active combat. Post-traumatic stress disorder might cause a patient to respond violently to unexpected or unwanted touch. One physical therapist warns of attempting to awaken a sleeping veteran by physically touching him or her. He notes that the veteran may awaken and understand you to be the enemy. Eye contact is highly recommended to gain the trust and respect of both military and veteran physical therapy patients.

Reflective Exercise

• How comfortable are you with physical touch from a stranger? • Imagine having served in combat and now having post-traumatic stress disorder. How might you react to unexpected physical touch?

Family Roles and Organization

Head of Household
The head of the household differs as vastly within military culture as it does within civilian culture; thus the physical therapist must recognize that the spouse of the active military person often needs to perform all the household responsibilities during times of deployment.

Gender Roles
Gender roles within the U.S. military, as within U.S. civilian society, aim for equality and yet statistically favor males. The first enlisted women in the U.S. military joined the Navy and Marines in World War I (1917–1918). They served as bilingual telephone operators in the Army Signals Corps, in administrative support positions in the Navy and Marine Corps, and as nurses for the Army and Navy Nurse Corps. However, these women were used only for the duration of the war and were discharged once the war was over. In World War II (1941–1945), approximately 400,000 women served at home and overseas in noncombat positions. President Truman granted women permanent status in the Army, Navy, Air Force, and Marine Corps in 1948. The Persian Gulf War in the early 1990s saw the deployment of 41,000 women overseas and into a myriad of combat

support positions ranging from reconnaissance to aircraft pilots.[21] Although women are still restricted from serving in specific positions that require direct engagement in fighting, such as infantry and Special Forces, they often become targets or victims of combat due to the blurred lines of combat and noncombat zones. Therefore, therapists may see similar medical and mental health issues in women that arise from exposure to violence and environmental hazards of a particular war and geographical region.

Currently, women account for 15% of active-duty, reserve, and guard units of the U.S. armed forces.[22] The number of female officers lags behind the number of male officers, and this very likely represents the recent acceptance of females into the rank of officers.[8] The April 2001 Department of Defense Almanac reports that females comprise 14.2% of officers for the four main branches of the military.[23] However, as the number of females who enter the military increases, one would expect the number of female officers also to rise.

Corresponding to the military's deemphasis of the individual and emphasis on group unity and oneness, gender differences within the military are vilified. The uniforms of all personnel are the same regardless of gender and are designed to downplay their differences. The guidelines for wearing hair, makeup, and jewelry minimize gender differences such that an observer would have a difficult time distinguishing a male from a female in a platoon lineup. Gender differences, however, are recognized when it comes to physical performance standards and weight measurement standards. In general, the military is consistent in its determination to minimize differences in individuals and to train personnel to respond with the best interests of the group in mind.

Goals and Priorities
Family is important within military culture, as demonstrated by programs such as Army Family Team Building, which has developed a "chain of concern"—a designated group of military spouses who shadow the chain of command in order to disperse information to family members of the deployed.[24] Likewise, service members are required to have "family care plans" in case of deployment.[25] While family is a priority within

the military, military families often make major sacrifices as their loved one demonstrates an overriding commitment to God and country and to the unit. The military culture operates more like a collectivist society than the individualistic society of the U.S. civilian culture; yet the collectivist commitment is not as much to family as it is to the military organization and the mission to defend the United States of America.

Role of the Aged

U.S. military culture, with its meritocracy and respect for rank and experience, innately promotes a respect for older persons. An older adult who has achieved a high officer rank or has significant experience and earned a high enlistment rank will be afforded greater respect among veterans than the same individual would in civilian society. Often, older military personnel are seen as valuable mentors and advisors.

Reflective Exercise

• In what ways is the military culture more individualistic and in what ways is it more collectivistic?
• What implications might these characteristics have on the physical therapy program?

Workforce Issues

Acculturation

U.S. military personnel are often bicultural to the degree that they interact within the military culture and yet come from and repeatedly return to the U.S. civilian culture. Sometimes these cultural lines may become muddled and lead to misunderstandings and confusion in a healthcare encounter.

Reflective Exercise

• Describe how someone with military experience might be bicultural. What tensions may develop as a result of this potential duality?

Military Model for Physical Therapists

The first formalized course of physical therapy instruction in the military began at Walter Reed General Hospital of Washington, DC, in 1922. This program evolved over several decades and was taken over by the combined forces of the U.S. Army and Baylor University. In 1971 the U.S. Army and Baylor University developed a Master of Physical Therapy program and in 2003 initiated a Doctorate of Physical Therapy program.[2] The program's development in 1971 coincided with a time in which there were a growing number of neuromuscular injuries caused by intense physical training and combat injuries in the Vietnam War. Also at this time a shortage of orthopedic physicians to evaluate and treat soldiers with these injuries existed. The U.S. Army responded to this problem by utilizing physical therapists as primary care providers, also known as physician extenders, for evaluation and treatment of neuromuscular complaints.

In the mid-1970s, the concept of physical therapists and physician extenders became more popular and widely implemented. Some Army facilities began to allow physical therapists the authority to prescribe certain medications. Over the next few decades, other military branches began to incorporate various forms of the "military model" into their health systems. Military physical therapists took on greater autonomy and enjoyed expanded privileges. These privileges, granted for specially trained and properly credentialed physical therapists, vary from branch to branch and from facility to facility. Examples of privileges a military physical therapist may have are ordering imaging and lab tests; prescribing anti-inflammatory medications, analgesics, and muscle relaxants; conducting electromyograph (EMG) and nerve conduction velocity (NCV) tests; making referrals to other healthcare providers; and restricting physical training or duty. Serving in this role, military physical therapists not only have taken on a greater responsibility, but have earned respect and high status among the military healthcare team.[2,26,27]

Primary Care Model for Physical Therapists

The "primary care model" of physical therapy is an emerging system in the VHA, with its foundation in the "military model" of physical therapy. Beginning as a pilot primary care internship program that took place in the VHA of Salt Lake City, UT, in the summer of 2000, this program was designed to improve upon the traditional physical therapy clinical internship by providing unique learning experiences and leadership opportunities. Physical therapist students and their attending physical therapists serve as direct care providers for neuromuscular disorders. Referrals may come directly from a telephone triage nurse or the emergency room. VHA facilities, such as the VHA Maryland Healthcare System and the VHA Salt Lake City, Utah, Healthcare System, have incorporated parts of the primary care model. The ultimate goal of this initiative is the expansion of the model throughout the entire VHA healthcare system as well as into the private sector.

Reflective Exercise

• Describe the military model and the primary care model for physical therapists. How are they different or the same from the model practiced outside the military? • What is your opinion of the military and primary care models?

High-Risk Behaviors

Tobacco

Tobacco is used by 35% of U.S. military personnel, a rate 9% higher than in the general population.[28] Tobacco is often used by military personnel as a stress management tool. Despite its perceived efficacy in stress management, tobacco use is strongly discouraged in the military. Smoking-related healthcare costs in the Defense Department are estimated at $530 million. The associated low-productivity costs are about $345 million.[29] Smoking cessation programs are available in military as well as in VHA hospitals.

Substance Abuse

Substance abuse, including use of illicit drugs such as marijuana, cocaine, and heroin, is an identified problem for some veterans. Often illegal substances are used by veterans with severe chronic pain and/or mental health issues. For example, results of the National Vietnam Veterans Readjustment Study showed that "73% of male Vietnam Veterans who met diagnostic criteria for PTSD also qualified for a lifetime diagnosis of alcohol abuse or dependence" and 15% qualified for a lifetime diagnosis of drug abuse.[30]

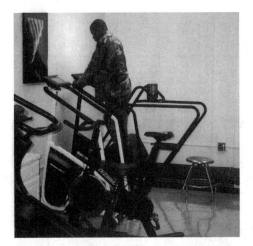

FIGURE 17.6 Those in the military are accustomed to physical fitness training. (Photo courtesy of Peter Glover.)

Physical Activity

Physical fitness is a recognized priority and value within the military. Physical readiness is essential for successful combat, and all military personnel undergo a form of regular physical training and fitness testing (Fig. 17-6). The physical therapist should find that the physical training of rehabilitation is understood and accepted by the client with military training.

Safety

The U.S. military dedicates personnel and funding to support research designed to prevent injuries in its uniformed men and women. Injury prevention and proper safety techniques are taught to ensure the long-term health of soldiers and to prevent unnecessary losses, which would deplete its active forces. As primary educators for safety, military physical therapists are often involved in job site analysis, demonstration of proper physical training techniques, and instruction in aerobics or weight lifting tasks.[27]

Reflective Exercise

• How might these high-risk behaviors positively or negatively affect the physical therapy program?
• What role or responsibility does the physical therapist have in encouraging positive behaviors?

Nutrition

An inadequate diet is a major contributing factor to the rising rate of type II diabetes in veterans. The October 2000 VHA Fact Sheet revealed that 16% of veterans had type I or type II diabetes; by 2003 the prevalence of diabetes had increased to 20%.[31,32] In contrast, 6.3% of the general U.S. population are diagnosed with diabetes.[33] Nutritionists are available within the VHA to assist veterans with their diets and to help with nutritional instruction in preventing or managing type II diabetes.

Reflective Exercise

• Why might the high rate of diabetes among veterans concern the physical therapist? • What impact might it have on the physical therapy program?

Death Rituals

Military funeral honors may be bestowed upon military members on active duty or in the Selected Reserve, or upon military veterans who served on active duty and departed under conditions other than dishonorable. Military funeral honors include draping the casket with the national flag, flag folding, flag presentation, and the playing of "Taps"[34] (Fig. 17-7).

The flag, for one who dies on active duty, is provided by the individual's branch of service. For the veteran, the flag is provided by the Department of Veterans Affairs. The flag covers the casket so that the union blue field is at the head and over the left shoulder. It is not allowed to touch the ground and is not placed in the grave. The flag folding ceremony follows, and the flag is usually presented to the next of kin by a military chaplain.[35]

"Taps" was composed by Union Army Brigadier General Daniel Butterfield in 1862 after a bloody battle. He felt that the traditional bugle call at the day's end was too formal. With the help of his bugler, he composed "Taps" and had it played to signal the day's end. In 1862, "Taps" was played at the burial of a soldier when the burial took place near enemy lines and it would have been too dangerous to fire the traditional 21-gun salute. "Taps" was officially adopted by the U.S. Army in 1874. The playing of "Taps" became a custom at military burials.[34,35]

The respective armed forces are responsible for the military funeral services of active service members, and the Department of Defense oversees the provision of military funeral honors

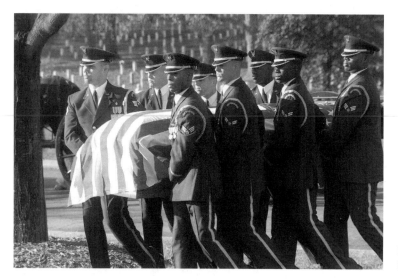

FIGURE 17.7 The honor of a military funeral. (Photo courtesy of U.S. Army.)

for eligible veterans. The National Defense Authorization Act of 2000 defined veterans' rights to military funeral honors.[36]

Reflective Exercise

• Why might it be helpful for a physical therapist working within the military and VHA system to understand military death rituals and traditions?

Spirituality

Individual Strength

The majority of active military servicemen and veterans are notable for their individual strength. This individual strength is made greater through their completing basic training, overcoming challenging military endeavors, and meeting the challenges of adjustment to post-military life and reintegration into civilian society.

Chaplain Services

The military as a whole places great value on spirituality, as demonstrated by its longtime commitment to chaplain services (Fig. 17-8). Chaplains have been a part of U.S. military battles since the Revolutionary War, when clergymen would often rally military units from their own congregations and accompany them into battle. Chaplains in the military were officially recognized on 29 July 1775 and were assigned the title and pay of a captain. In 1940, there were 137 Army chaplains on active duty. By 1945, the number had grown to 8,191, with 5,620 representing the Protestant faith, 243 the Jewish faith, and 278 the Roman Catholic faith.[37] Today the range of faiths represented by military chaplains has been expanded to include Hinduism, Buddhism, Islam, and others encompassing 290 endorsed agents.[37]

Qualifications to become a military chaplain include graduation from a 4-year college and a 3-year seminary, ordination, accreditation, good standing with a religious denomination, and active engagement in the ministry as one's principal occupation. The military provides additional training for qualified applicants to prepare them for service within the culture of the military.[37]

The Fort Gordon Ministry Team mission statement provides an overview of the role of the chaplain. The mission is to provide comprehensive pastoral care and unit-based religious support; to implement free exercise of religion; to advise and assist the command to care for soldiers and family members; and to accompany soldiers in peace, crisis, and war.[38]

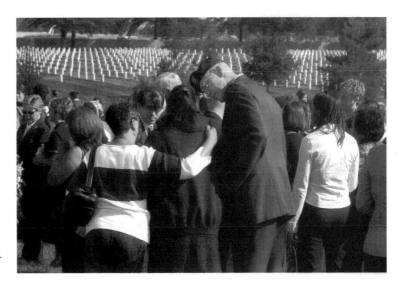

FIGURE 17.8 An Army chaplain comforts relatives and friends at a military funeral. (Photo courtesy of U.S. Army.)

The Army and Air Force staff and support their own respective chaplain services. The Navy provides chaplain services for the Navy, the Marines, and the Coast Guard. Each chaplain serves as a spiritual advisor to a commander and the corresponding unit of service personnel and their families. The chaplain is responsible for providing and performing religious ceremonies and spiritual encouragement and counseling. When one's faith is different from that of the chaplain, the chaplain is responsible for making appropriate arrangements to have the person's spiritual needs met.

Spirituality is an important part of a veteran's healthcare in the VHA. This is especially true for veterans dealing with serious medical issues. For this reason, chaplains are an integral part of the interdisciplinary healthcare team with the VHA, and chapels are present in VA hospitals for prayer, daily services, funerals, and even weddings.

Reflective Exercise

• What role do chaplains play in the military?
• Why does the military place such a high value on chaplain services? • How might a physical therapist employ the services of a chaplain on behalf of the client?

Healthcare Practices

Focus of Healthcare

Traditionally, the VHA has been more curative than preventive in its healthcare focus, but this appears to be changing. Preventive programs are emerging with regard to smoking cessation, diabetes management, and cancer screenings, to name a few. The VHA benefit program specifically endorses the following preventive services: periodic medical examination, health education including nutrition education, maintenance of drug use profiles, drug monitoring, drug use education, and mental health and substance abuse preventive services.[17]

The military also demonstrates a commitment to preventive services in its sometimes controversial practice of mandatory immunizations. In addition, the military has done a lot of research in efforts to prevent injuries. For example, they have researched how to avoid physical training–related injuries such as stress fractures, overuse syndromes, knee pain, and tendinitis. Many of these research articles are available on the U.S. Army Medical Department website, www.armymedicine.army.mil/default2.htm. Other preventive measures have been described in the Safety section of this chapter.

Reflective Exercise

• Is your practice of physical therapy focused more on curative or preventive care? • What role does the physical therapist have in preventive care?

The focus on healthcare differs in the VHA system compared with civilian systems. An informal survey of VHA physical therapists conducted by one of the authors (Beaman) in 2003 demonstrated that clients in the VHA system received a better-than-average continuum of care within the government system. In many instances, the array of services required by a patient is available on the local medical campus. If an off-site service is required, transportation is often provided. Physical therapists working in VHA hospitals often are able to follow the client from the intensive care unit to the acute care floor through transitional care or subacute care and outpatient care all within the same campus. For example, the physical therapist can follow a patient undergoing an amputation preoperatively, postoperatively, and through pre-prosthetic and post-prosthetic training. The VHA generally imposes no restrictions on the duration of physical therapy, unlike the third-party payers of the civilian system.

Reflective Exercise

• How closely connected is your physical therapy care of the client to other types of medical care of the client? • How might the physical therapist promote continuum of care across the disciplines?

Traditional Practices

Traditional practices vary between regions and cultural climates of the individual organizations within the military and VHA system. One example of the use of traditional practices is found in the VHA multidisciplinary pain clinic model. Pain has been identified as the fifth vital sign in the VHA system, and special pain clinics have been established to address this vital sign.[39] Services offered include hypnosis therapy, acupuncture, Reiki therapy, muscle relaxation therapy, progressive relaxation techniques, and guided imagery—practices that transcend the traditional biomedical model of practice. Primary care providers may refer patients with complex pain to the pain management clinic. Physical therapists treating patients with complex pain may make recommendations for referral of a patient to the pain management clinic.

Reflective Exercise

• Do you regard pain as the fifth vital sign? • What is your opinion of non-biomedical practices of controlling pain? • What is your opinion of the VHA's multidisciplinary pain clinic model?

Reflective Exercise

• In the initial vignette, what referral resource might the physical therapist recommend to assist with Sgt. Walker's pain management?

Responsibility for Health

One officer interviewed indicated that within active service, the military takes responsibility for the health of the troops. This is demonstrated by the mandatory administration of immunizations. He describes standing in line with his sleeves rolled up to receive the numerous shots, many of which had unknown purposes and side effects. In this case, he felt that the servicemen and women in a sense are required to rescind their responsibility for their own health and trust the military to take care of them (Sgt. Paul Morris, personal communication).

The VHA demonstrates responsibility for the health of veterans through financial compensation and provision of free healthcare services for service-connected disabilities. For example, veterans who are 70% service connected for their disability are entitled to long term care in a VHA nursing home or a contract nursing home.[40] A service-connected disability is defined as "a disability incurred in or aggravated during a period of active military service where the veteran did not receive a dishonorable discharge or disability was not due to willful misconduct of veterans."[17] The proportions of reported service-connected disabilities across the military branches according to the 2001 National Survey of Veterans are listed in Box 17-1.

Rehabilitation/Chronicity

The Paralyzed Veterans of America is a prominent advocacy group for disabled veterans, specifically those who have experienced spinal cord injury or dysfunction. Its mission is to be the leading advocate for quality healthcare for its members and to provide research and education for spinal cord injury and dysfunction, benefits based on its members' military service and civil rights, and opportunities that maximize the independence of its members.[41]

Reflective Exercise

• How familiar are you with the Paralyzed Veterans of America organization? • What resources are available through them? • How might you learn of other resources available to veterans with disabilities?

BOX 17.1

Service-Connected Disabilities across Military Branches	
Marine Corps	16.4%
Air Force	16.0%
Army	14.8%
Navy	10.7%

Source: Department of Veterans Affairs (2003)[17]

Pain/Sick Role

According to an informal survey by one of the authors in 2003 (Beaman), the consensus among physical therapists serving in the VHA and military systems is that active military members and veterans tend to have a higher pain threshold than civilians. This is likely due to the rigorous military training, which teaches servicemen to endure pain and other unpleasant sensations for the purpose of survival in wartime situations. This tolerance varies depending on one's military training, mental state, and morale. Army Rangers, Navy Seals, and Marines are among the military's toughest. The higher pain threshold reflects the intense training and indoctrination so that if the warrior should become distracted by pain in combat, it could result in fatalities.

Many veterans are dealing with chronic and debilitating pain. The NSV 2001 reported that 15.1% of veterans had severe, chronic pain.[39] In 1998 the VHA National Pain Management Strategy was initiated to reduce pain and suffering in veterans. Pain was designated as the fifth vital sign to stress the importance of routine screening, assessment, and prompt treatment for pain. Physical therapists as well as other VA healthcare professionals are responsible for documenting pain on a 0-to-10 numeric rating scale.[31] In patients who are unable to express themselves, pain can be assessed through nonverbal signs or body language such as facial expressions, muscle rigidity, and restlessness.

Mental Health

PTSD is a disabling condition that results from "the exposure to a traumatic event that involved actual or threatened death or injury (to self or others) or a threat to physical integrity."[42] Active military personnel engaged in warfare are more likely than not to experience a traumatic event or traumatic stressor(s) such as combat and rape. Vietnam veterans have the highest rate of PTSD due to their exposure to multiple traumatic stressors.[42] More than 150,000 veterans were service connected for PTSD in 2001.[42]

The Vet Center Program was established in 1979 out of recognition that a significant number of Vietnam veterans were still experiencing difficulties with readjustment. In 1991 the program was expanded to include veterans who served during other periods of armed hostilities. The VHA worked hard to reach as many veterans as possible, establishing 206 community-based Vet Centers located in all 50 states, Puerto Rico, the Virgin Islands, Washington, DC, and Guam offering readjustment counseling for veterans who served in certain war zones. Vet Centers offer comprehensive readjustment counseling by interdisciplinary teams composed of psychologists, nurses, and social workers.[30]

The VHA also operates a network of more than 140 specialized programs for the treatment of PTSD, including 8 specialized inpatient units, 18 residential rehabilitation programs, and 9 PTSD day hospitals. The National PTSD Center was established in 1989 to promote research, to train healthcare providers in the diagnosis and treatment of PTSD, and to serve as an informational resource.[30]

Special considerations should be made in performing evaluations or interventions for veterans with PTSD. A veteran who has undergone an invasive medical or surgical procedure or who is suffering from a life-threatening condition or experiencing any other type of emotional, physical, or psychological stress may be more susceptible to a triggering of the memory of a previous traumatic event.[42] Patient education and environmental modification are keys to successful interaction with a veteran in this situation. A therapist must obtain approval from the veteran before proceeding with the evaluation or intervention. This is especially important for any activity or technique that requires physical touch. A therapist should clearly explain the purpose and intent and allow ample time for the veteran to digest the information provided and become comfortable with the physical therapy procedure discussed. The therapist should continuously monitor the patient for signs of distress and ask the patient how he or she is tolerating the procedure. Respecting the patient's privacy while not making him or her feel confined is also important. Curtains may be better alternatives than closed doors for maintaining privacy.

A number of different services exist within the VHA system for sexual trauma/harassment victims, including readjustment counseling, referral for benefits assistance, liaison with community programs, marital and family counseling, and job counseling and placement. Mental health greatly influences physical health, and the effective physical therapist must respect the mental health challenges of veteran clients and consider the entire person when designing interventions in physical therapy.

Reflective Exercise

• Try to imagine the stress and difficulties of re-adjustment to civilian life for the military combatant. What challenges might one face? • What special considerations should a physical therapist make when conducting evaluations or interventions with a client who suffers from post-traumatic stress disorder or other mental health challenge?

Barriers to Healthcare

Barriers to healthcare for veterans include transportation, reduced social network, homelessness, distrust of government, and disability compensation issues. All can affect consistency or follow-through with physical therapy visits and compliance with home exercise programs. See Chapter 18 for additional perspectives regarding the homeless client.

Reflective Exercise

• In what ways can the physical therapist work to overcome barriers to care?

Healthcare Practitioners

Perceptions/Status of Practitioners

Healthcare professionals with a postgraduate degree who serve in the military are automatically awarded an officer title. This affords them higher status than enlisted men and women within the military hierarchy. In wartime, physicians possess particularly high status as they are the ones to determine whether the injured serviceman or woman may return to duty and in what capacity. This responsibility is increasingly being shoul-

dered by physical therapists when the disorder is neuromuscular in origin.

Gender and Healthcare

Due to the rising number of females in the U.S. military, a physical therapist should be prepared to treat issues specific to servicewomen. Physical therapy practitioners should be aware of the possibility of sexual trauma in the female military and veteran population. In 1996 the Defense Manpower Data Center reported that 78% of women in all branches reported having experienced some form of sexual harassment in a 12-month period.[39] In 2000, 23% of female veterans who had used VHA services reported being the victim of a sexual assault while in the military.[39] To increase the comfort level of female patients, a physical therapy department may implement specific procedures. Examples include asking if the patient has a gender preference for the evaluating or treating therapist, and modifying the environment to prevent direct contact with male patients while in an "exposed" situation, such as during aquatic therapy. In addition, the treating therapist can use the guidelines outlined in the previous section on treating patients with PTSD in treating sexual trauma victims.

Reflective Exercise

• In the initial vignette with Sgt. Walker, should the gender of the evaluating and treating therapist be considered in scheduling her appointments? • Why or why not? •How would you determine this?

Conclusion

Providing physical therapy care for our nation's military servicemen and women and veterans is a great honor and a privilege (Fig. 17-9). In order to do so effectively, however, the physical therapist must strive to gain an understanding, respect, and appreciation for the military culture characterizing both the individual clients and the institutions of service such as the military hospital or the VHA. The physical therapist has the opportunity to provide culturally competent care to

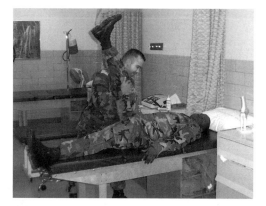

FIGURE 17.9 The honor and privilege of serving our nation's military servicemen and women. (Photo courtesy of Peter Glover.)

men and women who have served to defend our freedoms.

REFERENCES

1. Dorn E, Graves HD. *American Military Culture in the Twenty-first Century: A Report of the CSIS International Security Program.* Washington, DC: Center for Strategic and International Studies; 2000.
2. Bassett J. Mission critical: Military PT's strive to keep pace with an increasing demand on the armed forces. *PT Adv.* 2003;14:8.
3. Murphy B. Trended number of VHA therapists. October 20, 2003. E-mail message from head of the VA section of APTA.

CASE STUDY SCENARIO

*T*ho Nu, a new graduate from a DPT program, has taken her first job at a Veterans Hospital in rural Pennsylvania. Her family is from Vietnam, but she and her two brothers were born in the United States. Her first client, William "Billy" Howard, is a 52-year-old male who suffered a shrapnel wound to his right leg in Vietnam. He had a right transtibial amputation 32 years ago. He is admitted to the hospital at this time for a transfemoral amputation. He has diabetes and has developed an ulcer at the base of his stump that has not healed. The wound became gangrenous, necessitating the amputation. Billy also suffers from post-traumatic stress disorder and sometimes experiences hallucinations.

Two days ago Billy underwent the transfemoral amputation, and he has now been referred to physical therapy for acute post-amputation care and pre-prosthetic training. Tho Nu will be performing the evaluation. She enters the hospital room where Billy is sleeping. He is connected to a morphine patient-controlled analgesia (PCA) pump for pain control. Tho Nu closes the door for privacy. She is eager to start her examination and gently shakes Billy's shoulder to wake him up. Billy opens his eyes and sees Tho Nu standing next to his bed. His eyes widen and he begins to sweat. His eyes quickly search the room and detect that the door is closed. He sits bolt upright, pulls out his PCA pump, and tries to jump out of bed, which causes him to fall on his transfemoral stump. Blood begins to seep through the wound bandage over his stump, and Billy screams, "Vietnamese! Vietnamese!"

1. What just occurred?

2. What should Tho Nu do now?

3. What circumstances may have contributed to this reaction (prior to Billy's meeting Tho Nu)?

4. What might Tho Nu have done differently?

5. What could she do to successfully complete her evaluation?

4. Burke C. Military folk culture. In: Katzenstein MF, Reppy J, eds. *Beyond Zero Tolerance.* Lanham, Md: Rowman & Littlefield; 1999:53–63.

5. McCloy T, Clover WH. Value formation at the Air Force Academy. In: Moskos CC, Wood FR, eds. *The Military: More Than Just a Job?* Washington, DC: Pergamon-Brassey's International Defense Publishers; 1988:129–152.

6. Martin JA, McClure P. Today's active duty military family: The evolving challenges of military family life. In: Martin JA, Rosen LN, Sparacino LR, eds. *The Military Family: A Practice Guide for Human Service Providers.* Westport, Conn: Praeger; 2000:324.

7. Kier E. Discrimination and military cohesion: An organizational perspective. In: Katzenstein MF, Reppy J, eds. *Beyond Zero Tolerance.* Lanham, Md: Rowman & Littlefield; 1999:25–52.

8. Hosek SD, Tiemeyer P, Kilburn R, Strong DA, Ducksworth S, Ray R. *Minority and Gender Differences in Officer Career Progression.* Santa Monica, Calif: RAND; 2001.

9. Joseph N. *Uniforms and Nonuniforms: Communication through Clothing.* Westport, Conn: Greenwood Press; 1986.

10. Hillman EL. Dressed to kill? In: Katzenstein MF, Reppy J, eds. *Beyond Zero Tolerance.* Lanham, Md: Rowman & Littlefield; 1999:65–80.

11. Burk J. Military culture. In: Kutz LR, Turpin J, eds. *Encyclopedia of Violence, Peace and Conflict.* Vol 2. San Diego, Calif: Academic Press; 1999:447–461.

12. United States Army. The United States Army Seals. Available at: http://www.army.mil/ArmySeals.htm. Accessed January 31, 2004.

13. United States Navy. Navy organization: An overview. Available at: http://www.chinfo.navy.mil/navpalib/organization/org-over.html. Accessed March 3, 2004.

14. US Marine Corps. About the Marines. Available at: http://marines.com/about_marines/default.asp. Accessed January 31, 2004.

15. US Marine Corps. Marine Corps core values: Honor, courage, and commitment. Available at: http://www.marines.com/about_marines/corpsvalues.asp?format=flash. Accessed January 31, 2004.

16. Air Force History Support Office. Chronology: From Kitty Hawk to World War II. Available at: http://airforcehistory.hq.af.mil/PopTopics/Kitty.htm. Accessed March 3, 2004.

17. Department of Veterans Affairs. Enrollment in VA's health care system. Available at: http://www1.va.gov/Elig/page.cfm?pg=10. Accessed March 15, 2004.

18. Schohn M. Delivering integrated care. PowerPoint presentation at the Integrated Ambulatory Care Conference; June 24, 2003.

19. Department of Veterans Affairs. VA fact sheets: VA healthcare and the medical benefits package. Available at: http://www1.va.gov/opa/fact/enrollben.html. Accessed March 15, 2004.

20. Census 2000 Veteran Data. Veteran population in U.S. and Puerto Rico. Available at: http://www.va.gov/vetdata/Census2000/index.htm. Accessed March 3, 2004.

21. Bellafaire J. America's military women—the journey continues: Women in Military Service for America Memorial Foundation, Inc. Available at: http://womensmemorial.org/Education/WHM982.html#8. Accessed March 15, 2004.

22. Women in Military Service for America Memorial Foundation, Inc. History and collections: Questions and answers. Available at: http://www.womensmemorial.org/historyandcollections/history/learnmoreques.htm. Accessed March 15, 2004.

23. Department of Defense. DOD at a glance. Available at: http://www.defenselink.mil/pubs/almanac/. Accesssed March 15, 2004.

24. Army Family Team Building. The chain of command and the chain of concern. Available at: http://www.gordon.army.mil/aftb/chain.htm. Accessed March 3, 2004.

25. US Army Reserve. Family care plan resource guidebook. Available at: http://www.usarc.army.mil/90thrsc/directory/primaryStaff/dcsper/FamCarePlan/FCP_GuideIntro.pdf. Accessed March 3, 2004.

26. Benson D, Schreck R, Underwood R, Greathouse DG. The role of army physical therapists as nonphysician health care providers who prescribe certain medications: Observations and experiences. *Phys Ther.* 1995; 75:49–55.

27. Dinninny P. More than a uniform: The military model of physical therapy. *PT Mag.* 1995:42–48.

28. Johnson NA. Smoking: Why take the risk? Health Tips from Army Medicine. Available at: www.armymedicine.army.mil/hc/healthips/13/200309–10whyrisk.cfm. Accessed January 31, 2004.

29. West, G. Tobacco use affects military mission. Health Tips from Army Medicine. Available at: http://www.armymedicine.army.mil/hc/healthtips/13/20031022tobacco.cfm. Accessed January 31, 2004.

30. Department of Veterans Affairs. VA programs for veterans with post-traumatic stress disorder (PTSD): April 2002 fact sheet. Available at: http://www.va.gov/pressrel/ptsd402.htm. Accessed January 31, 2004.

31. Department of Veterans Affairs, Geriatrics and Extended Care Healthcare Group and National Pain Management Coordinating Committee. Pain: The 5th vital sign. Rev. ed. Available at: www1.gov/pain_management/docs/TOOLKIT.pdf. Accessed March 20, 2004.

32. Department of Veterans Affairs. VA achievements in diabetes care: January 2003 fact sheet. Available at: http://www1.va.gov/opa/fact/pressrel/diabtsfs.doc. Accessed March 20, 2004.

33. American Diabetes Association. National diabetes fact sheet. Available at: www.diabetes.org/utils/printthispage.jsp?PageID=STATISTICS_233193. Accessed March 20, 2004.

34. Military Funeral Honors. Who is eligible? Available at: http://www.militaryfuneralhonors.osd.mil/eligpage.htm. Accessed March 3, 2004.

35. Arlington National Cemetery. Military funeral customs. Available at: http://www.arlingtoncemetery.net/customs.htm. Accessed March 3, 2004.

36. Veterans Benefits and Services. Burial and memorial benefits: Military funeral honors. Available at: http://www.cem.va.gov/mhg.htm. Accessed March 3, 2004.

37. U.S. Army Chaplain Corps. Origins of the chaplaincy. Available at: http://www.usachcs.army.mil/history/brief/chapter_1.htm. Accessed March 1, 2004.

38. Fort Gordon Chaplain Services. Fort Gordon ministry team mission. Available at: http://www.gordon.army.mil/chaplain/. Accessed March 1, 2004.

39. Department of Veterans Affairs. Veteran data and information: Survey results. Available at: www.va.gov/vetdata/SurveyResults/. Accessed March 3, 2004.

40. Wilson, A. Veterans' long-term care needs. *DAV Mag.* Available at: http://www.dav.org/magazine/magazine_archives/2002–4/From the Nationa2046.html. Accessed March 20, 2004.

41. Paralyzed Veterans of America. About us. Available at: www.pva.org/aboutPVA/aboutpva.htm. Accessed January 31, 2004.

42. Department of Veterans Affairs. Veterans health initiatives: Post traumatic stress disorder: Implications for primary care. Available at: http://www.va.gov/vhi. Accessed January 31, 2004.

Chapter 18

The Challenge and Culture of Poverty and Homelessness

● Jill Black Lattanzi, PT, EdD

Randal, a 34-year-old of Polish descent, injured his back working on the docks in his home port city of Philadelphia. Randal is divorced and the father of two, and he has a mother who is not well and is in an assisted living facility. Randal lost his job, possibly due to his back injury, but this was difficult to prove. Although he is collecting unemployment compensation, he found it difficult to make rent payments and was evicted from his apartment. He no longer has health insurance and yet has debilitating back pain.

Introduction

Homelessness is a social phenomenon affecting, by conservative estimates, 3.5 million people in the United States, of whom 1.4 million are children.[1] Estimates vary because of the transient nature of the homeless, difficulty in finding them for a census count, and the changing status of the homeless. In most cases, homelessness is a temporary circumstance rather than a permanent situation; therefore, a more appropriate measure of homelessness is the number of people homeless over a certain period of time.

Today, the tragedy of losing one's home befalls people of all races, ethnicities, genders, and ages. Homelessness is a subculture in which people share the characteristics of low socioeconomic status, lack of a permanent shelter, social stigmatization, and exclusion from the dominant society. On the surface, the homeless appear to conflict with the traditional societal values of family and work; but in reality, this may not be the case. In order to better understand clients who experience homelessness, the physical therapist needs to understand the sociopolitical interconnections and complicating circumstances that surround those who become homeless. The culture of homelessness is complex and must be understood if the physical therapist is to provide culturally competent care for those who are homeless.

Overview/Heritage

Origins/Residence/Economics/Politics

Up until the mid-1970s the homeless more closely fit the traditional stereotype of the old, white, male, single, alcoholic, nomadic bum who fell into a state of social ostracism. These outcast men typically found a haven in the skid rows of major cities, living in abandoned apartment buildings or hotels. In the 1980s, the faces of the homeless changed dramatically and homeless people grew rapidly in number. A 1997 review of shelter statistics from 11 communities in 4 states reported that shelter capacity more than doubled in 9 communities and 3 states from 1987 to 1997. Shelter capacity tripled in 2 communities in 2 different states.[2]

Today the homeless are younger, are more ethnically diverse, and are more likely to be members of families compared with 1965, when 90% of the homeless in shelters were white males.[3] A survey of 27 cities found that the homeless population was 50% African American, 35% Caucasian, 12% Hispanic, 2% Native American, and 1% Asian (Fig. 18-1).[4] Additionally, families with children are among the fastest-growing segments of the homeless population, constituting approximately 40% of the people who become homeless (Fig. 18-2).[5] What led to the increased relocation to the streets of families with children, youth, and people of all ethnicities? Sociologists

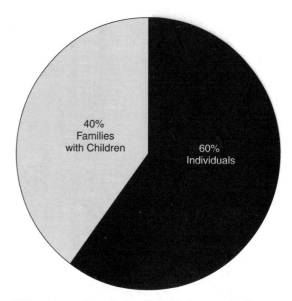

FIGURE 18.2 Percentages of individuals versus families with children who are homeless. (Data from Shinn, M., & Weitzman, B. C. (1996). Homeless families are different. In J. Baumohl (Ed.), *Homelessness in America* (pp. 109–122). Phoenix, AZ: Oryx Press.)

divide the causes of homelessness into two categories. The first category represents the social, institutional, and structural causes that arise from broad political concerns. The second encompasses individual, personal causes such as alcohol and substance abuse, family violence, broken marriages, and mental health problems.[6-8]

Reflective Exercise

• What stereotypes do you hold about those without a home? • From where do those stereotypes come?

Societal Causes

Deinstitutionalization of the mentally ill occurred in the 1960s and 1970s when asylums began to discharge their clients to the community. The relocation was based on the premise that integration into societal and community-based programs was more humane than continued institutionalization.[6,9] The community, however, was not adequately prepared or engaged to meet

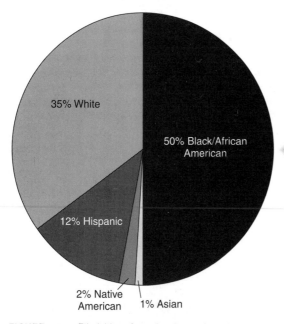

FIGURE 18.1 Ethnicities of people who are homeless. (Data from U.S. Conference of Mayors. (2001). *A status report on hunger and homelessness in America's cities.* Washington, DC: Author.)

the needs of those with mental illness. Within 10 years, many individuals struggling to maintain their medical regimens found it nearly impossible to assimilate into an unreceptive community. They landed on the streets.

In the 1980s, the United States experienced a global recession and implemented cutbacks in public assistance programs, including low-income housing. At the same time, unemployment rates were increasing and the traditional manufacturing industry declined, leaving many industrial workers unemployed.[10] A tightening of the eligibility criteria for public assistance programs and low-income housing ensued, while the number of people living in poverty increased.[6,8,11]

Gentrification also contributed to the lack of affordable housing. Popular in the 1970s and 1980s, gentrification involved the beautification and rehabilitation of inner cities, meaning that old, abandoned buildings—"home" for many of the homeless—were torn down. Gone were the skid rows, the abandoned warehouses, and single-room-occupancy (SRO) housing. From 1970 to 1985, an estimated 1 million SRO units were demolished, most notably in large cities such as New York, Chicago, and Los Angeles.[12,13] Those without a home moved to the streets and subway stations, becoming more visible to a society unwilling to see them.

Reflective Exercise

• What is the incidence of homelessness in your community? • How has this changed over the last 10 to 20 years? • What is your community doing to help remedy the situation? • What might you as a physical therapist do to help?

Individual Causes

While societal policies and conditions contribute to the homeless state, personal and individual factors, which are numerous and varied, also drive some to homelessness. Alcohol abuse is the most prevalent factor (comprising approximately 50% of homeless people), with drug abuse the next most common (approximately 33%) reason for homelessness. Substance abuse traps the in-

dividual in an expensive addiction and quickly robs one of home and stability. In addition to its effect on the individual user, studies show that many women and children become homeless as the result of a husband's or boyfriend's drug addiction. Domestic violence also drives some to homelessness.[11,13,14]

Victims of domestic violence flee to the streets in an attempt to protect themselves and their children from an unsafe home environment. In a study of 777 homeless parents, the majority of whom were mothers, 22% said they had left their last place of residence because of domestic violence.[15] Forty-six percent of the cities surveyed by the U.S. Conference of Mayors identified domestic violence as a primary cause of homelessness. An estimated 32% of requests for shelter from homeless families were denied in 1998 due to lack of resources.[16]

The breakdown of the family in recent decades has contributed to the rise in homelessness among women and children. With the increased incidence of divorce and unwed mothers, single mothers find themselves burdened with financially caring for themselves and their children without help. Often this leaves them unable to pay for housing or meet other financial needs.[6,9,11] Moreover, the personal, individual causes of homeless are often intertwined with broader societal issues.

A substantial number of homeless people are veterans. According to the Veterans Administration, an estimated 275,000 veterans are homeless each night, and more than a half-million experience homelessness over the course of the year. Approximately 47% of homeless veterans served during the Vietnam era, more than 67% served our country for at least 3 years, and 33% were stationed in a war zone.[17]

Vietnam veterans constitute a large segment of the homeless society. They bravely fought a war at their country's command; witnessed and participated in atrocious horrors; and returned to an unwelcoming, unreceptive country, ready to forget the war and thus forget them. They met a resistant culture at home, both from civilians and from older vets who had fought and achieved definitive victories in World Wars I and II. In addition to the general causes of homelessness,

---

Reflection 18.1

By conservative estimates, "one out of every four homeless males who is sleeping in a doorway, alley, or box in our cities and rural communities has put on a uniform and served our country ... now they need America to remember them."[19]

---

combat exposure, particularly post-traumatic stress disorder, may contribute to veteran homelessness.[18]

Educational/Occupational Background

Those who are homeless in the twenty-first century come from all levels of education and all occupations. A year-long cross-sectional study of 1,437 homeless adults in northern California found that 68% of the homeless had completed high school and 30% had attended college.[20] People of all backgrounds, educations, and occupations can fall prey to unfortunate circumstances such as substance abuse, divorce, and domestic violence. Hard financial breaks befall people indiscriminately. One need only visit a homeless shelter and listen to the stories of the residents to learn of the diverse life histories and unfortunate scenarios that led them to be without a home.

Reflective Exercise

• What are common causes of homelessness in your community? • What circumstances threaten the stability of your home life or those of the people around you?

Communication

The domain of communication includes verbal and nonverbal language, volume of speech and tone, spatial distancing, physical touch, and the meaning of time. People without a home vary in their communication habits and patterns according to the length of time they have been without a home and their individual culture.

Temporality/Time

While mainstream U.S. society views time linearly and pays close attention to the clock, those who have been homeless for some time come to view time as cyclical, marking their days by various events such as the opening and closing of a shelter or the time at which meal or bed tickets are distributed, rather than living by an arbitrary clock.[21] Indeed, many homeless people do not own or wear watches, which are a target for thieves.

Homeless people may have great difficulty meeting the demands of a daily schedule. Though one might typically think of the homeless as having lots of time on their hands, with no job and no home for which to care, in reality they often must juggle many different schedules to meet their basic needs. Shelters open and close and meals are served at specified times. Employment offices and medical clinics may be far away from a shelter, and the homeless person may need to rely on his or her feet for transportation. Schedule demands and the stress of meeting basic needs can take a great toll on the homeless person and make compliance with medical instructions very difficult or impossible. The culturally competent physical therapist must appreciate the demands of the homeless lifestyle.

Because people without a home present with a myriad of immediate needs, they tend to be present oriented rather than future oriented. While

---

Reflection 18.2

A student's response when asked about her experience volunteering at the homeless shelter: "I first noticed the odor. The whole place smells like sweat. And I felt that I really stood out. I was definitely out of my comfort zone. It was really shocking—like having to put my car behind a locked gate—I definitely was not prepared. Within half an hour I felt more comfortable. I just started to talk to people like the other students were. I came to realize that these guys were just like anybody else—they had just come across some hard times. It gave me a new perspective.

the physical therapist looks ahead and strives to prevent future medical problems, the homeless person focuses on overwhelming present needs and may be unable to embrace preventive measures. Physical therapists need to understand the client's perspective and adjust treatment and expectations accordingly.

Reflective Exercise

• Are you more present oriented or future oriented? Does this change according to circumstances? • How have you felt when you were pressed with present demands and someone pushed you to consider future goals and expectations?

Spatial Relationships/Touch

Physical touch can be a powerful communicator of respect or disrespect and has the capacity to both heal and harm. Physical touch is an integral part of physical therapy practice, and students in physical therapy schools soon become accustomed to other students poking and pressing on them as they learn and practice on each another. In contrast, homeless people may not have experienced physical touch in a long time, and their last experience may have been a harmful or threatening touch. Because of the possible negative associations with touch, the physical therapist should always explain procedures thoroughly and obtain verbal agreement before proceeding (Fig. 18-3). Physical touch must also be performed in a respectful and professional manner. Respectful, professional touch is characterized by purposeful, nonthreatening contact such as a handshake or a firm hand on one's shoulder. In a study of physical therapy students serving in a homeless shelter clinic, Black[22] observed students interacting in various ways with respectful physical touch and found that it enhanced their rapport with the clients.

Cultures identify appropriate respectful distances when communicating, and appropriate spatial distancing for people who are homeless will also differ according to their primary culture. In general, however, physical therapists should allow adequate, respectful spatial distance initially because homeless clients may be uncomfortable with what they may perceive as aggressive, threatening advances. With the development of

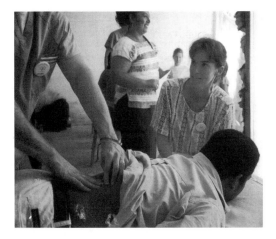

FIGURE 18.3 Physical touch may sometimes be perceived as threatening or harmful. The physical therapist should always obtain consent from the patient before proceeding with physical touch.

mutual rapport and respect, the physical therapist will build trust and earn the right to approach more closely.

Reflective Exercise

• How comfortable are you with physical touch and spatial distancing? • How comfortable were you before entering the physical therapy profession? • Have you ever experienced abusive or harmful touch?
• How would that change your response to touch?

Family Organization

Family organization varies among homeless people. The fastest-growing segment of the homeless

---

Reflection 18.3

"At first I felt uncomfortable asking them about their homelessness. I was hesitant and afraid of offending them. I am from suburbia and was nervous about what to say. Then I learned to relax and interact just like I would with anyone else."

within the United States is families with children, usually consisting of a single mother and her children.[23] The actual number of families who are homeless on a given night is extremely difficult to count, as many families move in and out of homelessness, shifting between relatives' and friends' homes and family shelters. Homeless mothers are more likely to have been hospitalized for a mental disorder than are mothers who are poor but have a permanent home. McChesney[11] reports an 8% to 50% prevalence of substance abuse among homeless mothers, which is two to eight times higher than the rate for poor housed mothers. A history of physical and/or sexual abuse is more common among homeless mothers. Moreover, approximately 25% to 35% of homeless mothers leave home to flee domestic violence.[24]

The plight of homeless children is perhaps even more complicated and life altering than that of the adult. Social learning theorists confirm that children learn behaviors, societal expectations, and relationships from the people with whom they live and the environment in which they grow up. Moving among crowded shelters without the stability of a home has far-reaching effects on the development of the child. Adequate nutrition is a major concern for the growing child, and nutritional deficiencies abound among homeless children.[23]

Studies have consistently found that homeless children are more prone to illness than children who have a permanent home. Common illnesses include upper respiratory disorders, gastrointestinal problems, trauma, eye disorders, ear disorders, skin diseases, and infestations of lice.[25,26] Developmental delays and immature behaviors such as short attention spans, withdrawal, aggression, and sleep disorders are common among homeless preschool children, as are cognitive and motor delays.

Reflective Exercise

• As a physical therapist working with a homeless pediatric clientele, what difficulties might you encounter? • How could you make a difference in regard to the child's health, wellness, and development?

High–Risk Behaviors

Factors related to high-risk behaviors often contribute to homelessness. The incidence of drug and alcohol abuse for the homeless population exceeds that for the general population. Alcohol and substance abuse contributes to health problems such as hypertension, stomach and liver disorders, and respiratory disease. High-risk behaviors also perpetuate financial and relationship problems, ensnaring one in a homeless state.

Alcohol and illegal substances are used for self-medication. Psychologically tortured Vietnam veterans sometimes find solace in the numbing effects of mind-altering drugs or alcohol. They acknowledge that to become sober means being plagued with their searing memories as well as awareness of their present state of need.[27]

Reflective Exercise

• How do you feel about working with someone who has an alcohol or drug addiction?

Nutrition

Poor nutrition leads to a worsening of health conditions. Obtaining adequate food, let alone a nutritional balance, is a major challenge for one who is living on the street without access to storage facilities, stove, microwave, refrigerator, or the finances to purchase food. Those with special dietary needs, such as people with diabetes or hypertension, have great difficulty complying with prescribed recommendations. Homeless shelters and soup kitchens attempt to provide adequate nutritional meals but are limited in resources and the ability to meet specific dietary requirements.

Reflective Exercise

• What challenges do you encounter in attempting to adhere to a well-balanced diet? • How would that be complicated if you were homeless?

Healthcare Practices

Common health problems among homeless people include physical illnesses or injuries that may have contributed to their homelessness, especially if the infirmity caused the loss of a job or depletion of financial resources. In such cases, the homeless person continues to face the challenges and difficulties of the physical illness or injury in addition to the complicated demands of homelessness. The homeless lifestyle itself poses the following health threats: (a) exposure to the elements, potentially resulting in hypothermia; (b) vascular and skin disorders from not being able to lie down; (c) diabetic complications with the difficulties involved with insulin regulation; and (d) orthopedic foot, knee, hip, and back problems resulting from extensive walking and complicated by a lack of appropriate footwear. Other threats to physical health include trauma from muggings or rapes and injury from gun and knife violence. Ironically, battered women fleeing violence at home find themselves at high risk for violence on the streets.

Focus on Healthcare

While physical therapists tend to view healthcare decisions from the perspective of medical practice, homeless people make healthcare decisions from the perspective of daily survival. A threat to one's physical health may be secondary to needs for food and shelter, particularly when the physical threat is without symptoms, such as hypertension. The physical therapist may become frustrated when the homeless person fails to take his or her hypertensive medications, when in reality, the priority for the homeless person is to feed his or her family.

Similarly, the homeless person may view a "minor" health concern with more gravity than a "major" health concern when the minor concern affects his or her immediate circumstances. For example, an infected toe may be of greater concern than the risk of a future heart attack when the painful toe interferes with the person's main form of transportation. The physical therapist should first communicate respect for the client's main concern, and afterward the client may be

---

Reflection 18.4

"I felt fear. Just walking into the shelter and the smell and everyone looking at you... I realized how different I was... but by observing the way that the other students interacted, you just knew that they were safe and that you would be safe. In fact, I now know that if anyone tried to bother us, the guys that come into the clinic would not allow it."

---

more willing to listen to the physical therapist's additional recommendations.

Physical Rehabilitation

Those in poverty often struggle to meet basic healthcare needs involving life and death, illness, and disease. Survival is the goal; rehabilitation is the luxury. Rehabilitation is also difficult because it requires time and consistency. Homeless people tend to be present oriented and time commitments may be difficult due to lifestyle demands. Commitment to regular physical rehabilitation sessions as well as compliance with "home" exercise programs is difficult. Yet a physical illness or injury that may have prompted homelessness will still be present and in need of rehabilitation in order for the person to overcome the homeless state.

Reflective Exercise

• How do you prioritize your health concerns?
• Do your health concerns sometimes come second to other concerns in your life? Why or why not?

Mental Health

Mental health problems dominate the homeless society and remain one of the major health concerns of the homeless. Deinstitutionalization has left many mentally ill patients without the medical care and support structures they need to function. Studies estimate that 20% to 50% of homeless people in the United States suffer from

---

Reflection 18.5

"I think I've learned that when it comes down to it you are really not all that different, and I think that's probably the biggest thing. That at first I think people may seem very foreign and their ideas may seem very different, but when it comes down to it, it is very similar."

---

a severe mental illness such as schizophrenia, major affective disorders, paranoia, and other psychoses. Only 1% of the general U.S. population suffer from these mental illnesses.[14]

Approximately 1 million Vietnam veterans suffer from post-traumatic stress disorder, a progressive mental illness arising from the atrocities witnessed and executed in Vietnam. Early symptoms are depression, withdrawal, and sleeplessness, and these often go undiagnosed until later symptoms of psychosis, manic violence, and suicide erupt, devastating both the afflicted veterans and their families. Many end up on the streets due to family breakdown and their inability to hold a job. Vietnam veterans with PTSD are five times more likely to be unemployed than those without it, and up to six times more likely to abuse drugs and alcohol.[17,18,27]

Barriers

Health problems of the homeless are often complicated by the fact that the person does not have a home, a refrigerator, or financial resources. Storing medications is often a problem, and the possession of prescription drugs makes the homeless a target for theft. Moreover, syringes are desirable items on the street, so a person with diabetes might have trouble retaining the supplies needed to deliver daily doses of insulin.

Some of the homeless who are dealing with alcoholism or other addictions may be reluctant to seek formal medical care, thus establishing a barrier to care. Likewise, the physical therapist must consider the addiction in the treatment of the client, as it is often intertwined with the health-related complaint. The implication, then, is that physical medical care, mental health care, and substance abuse treatment must be integrated. Unfortunately, addiction may be the barrier that prohibits the homeless individual from ever seeking medical services.

Inaccessibility to appropriate healthcare poses another barrier. Wood[8] cites a comprehensive report stating that the primary health-related problem for the homeless person is access to healthcare. "The traditional medical model, in which the client comes to the outpatient clinic or hospital or hospital emergency department, often poses a formidable barrier for the homeless in need of medical care"[21] (p. 48). The homeless client may have experienced discrimination or misunderstanding in such settings in the past. They may have encountered healthcare professionals who were insensitive to their needs, priorities, or values. Smith[28] recommends meeting homeless people in their own environment. "Meeting people in their own living situation, whether on the streets or in lunch lines, communicates to them a willingness to meet their health needs"[28] (p. 48).

Reflective Exercise

• How might you as a physical therapist help break down some of the barriers for the homeless in obtaining physical therapy?

Healthcare Practitioners

Those who experience homelessness share a subculture that may also cross dominant cultural lines. The nature of existing without a home and surviving without stability leads to specific attitudes, values, priorities, and time orientation that differ from those who have homes. Because most physical therapists interacting with the homeless have homes, the interaction between the therapist and the homeless client is culturally misaligned to begin with. Often aspects of this misalignment may go undetected by the physical therapist. Koegel and Gelberg[21] note

Because the homeless population includes people from so many backgrounds, and because this group lacks the clear boundaries (like language and ethnic identity) that signal the potential importance of cultural sensitivity, health practitioners can all too easily ignore the possibility

that cultural factors influence their relationships with homeless clients…. The attitudes of homeless people toward services, their priorities, and their view of concepts such as time may differ from those of providers, setting up the possibility of conflict and failure.[21] *(p. 26)*

Housing is such a basic need that few people with homes consider all the ramifications of not having one. Homelessness requires that physical therapists consider carefully their instructions and recommendations, as they might not be meaningful or appropriate to someone without a home. For example, a physical therapist working with someone with back pain will make recommendations for daily living. Those recommendations typically include sleeping on a firm mattress, sitting in supportive chairs with a lumbar support, and alternating periods of activity and rest. Someone who is without a home may be sleeping on a grate at night or on a worn cot at a shelter. Rarely will they find a chair on which to sit, especially a supportive chair with a lumbar pillow. Alternating periods of activity and rest

Reflection 18.6

"I think the biggest thing I have learned is to leave your stereotypes at home. Everybody's got their own story. There is so much potential locked up in many of the people I have met. I think stereotypes are about the worst thing you could carry with you into any situation."

may not be an option given the demands of the day and night. The culturally sensitive physical therapist must consider the ramifications of homelessness and adjust instructions accordingly if care is to be effective.

Reflective Exercise

• How might you adjust your instructions for proper body mechanics and positioning or exercise for someone who is without a home?

CASE STUDY SCENARIO

*M*r. Paul Lombardo worked in general maintenance for a large apartment complex. He is 52 and is of Italian and German descent. One of the benefits of his job was free housing and electricity in one of the units. Mr. Lombardo had been married, but his wife died of breast cancer at a young age. They had no children. Living rent free, he was able to save a significant amount and invested a good portion of it in the stock market.

Six years ago, he was helping to move a heavy refrigerator down a set of steps when he felt a crippling, shooting pain in his back and legs. His legs gave way and the refrigerator tumbled down the steps, landing on him at the bottom of the steps. Mr. Lombardo was taken to the hospital and treated for his back injury. After a year of being out of work and extensive physical therapy, he was able to return to the job only to find that his back pain would flare with the least amount of physical labor. He had to leave his job completely, which meant assuming responsibility for the rent payment and the electric bill for his apartment. He lived on worker's compensation, disability, and his savings for a while and continued physical therapy. Pool therapy seemed to work best for him. Soon, however, the worker's compensation and disability income ended and his medical insurance expired. When the stock market dropped, Mr. Lombardo found that he could no longer make the rent payments and was evicted. He qualified for Medicaid, but it still wasn't enough to find affordable housing. No low-income housing was available at the time. He wound up on the streets and found his way to a shelter, with chronic back pain still precluding him from returning to work.

(continued)

Case Study Scenario Continued

The homeless shelter houses a physical therapy clinic manned by student volunteers and supervising volunteer faculty from a local physical therapy program. The clinic is open on Tuesday evenings and is sparsely equipped. He goes in the first Tuesday for an evaluation.

1. How will Mr. Lombardo's evaluation differ from an evaluation in a traditional clinic?

2. What questions should the physical therapist ask?

3. What approach should the physical therapist take?

4. What considerations does the physical therapist need to make in helping Mr. Lombardo set goals?

5. What considerations does the physical therapist need to have in giving instructions?

6. How can the physical therapist best address the situation with the limited resources available?

7. How might the physical therapist act as an advocate for Mr. Lombardo's physical therapy needs?

REFERENCES

1. Urban Institute. What will it take to end homelessness? Martha R. Burt Urban Institute. Available at: http://www.urban.org. Accessed July 27, 2005.
2. National Coalition for the Homeless. *Homelessness in America: Unabated and Increasing.* Washington DC: Author; 1997.
3. Barak G. The epidemiology of homelessness in Black America. In: Livingston I, ed. *Handbook of Black American Health: The Mosaic of Conditions, Issues, Policies, and Prospects.* Westport, Conn: Greenwood Press; 1994:285–299.
4. US Conference of Mayors. *A Status Report on Hunger and Homelessness in America's Cities.* Washington DC: Author; 2001.
5. Shinn M, Weitzman BC. Homeless families are different. In: Baumohl J, ed. *Homelessness in America.* Phoenix, Ariz: Oryx Press; 1996:109–122.
6. Glasser I, Bridgman R. (1999). *Braving the Street: The Anthropology of Homelessness.* New York: Berghahn.
7. Seltser BJ, Miller DE. *Homeless Families: The Struggle for Dignity.* Urbana: University of Illinois Press; 1993.
8. Wood D. *Delivering Health Care to Homeless Persons.* New York, NY: Springer; 1992.
9. Bowdler JE. Health problems of the homeless in America. *Nurs Pract.* 1989;14:44–51.
10. Hutson S, Clapham D. *Homelessness: Public Policies and Private Troubles.* New York, NY: Cassell; 1999.
11. McChesney, KY. A review of the empirical literature on contemporary urban homeless families. *Soc Serv Rev.* 1995;69:429–460.
12. Dolbeare CN. Housing policy: A general consideration. In: Baumohl J, ed. *Homelessness in America.* Phoenix, Ariz: Oryx Press; 1996:34–45.
13. Koegel P, Burnam A, Baumohl J. The causes of homelessness. In: Baumohl J, ed. *Homelessness in America.* Phoenix, Ariz: Oryx Press; 1996:24–33.
14. Burt MR. Homelessness: Definitions and counts. In: Baumohl J, ed. *Homelessness in America.* Phoenix, Ariz: Oryx Press; 1996:15–23.
15. Homes for the Homeless. *Ten Cities 1997–1998: A Snapshot of Family Homelessness across America.* New York, NY: Author and Institute for Children and Poverty; 1999.
16. US Conference of Mayors. *A Status Report on Hunger and Homelessness in America's Cities.* Washington, DC: Author; 1998.
17. National Coalition for Homeless Veterans. Background and statistics. Available at: http://www.nchv.org/background.cfm. Accessed July 14, 2003.
18. Rosenheck R, Leda CA, Frisman LK, Lam J, Chung A. Homeless veterans. In: Baumohl J, ed. *Homelessness in America.* Phoenix, Ariz: Oryx Press; 1996:97–108.
19. National Coalition for Homeless Veterans. Homeless veterans: Questions and facts. Available at: http://www.nchv.org/qa.html. Accessed April 18, 2001.

20. Winkleby MA, Rockhill B, Jatulis D, Fortmann SP. The medical origins of homelessness. *Am J Public Health.* 1992;82:1394–1398.

21. Koegel P, Gelberg L. Patient-oriented approach to providing care to homeless persons. In: Wood D, ed. *Delivering Health Care to Homeless Persons.* New York, NY: Springer; 1992:16–29.

22. Black JD. "Hands of Hope": A qualitative investigation of a student physical therapy clinic in a homeless shelter. *J Phys Ther Educ.* 2002;16:32–41.

23. Sullivan L. *The Impact of Homelessness on Children.* New York, NY: Garland; 1997.

24. McChesney KY. Homeless families since 1990: Implications for education. *Educ Urban Soc.,* 1993;25:361–380.

25. McNamee MJ, Bartek JJ, Lynes D. Health problems of sheltered homeless children using mobile health services. *Issues Compr Pediatr Nurs.* 1994;17:233–242.

26. Wright JD. Poverty, homelessness, health, nutrition, and children. In: Kryder-Coe JH, Salamon LM, Molnar JM, eds. *Homeless Children and Youth: A New American Dilemma.* New Brunswick, NJ: Transaction; 1991:71–103.

27. Solotaroff P. *The House of Purple Hearts: Stories of Vietnam Vets Who Find Their Way Back.* New York, NY: HarperCollins; 1995.

28. Smith M. General guidelines for health care delivery to homeless adults and families in shelter and outreach sites. In: Wood D, ed. *Delivering Health Care to Homeless Persons: The Diagnosis and Management of Medical and Mental Health Conditions.* New York: Springer; 1992: 47–60.

Chapter 19

Physical Therapy Cultural Encounters in Pediatrics

● Robin L. Dole, PT, EdD, PCS

Louis and his single mother have traveled from their home, their family, and their community in Puerto Rico to the Hudson Valley region of New York to seek medical care. They have extended family here, and Louis is very ill. Louis's mother was only 16 years old when he was born, and the birth was very complicated. Louis did not want to nurse, he was difficult to console, and he developed seizures as an infant. Physicians in Puerto Rico did not give Louis very long to live, a few months to a few years. When Louis was 5 years old, he and his mother moved to the United States and settled in a small community of other immigrants from Puerto Rico. The community assisted Louis and his mother in applying for medical assistance and referral to an American physician. The physician diagnosed Louis with a severe seizure disorder and significant developmental delays, and referred the child to physical therapy. Louis's mother is learning English, but she is still reliant on family members or an interpreter for assistance in communicating her needs, questions, and concerns for her son.

An old African proverb admonishes, "It takes a village to raise a child." "Wealth and children are the adornment of life" is one of the teachings of the Koran. A Chinese proverb states, "To understand your parents' love, you must raise children yourself." How is this interpreted in the mainstream Western culture of the United States? How is this interpreted in the small community in Puerto Rico where Louis's mother spent her entire life? How is this interpreted in other communities of immigrants to the United States (Fig. 19-1)? Physical therapists who serve the needs of

children and their families should be aware of the various ways in which cultural heritage and experience shape the way children are viewed—including the social role of children within families and communities and the way decisions are made about child rearing and seeking health care.

The Purnell Model for Cultural Competence provides a helpful framework for understanding and developing culturally sensitive and competent therapy practices for children and families. Several domains within the model are discussed

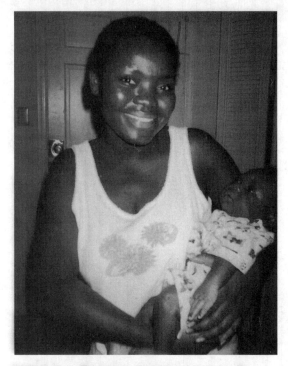

FIGURE 19.1 This woman recently immigrated to the United States from Togo, a small country on the southwest coast of Africa. She gave birth to her son in the United States.

here, with detail given to particular issues that may affect the practice of pediatric physical therapy.

Overview/Heritage

In the United States, infants, children, and adolescents make up approximately 27% of the total population. Adolescents (children between ages of 10 and 19), who represent 13% to 15% of the total population, are a more ethnically and racially diverse group than the population at large.[1] The 2000 census reported that 64% of all children living in the United States are of white, non-Hispanic origin. This represents a 10% decrease over the last two decades. Children of various ethnic backgrounds, however, continue to increase as a percentage of the total population of individuals less than 18 years of age (Fig. 19-2). The greatest increases have been in the Asian/

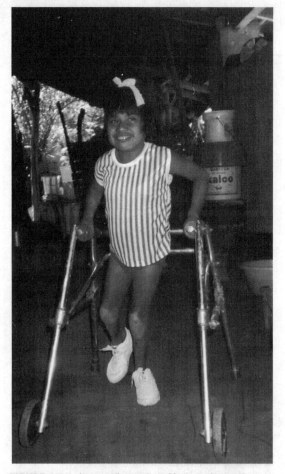

FIGURE 19.2 In countries such as Mexico, where values emphasize physical labor and productivity, this disabled child might be more stigmatized than in a country that puts more value on education and cognitive ability.

Pacific Islander and Hispanic categories, as identified by the census. By the year 2020, one in five children living in the United States will be of Hispanic heritage.[2]

While statistics vary based on race/ethnicity, the number of children living in two-parent households continues to decrease. Children who live in single-parent households, usually with their mother, are five times more likely to live in poverty than those who live with both parents. Overall estimates are that one in five children lives in poverty.[1] The 2000 census also indicates that 6.3% of the nation's children do not live with either parent, but are being raised in their grandparents' household.[3]

The U.S. Census Bureau predicts a world population of 7.5 billion or more by the year 2020. Infant mortality, in both more and less developed countries, is expected to decrease and life expectancy is expected to increase.[4] Thus, the population of children will increase in the United States and abroad. The needs of children will also increase. Those needs are even greater for children with disabilities. Of children between the ages of 5 and 15 years, 5.8% will have some form of disability. In terms of the ethnic categories used by the Census Bureau, (a) African Americans/blacks and (b) Native Americans and Alaska Natives had the highest percentage of children with disabilities (7.0% and 7.7%, respectively). Children of white, non-Hispanic; Native Hawaiian and other Pacific Islander; and Hispanic/Latino origin each experienced a disability rate of 5% to 6%.[5]

Reflective Exercise

• With the changing nature and demography of individuals living in the United States, how important will it be to increase the cultural and ethnic diversity of pediatric physical therapists?

Communication

One of the most important of Purnell's domains of culture to consider in physical therapy interventions for children is communication. It is well accepted in the literature of child development that the younger a child is when he or she learns a second language, the more successful he or she will be in learning it. Many children hear and communicate using one language at home and in the community, and another when at school. As a result, children who are bilingual may be put in the uncomfortable position of acting as interpreters of information traveling from the healthcare practitioner to the family or caregivers.[6] A child should never be placed in the position of being an interpreter except for the purpose of obtaining initial admission information. In the report America's Children: Key National Indicators

of Well-Being,[2] the number of children who exhibited difficulty with English and spoke a language other than English at home doubled between the years of 1979 and 1999 (totaling 2.6 million school-age children).

In a systematic review of the literature, Timmins[7] determined that language represented a major barrier to the receipt of quality medical care, including adequate prenatal care, by Latinos in the United States. Communication, regardless of the need for an interpreter, can be facilitated with the development of rapport and trust that come from recognizing the interrelationship of the culture of the child and family and the culture of the therapist.[8]

Reflective Exercise

• Louis's mother is learning English but is having difficulty communicating their needs to healthcare professionals. What strategies are available (and what is legally required) for facilitating communication?

Physical therapists also need to consider the impact of nonverbal communication when interacting with patients and their families. Physical touch, as part of nonverbal communication, is often a significant part of therapeutic interventions. Across cultures there are many ways in which proximity in one's personal space and physical touch are components of communication—sometimes welcome and sometimes not. For example, in Singapore, China, and Vietnam the head is considered sacred, and an act as seemingly innocuous as touching a small child on the head could be interpreted as intrusive or offensive.[9,10] Likewise, in parts of Mexico, it is offensive to indicate the growth or height of a child by gesturing with a flat hand and forearm pronated. This is the indication for the height of an animal. Instead, one should indicate the height of a child by supinating the forearm, flexing the wrist, and extending the index finger upward. This gesture should be used by the clinician to comment on the height or growth of a child (Jill Lattanzi, personal communication, March 2004).

Information that health professionals provide to individuals from cultures other than their own needs to be provided in a way that is acceptable and understood within a context that is meaningful to the individual.[6,7] One of the ways communication impacts pediatric physical therapy is in the use of standardized instruments to gain information about the developmental and functional skills of a child. Assessment tools should not be culturally biased, but should reflect the developmental and functional expectations that are consistent with the child's cultural heritage and experiences. The assessments also need to be conducted and the results communicated in a manner that brings meaning to the child and his or her family.

Modification of test items and instructions and creating realistic norms or criteria so that the test is a true reflection of the child's ability and not of the child's assimilation to Western culture should occur. Examples include the use of the Denver Developmental Screening Test and the Denver II for Armenian Americans, Alaska Natives, Southeast Asian refugees living in the United States, as well as children living in the Netherlands, Tokyo, Okinawa, and the Philippines.[11] In their review of studies on cross-cultural variability in child motor development, Suske and Swanson[11] discuss the modifications that were made by various researchers and the implications of not modifying developmental tests to limit cultural bias. The most common problems identified were over- or underreferral of children for services to address delays in motor performance and the need for translation of items (for both language and cultural significance) to ensure valid use of the test.

Reflective Exercise

• Who "owns" the therapeutic goals that shape the relationship and intervention between therapists and the children and family they serve? • In what ways do you communicate this implicitly and explicitly?

Family Roles and Organization

The first relationships that a child forms are those they share with their caregivers. Depending on cultural heritage and family beliefs and practices, those early relationships can include parents,

siblings, extended family, and community members. The structure of a family can take on a myriad of forms depending somewhat on the constitutional makeup of the members and on the level of cultural influence that is present. For families who are bicultural, the members may need to find ways to support and retain their traditional beliefs and practices while also assimilating into the dominant culture of the country in which they live. This can cause generational stress as younger members seek to incorporate both cultures into their lives and older members try to hold strongly to their traditions.[8] This impacts both family dynamics and child rearing practices for children with and without disabilities.

While the importance of family and the role of the members of a family may differ from culture to culture, within a given culture the family may also function as a subculture. Sparling[12] considers the family a "unique cultural unit," stating that "families are a diverse mixture of characteristics which when occurring together define a unique culture" (pp. 18–19). Specific issues related to the family structure can be influenced greatly by cultural heritage. Hmong families, who moved from Laos to Thailand and then later immigrated to the United States and Australia, are typically large and associated with one of several "clans." These clans help to form the basis of the family name and the names given to children.[13] Children in Hmong society are valued for their role in the community; males, specifically, perform specific rituals such as tending the family altar, caring for their ancestors, and bringing on the next generation.[13]

Reflective Exercise

• Louis and his mother have come a long way from their home to seek medical care. This is made possible by the close family connections within this Latino family. In what ways may his therapy services be impacted by the involvement and influence of his extended family?

Families of children with disabilities may face unique challenges, and the way that the child is viewed within the family structure is also important.[14,15] The way in which a child's disability is defined and experienced can be associated with the role expectations of various members in a family or community. In cultures that place a high value on education and technology, cognitive disabilities may be viewed quite negatively, whereas for cultures that rely on labor and productivity, a physical disability may be more highly stigmatized[16] (Fig. 19-3).

Being sensitive to and aware of how parents and other caregivers view the child's disability and to what they attribute the cause of the condition is important. For some cultures, having a child with a disability is seen as a special calling or mission. For others, the child's disability is a manifestation of the child's or parent's own wrongdoing in this or a previous life. Families who refuse intervention for a child's disability may be doing so out of reverence for the blessing that has been given to them, or because doing so would be a statement that the disability was not divinely or spiritually ordained.[16] For example, in the Hispanic culture, some pregnant women believe that acts of God, such as an earthquake or hurricane, will result in a child being born with a disability.[17]

In their systematic review of articles published in the early childhood special education literature between 1996 and 1997, Taylor and Baglin[18] found that the majority of articles viewed the family in a positive light and stressed the importance of family involvement in the care of children with special needs. Of research-oriented articles, 38% stressed the importance and influence of diversity such as ethnicity and socioeconomic status. The authors caution, however, that issues of cultural diversity and the family need to be addressed and studied further to illuminate the importance of these factors to the delivery of special services to children (Fig. 19-4).

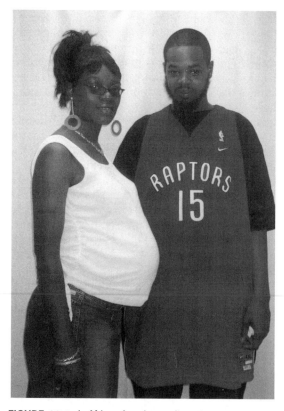

FIGURE 19.4 In African American culture, teenage pregnancy may not carry the stigma that it does in the prevailing white culture.

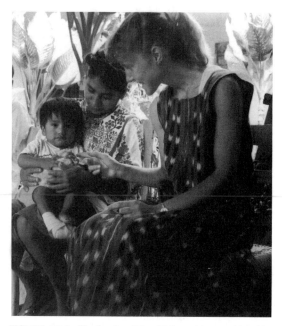

FIGURE 19.3 The family of the child must be considered in addition to the child.

Reflective Exercise

• A physical therapist working with Native American families on a reservation encounters a family who is "noncompliant" with a program of intervention designed for their 7-year-old daughter, who has cognitive delays and has been diagnosed with fetal alcohol syndrome. What might be some of the reasons the family has chosen not to embrace the therapy program? • What might the therapist do to help the child within the cultural context and spiritual beliefs of the family?

Nutrition

Nutritional practices are influenced by cultural heritage and experience.[19,20] Within this domain, it is important to consider the impact of nutrition on the health status of children at all ages, while also respecting the diversity of practices represented within the various cultures with which the physical therapist may interact. Two particular areas of concern, infant feeding practices and the problem of obesity in adolescence, will be discussed in detail.

Infant Feeding Practices

Infant feeding patterns have been the subject of significant cross-cultural research. In some cultures where breastfeeding is an expectation of all mothers, there is also a belief that the early milk, or *colostrum*, is not healthy for infants.[19–21] Western societies have a history of supporting the feeding of only breast milk for the first 4 to 6 months, and recognize the nutritional value of the colostrum. In other cultures, however, colostrum is viewed as detrimental or even "evil," and described as pus-like or stale from having sat in the breast for too long.[21,22] These beliefs tend to be stronger among immigrant mothers of similar cultural heritage who retain their traditional practices, compared with mothers who have been acculturated within countries or locales where Western or Anglo practices dominate.[19]

Where mothers have undergone strong acculturation to the new country, infant feeding practices are more likely to reflect those of the host culture. Common reasons for why mothers might initiate bottle feeding over breastfeeding or discontinue breastfeeding and begin bottle feeding include feeling embarrassed in public, the ease of use and availability of formula for bottle feeding, the need to return to work, and concern that the child isn't getting enough nourishment.[23]

For mothers who retain their traditional beliefs and practices regarding infant feeding, *prelacteal* feedings are common. This is true in the primary culture of India, where mothers feed their infants a diet of sugar water for the first 24 hours after birth and may not begin breastfeeding until 5 or 6 days after birth.[19,24] Mothers from India may also view foods ingested during pregnancy and lactation within the context of "hot" and "cold" foods. Food items are harmful or helpful depending on whether they are considered to be "hot" or "cold," which is defined not by the temperature of the food but rather by how the food is used in the body, by tradition, and by belief. Cold foods are preferred during pregnancy, while hot foods might be encouraged toward the end of pregnancy to assist in birth.[24,25]

Reflective Exercise

• Consider your own family's practices when it comes to breastfeeding or bottle feeding. What factors influence these decisions?

A variety of demographic factors influence the choice of whether to breastfeed or bottle feed a newborn. One study of mothers from Canada, representing both the dominant and minority cultures, showed that maternal education and age, socioeconomic status, and social support network/living status all impact the decision to breastfeed, to continue breastfeeding past the first month, and, if bottle feeding, whether to use formula or less expensive evaporated milk. Matthews and colleagues,[23] in a study that included mothers from Caucasian and aboriginal backgrounds, showed that younger, single, less educated, lower-income mothers tended to bottle feed and often used poorer-quality sources of nutrition for their infants. Ethnicity played a significant role and confirmed what others have shown: that when a mother remains faithful to her culture's traditional practices, breastfeeding is more common.

Other infant feeding practices of which therapists should be aware when planning culturally sensitive and competent intervention programs for young children and their families include the practice of breastfeeding on demand, the duration of breastfeeding (with extended breastfeeding believed to lengthen the interbirth interval), the use of wet nurses, the influence of the mother's social support network (especially female family members and the woman's husband/partner), and the appropriate timing for the introduction of solid foods.[13,26]

Reflective Exercise

• How might a pediatric therapist working in the neonatal intensive care environment support the ability of a young Indian mother as she attempts to bond with and breastfeed her preterm baby?

Obesity in Adolescence

The increasing incidence of children who are overweight to the degree of obesity has resulted in a significant health crisis in the United States. Ogden, Flegal, Carroll, and Johnson[27] determined that 15.5% of children ages 12 through 19 years had body mass indices that were above the 95th percentile, representing an increase of 5% over the level observed between 1988 and 1994. They also provided evidence that obesity is higher in children of non-Hispanic black and Mexican American backgrounds. This leads to concern that at least some of the factors influencing obesity in children may be culturally mediated; for example, being overweight, at least by U.S. standards, is seen as positive[28,29] (Table 19-1).

Melnyk and Weinstein[30] discussed obesity among African American women and adolescents. The concern that African American women were at increased risk for obesity and associated health problems (hypertension, diabetes, cardiovascular disease) and the disproportional increase in the rate of obesity among adolescent black females prompted these researchers to review the literature and make recommendations regarding programs to address the issue. They

found that the most successful programs involved support from the community (namely church organizations and community leaders), incorporated culturally appropriate and acceptable diets, and encouraged mutual participation by mother and daughter.[30]

Reflective Exercise

• What role might physical therapists play in addressing the growing health concerns associated with obesity in childhood and adolescence? • What responsibility does the physical therapist have?
• What resources might the physical therapist use?
• What concerns might the physical therapist have in combating this growing problem in a culturally sensitive manner?

Pregnancy and Child Rearing Practices

Pediatric physical therapists must explore and understand the impact of cultural heritage and experience on the process of pregnancy, delivery, and early care of the infant. What women believe, the foods they choose to eat, and who they select to assist in the birthing process are all influenced by cultural and social practices. For example, in India pregnancy is not considered a health issue and women may not seek prenatal or antenatal care from a health professional.[24] The birthing process may involve a special birth attendant and may occur in the squatting position rather than supine, as is the customary practice in American hospitals.

Practices may differ from culture to culture and from individual to individual within the culture. Specific issues discussed in this section include how culture influences the rates of teenage pregnancy among minority groups and how child rearing and child development are impacted by cultural practices.

Teenage Pregnancy

The age when women typically begin having children can vary among different geographical regions and among individuals from various religious, cultural, and ethnic backgrounds. Adolescent pregnancy, the incidence of which

TABLE 19.1

Incidence of Childhood Obesity

	TOTAL			MALE			FEMALE	
	1976–1980	1988–1994	1999–2000	1976–1980	1988–1994	1999–2000	1976–1980	1988–1994
Children ages 6–18								
Total[a]	5.7	11.2	15.3	5.5	11.8	15.9	5.8	10.6
Race or Hispanic origin								
White, non-Hispanic	4.9	10.5	11.6	4.7	11.3	12.0	6.1	9.6
Black, non-Hispanic	8.2	14.0	21.5	5.8[b]	11.5	19.0	10.7	16.5
Mexican American	-	15.4	24.5	-	16.1	28.5	-	14.7
Children ages 6–11								
Total[a]	6.1	11.3	15.3	6.2	11.6	16.0	6.0	11.0
Race or Hispanic origin								
White, non-Hispanic	6.6	10.2	11.8	6.1	10.7	12.0	5.2	9.8
Black, non-Hispanic	9.0	14.6	19.5	6.8[b]	12.3	17.1	11.2	17.0
Mexican American	-	16.4	23.7	-	17.5	27.3	-	15.3
Children ages 12–18								
Total[a]	4.7	11.1	15.3	3.7	12.0	15.9	5.7	10.2
Race or Hispanic origin								
White, non-Hispanic	4.3	10.8	11.3	3.6	12.0	12.1	5.0	9.5
Black, non-Hispanic	7.5	13.3	23.6	*	10.7	21.3	10.3	16.0
Mexican American	-	14.2	25.4	-	14.4	30.3	-	14.0

− = not available

* = Estimates are considered unreliable (relative standard error greater than 40 percent)

[a] Total include data for racial/ethnic groups not shown separately.

[b] Estimates are unstable because they are based on a small number of persons (relative standard error greater than 30 percent)

NOTE: Overweight is defined as body mass index (BMI) at or above the 95th percentile of the 2000 Centers for Disease Control and Prevention BMI for age growth charts (http://www.cdc.gov/growthcharts). BMI is calculated as weight in kilograms divided by the square of height in meters.

SOURCES: Centers for Disease Control and Prevention, National Center for Health Statistics, National Health and Nutrition Exam Survey.

has been increasing among minorities, is a major health concern in the United States and the world at large.[4] Talashek and colleagues[31] attribute the rate of adolescent pregnancy among African Americans and Latinas to demographic (race/ethnicity), physiological (age at menarche and sexual maturity), and sociocultural (history of sexual activity and contraceptive practices) factors. Their model for predicting the age of first pregnancy among these ethnic minority groups suggests that the longer the duration between a young woman's first menstrual period and her first sexual experience, the older she will be at the time of her first pregnancy. Interestingly, their research also revealed that using contraception at first intercourse was associated with younger age at first pregnancy.

Yoos and co-workers[32] explain that in the African American culture, teenage pregnancy may not carry the same stigma that it does in the

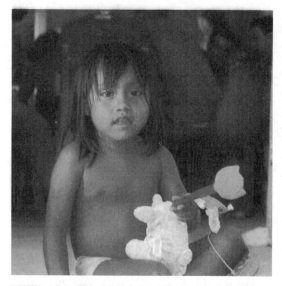

FIGURE 19.5 This child has been left to play alone while the adults socialize.

Anglo-European American culture (Fig. 19-5). In some African American communities, the concept of family extends well beyond the parent or parents and child, and young mothers may be well supported by multi-generation households.[28] The number of grandparents who provide a home for their grandchildren is tracked by the U.S. Census Bureau and has increased by almost 30% between the years of 1990 and 2000.[2]

Reflective Exercise

• How do the religious and cultural influences in your life shape the way you view issues of teenage pregnancy, contraception, and inter-generational caregiving?

Child Rearing and Child Development

Cultural heritage and traditional beliefs impact child rearing practices, expectations for child development, and views on health and disability. The home environment and the relationship between child and caregiver, which can vary both within and across cultures, have been shown to influence cognitive and motor development.[32–34] Moreover, parent and caregiver expectations for

child development are influenced by cultural heritage (Figs. 19-6 and 19-7). Communities and groups who value independence and autonomy have developmental expectations, engage children in activities, and use disciplinary practices that are consonant with this philosophy about the social role of children and adults. Conversely, when a family, group, or culture's expectations of children emphasize interdependence, cooperation, and interpersonal relationships, the expectations, activities, and disciplinary practices reflect this philosophy.[32] For example, children from the former Soviet Union are expected to be toilet trained and dress themselves by 18 months of age,[35] whereas children from Puerto Rico might still have their mothers feeding them with a fork at 4 to 6 years of age.[15]

Mothers' and caregivers' expectations for the development of their children, and subsequently the activities in which the child engages as well as the timing of milestone achievements, vary among cultures. Parents in Puerto Rico, when interviewed about their expectations, reported that their children are more dependent on caregivers for skills that are typically mastered by similar-age American children. Gannotti and colleagues,[15] in their study to support the cultural interpretation of a Spanish translation of the Pediatric Evaluation of Disability Inventory, also found that Puerto Rican parents might choose to do more for their children, things that the children might be able to do on their own, out of protection of the child or because they wanted the child to feel special.

Reflective Exercise

• Investigate the standardized and nonstandardized assessments that you typically use to evaluate the needs of children and families. Are testing or interview items potentially culturally biased? • What considerations should a physical therapist make when using screening tools with children from other cultures? • How might a physical therapist ensure that a screening tool is culturally valid?

Despite the evidence from the literature, most authors who have studied or reviewed published

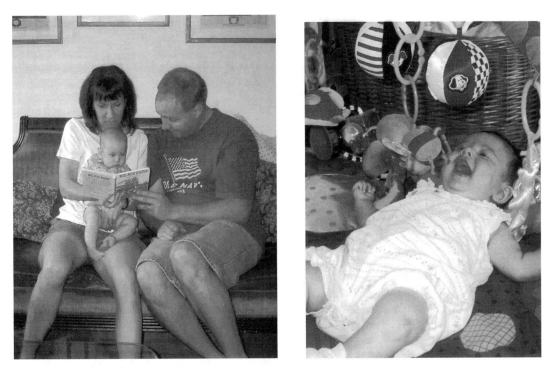

FIGURE 19.6 (*A*) This couple from the United States focuses on reading and with their infant daughter. (*B*) This 3-month-old infant participates in developmental play.

works on the impact of culture on child development caution that many studies do not control for or recognize the influence of socioeconomic status on the developmental variations found in various minority groups, or they tend to confuse the concept of culture with issues of ethnicity and/or race. For this reason, research on child development and interventions implemented for children with special needs must be considered.

Spirituality

Religious and spiritual practices are integral to the life experiences of many children and families; religious beliefs may lead some individuals to refuse certain aspects of Western medicine. For example, Jehovah's Witnesses may not accept blood transfusions because of specific biblical teachings; and although the Amish strongly favor health prevention activities, they do not always participate in immunization for children as it would demonstrate a lack of faith in God.[36] Whiteford and Wilcock[37] remind us that occupational and physical therapy services are products of Western medicine, and the culture that these professions arose from may be in direct or indirect conflict with other views of health, wellness, illness, disease, and rehabilitation. An example of how the religious/cultural practices of the Hasidim influenced the development of an aquatic physical therapy program for a young boy with cerebral palsy is presented in the case study at the end of this chapter.

Reflective Exercise

• How do you view the families and children who come to the United States to receive medical care that can't be obtained in their home country? • How do you view the "medical missions" that take Western medicine to less developed countries and to villages and communities in poverty?

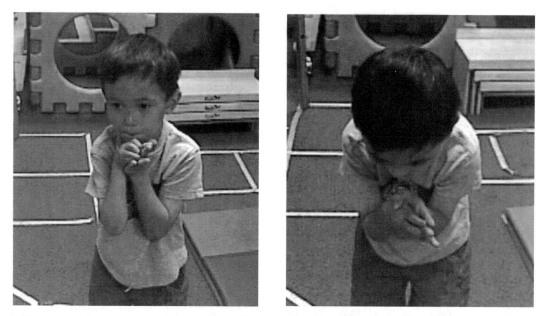

FIGURE 19.7 This 5-year-old boy's mother is from Thailand and his father is from the United States. Though he is living in America, he is learning the traditional practices of Thai culture, including the language and customs associated with greeting another person. Here he is shown performing the *sawasdee khrap*, which requires that he bring both his hands together to bow and accompanies a greeting. His therapist uses this practice to help him meet his therapeutic goals related to a diagnosis of hemiplegic cerebral palsy. (Photo courtesy of Robin Dole.)

Healthcare Practices

As healthcare professionals, physical therapists must be cognizant of the fact that healthcare settings in themselves are a culture, and those people not attuned to the practices of that culture can be marginalized. This is especially true in the area of early intervention and special education, where various professionals from many disciplines gather to make decisions about the services a child will need. The parents or other family members are generally present at these meetings, but far too often they are not fully incorporated as members of the team. Philosophies of family-centered interventions in pediatrics help to identify alternative practices that can facilitate participation of the child and his or her family in decision-making processes to bring meaning to intervention that is simply not possible when decisions are made independently.[18]

By engaging the child's family and caregivers in goal setting and intervention planning, issues and activities that are important to the child can be incorporated. Social, spiritual, and family practices may need to be both respected and included in culturally congruent therapy interventions. An example of how a pediatric physical therapist included a cultural custom of greeting in the therapeutic goals and interventions for a young boy with a physical disability is depicted in Figure 19-7.

Reflective Exercise

• How are the principles of family-centered care influenced by the way that individuals and communities define the concept of family?

Health professionals may find that strong belief in and emphasis on folk medicine and rit-

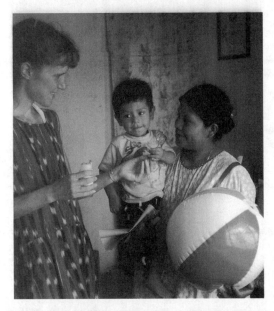

FIGURE 19.8 People in some cultures believe that the "evil eye" can be transmitted to a child when someone compliments the child without touching him or her.

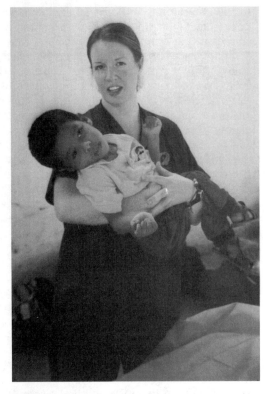

FIGURE 19.9 The physical therapist must be prepared to work with children from different cultures.

ual healing may contradict or interact with contemporary Western medicine. Salas-Provance, Erickson, and Reed[38] interviewed a four-generation Hispanic family to investigate the way cultural and spiritual beliefs influenced their opinions about health and disability. These authors found that in this family, members of all ages (21 to 96 years) discussed traditional medical beliefs more often than folk medicine beliefs. Folk medicine practices, however, had some influence over their health beliefs regardless of generation. They also described the folk illnesses of *mal de ojo* (evil eye), *susto* (sickness caused by fright), and the ritual purification and healing practices performed by the *curandero*. The evil eye is cast when a person looks too directly or too longingly at another, which can lead to ill health; *susto* is the belief that an intense emotional experience can cause illness[15] (Fig. 19-9).

The malady of the evil eye can be found across many cultures and religious practices, and may involve excessive praise of an individual. In Kuwait, parents may well prefer public denigration of themselves or their children over recognition and compliments in order to avoid the evil eye.[9] In some Central American cultures, babies may wear a red *bolsita,* which is a little bag of herbs worn around the neck to protect the baby from harm. Red is recognized as a strong color, and some female children wear red earrings to ward off the *mal de ojo*. Physical therapists should check with the parents before removing any red item from the child.[39] Kalofissudis[40] suggests that allowing and encouraging rituals or procedures for ridding patients of folk illness (like the evil eye) may have a real therapeutic value; such practices should not be discounted, even in traditional healthcare settings.

Healthcare Practitioners

The importance of understanding the diversity among families and children from various cultural backgrounds has been echoed throughout this chapter. An important concept for therapists to understand and respect is reflected in an article discussing the importance of parent/family-practitioner partnerships in the delivery of care to young children with disabilities. Bruns and Steeples[41] state that therapists should not "emphasize differences" but "highlight the need to tailor practices to individual preferences and move away from a 'one size fits all' approach" (pp. 241–242).

Another important concept for physical therapists is the need to understand one's own culture before attempting to understand that of another. Leonard and Polotnikoff[42] tell a powerful story of how healthcare students who viewed a film and discussed healing practices with a Hmong shaman considered the experience to be an unnecessary intrusion on their time (which they undoubtedly wished had been spent learning things they really needed to know!). The authors pointed out that many of these future healthcare practitioners were likely to experience patients of Hmong background and clearly dismissed an important experience that might have helped them tremendously in their practice. Whiteford and Wilcock[37] warn of this kind of *cultural blindness*, which can occur in therapists who represent the dominant culture or social group. Carnevale[14] argues that Western philosophies of health and medicine, especially mental health, are "based on an ethnocentric conception of the self" (p. 26). Physical therapists whose own culture is consistent with traditional Western medicine, where the right to self-determination and the quest for independence and cure are paramount, may not realize that another individual's choices or actions may be mediated by a culture and tradition that is not "right" or "wrong" but is just another way of viewing the situation. Being aware of one's own beliefs and biases will help one recognize when they might interfere with the provision of culturally sensitive and competent care.

Reflective Exercise

• How might the physical therapist working with Louis in the initial vignette exhibit cultural blindness?
• How might the physical therapist work to overcome cultural blindness?

Reflective Exercise

• Take time to think about your own beliefs regarding health, wellness, illness, and disease. How do your personal and professional experiences influence these beliefs? • How best can you recognize when your beliefs may be in conflict with those of your colleagues? • Those of your patients and their families?

When planning interventions for a child with disabilities and his or her family, therapists may consider completing an individual cultural assessment.[8] Avoid the common mistake of stereotyping an individual based on the automatic attribution of characteristics common to a group, whether an ethnic or minority group or a specific culture or heritage. See Table 19-2 for suggestions for an individual cultural assessment based on the literature. Krefting[8] discusses three main ways in which culture is misinterpreted

TABLE 19.2

Considerations for Conducting an Individual Cultural Assessment with Families and Caregivers of Children with Disabilities

• Solicit permission to discuss issues related to the child's illness and care, and inquire as to who is most appropriate to provide that information.
• Provide for a language or cultural interpreter to assist when necessary, or a therapist with the same cultural background or who speaks the same language as the child and family.[6,7]
• Determine if there are others in the community who may need to approve or supervise the interventions on behalf of the child.

- Ask why the family or caregiver is seeking your help.
- Ascertain the extent of the family's or community's expectations of children, and the child's social role in the family or community.[32]
- Understand to what the family or caregivers attribute the cause of the child's illness or disability.[6,16]
- Collect information on how the family typically seeks help for its children.[8,42]
- Discuss the individuals or practices that the family uses when someone is ill or experiencing difficulties with health.[8,42]
- Find out if the child is receiving or participating in any other interventions or alternative care for the illness or disability.[8]
- Pay attention to your own body language and nonverbal behaviors; be aware of the cultural meanings of eye contact, touch, etc.[6]
- Inquire as to the type and extent of disciplinary and behavior management strategies (authoritarian, permissive, or a combination) that are preferred/accepted and who is typically responsible.[32]

TABLE 19.3

Helpful Readings for Pediatric Physical Therapists Providing Care to Culturally Diverse Families

- *Amazing Grace: The Lives of Children and the Conscience of a Nation* (1995) by Jonathan Kozol
- *The Spirit Catches You and You Fall Down* (1997) by Anne Fadiman
- *Our Babies, Ourselves: How Biology and Culture Shape the Way We Parent* (1998) by Meredith Small
- *Kids: How Biology and Culture Shape the Way We Raise Our Children* (2001) by Meredith Small

in healthcare: (a) using concepts of culture and race/ethnicity interchangeably, (b) associating culture with a geographical area or area of origin, and (c) considering only the issues of immigrants when discussing the influence of culture. Advice to physical therapists can be garnered from her statement, "The idea of culturally sensitive treatment should not come to mind only when a therapist hears an unfamiliar accent or sees a note on the patient history indicating that the person in the treatment room is a recent immigrant. It should come to mind *every time* the therapist enters that treatment room"[8] (p. 7). Table 19-3 provides a list of helpful readings for the pediatric physical therapist.

CASE STUDY SCENARIO

Joel is an 11-year-old boy whose family and community are part of a particular sect within the Jewish faith. The Hasidim in the United States typically live and work in defined, segregated areas and are identified by their traditional dress and religious practices. Men and women wear dark, conservative clothing that covers the extremities. A head covering—a wig or a hat of some sort—is common for men and required for women. A man is not permitted to touch a woman unless she is his wife.[43] Joel's father is a rabbi, and one of his responsibilities in the community is to help children with disabilities and their families obtain the care they need. Joel's father knows too well the importance of this because Joel has cerebral palsy.

(continued)

The rabbi has raised funds to build a therapeutic pool in the community and enlists the services of a private physical therapist to begin sessions in the pool, with his son as the first recipient. While the therapist has many years of experience with aquatic therapy, she is not prepared for the restrictions that Joel's faith and culture place on the services she can provide. As a female, she is able to have direct contact with Joel because he has not yet been called to the *Torah* for the bar mitzvah; however, to be respectful of Joel's cultural practices, she must not reveal her body. This means wearing, even while in the pool, clothing that covers her arms to the wrists, her trunk up to the clavicles, and her legs to the ankles. In a therapeutic pool environment over 85 degrees, the clothing needed to be breathable so as not to overheat the therapist, and loose fitting so as not to "reveal" her body when the clothing was wet.

The answer to the dilemma was a successful collaboration between Joel's mother and the therapist. The therapist found a style of clothing that would meet the needs of the culture, but the material was too restricting and created heat, rather than dispersing it. Joel's mother found material that "breathed" and resisted clinging when wet, and used the clothing example to fashion a pattern. She sewed the "suit," and the therapist tried it out in the therapeutic pool outside of view of the males in the household. When Joel's mother approved of the "suit," therapy sessions began in the new community pool.

The success of this collaboration was significant in the development of a trusting therapeutic relationship between Joel's family and the therapist. Several years after the therapist had moved away from the area and was practicing more than 300 miles away, the rabbi tracked down the therapist and asked her to return and provide training and consultation to therapists assisting in the opening of another pool in a distant Hasidic community. The therapist was pleased to see that the "suit" she once wore to provide Joel's therapy was still used by the therapists at the new site.

1. What cultural barriers were present in this scenario?

2. How did those involved overcome the cultural barriers?

3. Why was the collaboration between the therapist and Joel's mother so successful?

4. If Joel was older than 13 years and had received the bar mitzvah, how might this scenario have been different?

5. What is the significance of gender in this scenario? Would it have been easier to just find a male therapist?

6. In what ways did the physical therapist demonstrate cultural competence?

7. How might the physical therapist have learned more about the Hasidic Jewish culture?

8. What specific training do you think the physical therapist provided for the new therapists?

9. Which of the 12 domains of Purnell's model of cultural competence were influenced or impacted by the actions of the therapist? The rabbi? Joel's mother?

REFERENCES

1. National Adolescent Health Information Center. Fact sheet on adolescent demographics. San Francisco: National Adolescent Health Information Center, University of California. Available at: www.youth.ucsf.edu/nahic/. Accessed June 1, 2004.

2. United States Interagency Forum on Child and Family Statistics. America's children: Key national indicators of well-being. Available at: http://www.childstats. gov/ac2003/highlights.asp. Accessed June 1, 2004.

3. US Census Bureau. 2000 census: Profiles of general demographic characteristics. Available at: http://www. census.gov/main/www/cen2000.html. Accessed June 1, 2004.

4. US Department of Commerce. World population at a glance: 1996 and beyond. Available at: http://www. census.gov/ipc/prod/ib96_03.pdf. Accessed June 1, 2004.

5. Waldrop J, Stern SM. Disability status 2000. Available at: http://www.census.gov/prod/2003pubs/c2kbr-17.pdf. Accessed June 1, 2004.

6. Lester N. Cultural competence: A nursing dialogue— Part 1. *Am J Nurs.* 1998;98:26–34.

7. Timmins CL. The impact of language barriers on the health care of Latinos in the United States: A review of the literature and guidelines for practice. *J Midwifery Womens Health.* 2002;47:80–96.

8. Krefting L. The culture concept in the everyday practice of occupational and physical therapy. In: Campbell SK, Wilhelm IJ, eds. *Meaning of Culture in Pediatric Rehabilitation and Health Care.* Binghamton, NY: Haworth Press; 1991:1–16.

9. Geissler EM. *Mosby's Pocket Guide: Cultural Assessment.* 2nd ed. St Louis: Mosby; 1998.

10. Nowak T. People of Vietnamese heritage. In: Purnell L, Paulanka B, eds. *Transcultural Health Care: A Culturally Competent Approach.* 2nd ed. Philadelphia, Pa: FA Davis; 2003:327–345.

11. Suske KS, Swanson MW. Cross-cultural variability in early childhood motor development: An annotated bibliography. *Phys Occup Ther Pediatr.* 1997;17:87–96.

12. Sparling JW. The cultural definition of the family. In: Campbell SK, Wilhelm IJ, eds. *Meaning of Culture in Pediatric Rehabilitation and Health Care.* Binghamton, NY: Haworth Press; 1991:17–29.

13. Liamputtong Rice PL. *Hmong Women and Reproduction.* Westport, Conn: Bergin & Garvey; 2000.

14. Carnevale F. Toward a cultural conception of the self. *J Psychosoc Nurs.* 1999;37:26–31.

15. Gannotti ME, Handwerker WP, Groce NE, Cruz C. Sociocultural influences on disability status in Puerto Rican children. *Phys Ther.* 2001;81:1512–1523.

16. Zhang C, Bennett T. Multicultural views of disability: Implications for early intervention professionals. *Infant Toddler Intervent.* 2001;11:143–154.

17. Risser A, Manzur L. Use of folk remedies in the Hispanic population. *Arch Pediatr Adolesc Med.* 1995;149: 978–981.

18. Taylor JM, Baglin CA. Families of young children with disabilities: Perceptions in the early childhood special education literature. *Infant Toddler Intervent.* 2000; 10:239–257.

19. Kannan S, Carruth BR, Skinner J. Cultural influences on infant feeding beliefs of mothers. *J Am Diet Assoc.* 1999;99:88–90.

20. Monti D. Food customs and their role in pregnancy and infant feeding. *J Child Educ.* 2000;15:18.

21. Riordan J, Gill-Hopple K. Breastfeeding care in multicultural populations. *J Gyn Neonatal Nurs.* 2000;30:216–223.

22. Liamputtong P. Infant feeding practices: The case of Hmong women in Australia. *Health Care Women Int.* 2002;23:33–48.

23. Matthews K, Webber K, McKim E, Banoub-Baddour S, Laryea M. Maternal infant-feeding decisions: Reasons and influences. *Can J Nurs Res.* 1998;30:177–198.

24. Choudhry UK. Traditional practices of women from India: Pregnancy, childbirth, and newborn care. *J Gynecol Neonatal Nurs.* 1997;26:533–539.

25. Jambanathan J. People of Hindu heritage [chapter on CD-ROM]. In: Purnell L, Paulanka B, eds. *Transcultural Health Care: A Culturally Competent Approach.* 2nd ed. Philadelphia, Pa: FA Davis; 2003.

26. Sellen DW. Weaning, complementary feeding, and maternal decision making in a rural East African pastoral population. *J Hum Lactation.* 2001;17:233–244.

27. Ogden CL, Flegal KM, Carroll MD, Johnson CL. Prevalence and trends in overweight among US children and adolescents, 1999–2000. *JAMA.* 2002;288: 1728–1732.

28. Glanville C. People of African American heritage. In: Purnell L, Paulanka B, eds. *Transcultural Health Care: A Culturally Competent Approach.* 2nd ed. Philadelphia, Pa: FA Davis; 2003:40–53.

29. Zoucha R, Purnell L. People of Mexican heritage. In: Purnell L, Paulanka B, eds. *Transcultural Health Care: A Culturally Competent Approach.* 2nd ed. Philadelphia, Pa: FA Davis; 2003:264–278.

30. Melnyk MG, Weinstein E. Preventing obesity in black women by targeting adolescents: A literature review. *J Am Diet Assoc.* 1994;94:536–540.

31. Talashek ML, Montgomery AC, Moran C, Paskiewicz L, Jiang Y. Menarche, sexual practices, and pregnancy: Model testing. *Clin Excell Nurs Pract.* 2000;4:98–107.

32. Yoos HL, Kitzman H, Olds DL, Overacker I. Child rearing beliefs in the African-American community: Implications for culturally competent pediatric care. *J Pediatr Nurs.* 1995;10:343–353.

33. Abbott A. Bartlett D. The relationship between the home environment and early motor development. *Phys Occup Ther Pediatr.* 1999;19:43–57.

34. Wallace IF, Roberts JE, Lodder DE. Interactions of African American infants and their mothers: Relations with development at 1 year of age. *J Speech Lang Hear Res.* 1998;41:900–912.

35. Liebert R, Wicks-Nelson R. (1981). Cross-cultural differences in parenting. In: Schultz J. ed. *Developmental Psychology.* 3rd ed. Rutherford, Conn: Prentice-Hall.

36. Wenger AF, Wenger M. The Amish. In: Purnell L, Paulanka B, eds. *Transcultural Health Care: A Culturally Competent Approach.* 2nd ed. Philadelphia, Pa: FA Davis; 2003:54–73.

37. Whiteford GE, Wilcock AA. Cultural relativism: Occupation and independence reconsidered. *Can J Occup Ther.* 2000;67:324–336.

38. Salas-Provance MB, Erickson JG, Reed J. Disabilities viewed by four generations of one Hispanic family. *Am J Speech Lang Pathol.* 2002;11:151–162.

39. Andrews M, Boyle J. *Transcultural Concepts in Nursing Care.* 3rd ed. Philadelphia, Pa: Lippincott; 1999.

40. Kalofissudis IA. Evil eye, creative metaphors and the postmodern nursing paradigm (Editorial). *ICUs Nurs Web J.* 2003:13.

41. Bruns DA, Steeples T. Partners from the beginning: Guidelines for encouraging partnerships between parents and NICU and EI professionals. *Infant Toddler Intervent.* 2001;11:237–247.

42. Leonard BJ, Polotnikoff GA. Awareness: The heart of cultural competence. *Am Assoc Crit Care Nurs Clin Issues.* 2000;11:51–59.

43. Selekman J. People of Jewish Heritage. In: Purnell L, Paulanka B, eds. *Transcultural Health Care: A Culturally Competent Approach.* 2nd ed. Philadelphia, Pa: FA Davis; 2003:234–248.

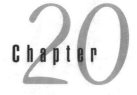

Chapter 20

Physical Therapy Cultural Encounters in Geriatrics

● Jill Black Lattanzi, PT, EdD

*M*r. Edmondson had just celebrated his ninetieth birthday and had the misfortune of falling and breaking his hip. He underwent surgery and is now in rehabilitation. He lives alone in a two-story farm home and is determined to return home upon completion of his rehabilitation. He grew up in a farming community in the heartland of Pennsylvania and has been widowed for 10 years. He suffered a heart attack shortly after his wife passed. He also has hypertension and diabetes, both of which are controlled by medicine. His daughter lives in the same town but his grandchildren all live out of state.

Introduction

Old age is a relatively recent phenomenon in the United States and is destined to have a great impact on U.S. society over the next 50 years. In 1776 the average life span was 35 years, in 1900 it was 47 years, and in 1970 it was 68 years.[1] As of the year 2000, the average life expectancy for the general population is 76.9 years. The average life expectancy for males is 74.1 years and for females 79.5 years.[2] In the year 2000, people 65 years of age had an average remaining life expectancy of 19.2 years for women (a total of 84.2 years) and 16.3 years for men (total 81.3 years).[3] The average life expectancy is expected to increase to 81 years by 2050. Because of this increased life expectancy,

old age has been redefined. With people now living to age 90 and beyond, someone age 65 is from a completely different generation and most likely will present with different needs and perspectives. Therefore, old age has been redefined into three categories: the young-old, ages 65–74; the middle-old, ages 75–84; and the oldest-old, ages 85 and above (Box 20-1). From 1990 to 2000, the oldest-old group demonstrated the most rapid growth, from 3.1 million to 4.2 million, an increase of 38%.[4]

It is also important to consider one's physiological age versus one's chronological age. Chronological age is the actual number of years, or the *quantity* of life, while physiological age is the measure of one's physical fitness, or *quality* of life. In the initial vignette to this chapter,

BOX 20.1

Old Age Redefined

Young-old are ages 65–74
Middle-old are ages 75–84
Oldest-old are ages 85 and above

Reflection 20.2

Most older people are young people in old bodies. Some younger people are old people in young bodies.[5]

Mr. Edmondson's chronological age is 90 years, but his physiological age before his hip fracture was likely much less. Physical therapists are wise to note a person's chronological age but will demonstrate greater wisdom by considering the person's physiological age and other functional measures when taking the person's history.

Advances in medicine and improvements in medical technology account for the dramatic increases in life span. In the last century, medicine has been better able to manage acute epidemic outbreaks, and the discovery of penicillin and other antibiotics has improved the management of bacterial infections. These advances have allowed for longer life spans, resulting in an increase in chronic diseases, disabilities, and physical decline or senescence that often accompanies older age. The physical therapy professional excels in the management and intervention of chronic disorders, disabilities, and physical decline; physical therapists must be prepared to meet the challenges specific to the culture of aging.

Not only is the average life expectancy increasing, but the number of persons over age 65 is increasing dramatically. Actually, between 1990 and 2010, there is projected to be a slight decline in the number of persons over age 65. This is due to lower birth rates during the years of the Great

Reflection 20.1

The characteristic feature of older people is diversity. There is no homogeneous biomass called "the elderly."[5]

Depression. However, the period following the Great Depression, 1945–1964, are the years of the baby boomers. Figure 20-1 depicts the expected population increases through the year 2020. The baby boomers will begin to turn 65 years of age in the year 2011, resulting in dramatic increases in the number of persons over the age of 65. According to the U.S Bureau of the Census, people over age 65 represented 12.4% of the population (or 35 million) in the year 2000. One of every eight persons in the United States is over the age of 65. By the year 2030, the population over age 65 is expected to double to 70 million people, and the oldest-old segment (85+ years) is projected to increase from 4.2 million in the year 2000 to 8.9 million in the year 2030[4] (Fig. 20-2).

The number of older minority representatives is also growing and expected to continue to do so. Minority populations represent 16.4% of people 65 years and older. By the year 2030, the U.S. Bureau of the Census projects this will increase to 25.4%. The white population of older people is expected to grow by 81% while the minority population of older people is projected to grow by 219%. The minority projection includes Hispanics (328%); African Americans (131%); American Indians, Eskimos, and Aleuts (147%); and Asians and Pacific Islanders (285%).[3]

Globally, Asia has the largest number of persons age 65 years and older (54%), with Europe second (24%). For the year 2000, the number of people worldwide 65 years and older was estimated to be 629 million, with a projection of growth to almost 2 billion by the year 2050.[6] The competent physical therapist not only must be prepared to work with the dominant culture of older persons, but must also be competent in working with ethnically and culturally diverse older clients.

Population Age Structure
1960 to 2020

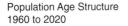 Baby Boom

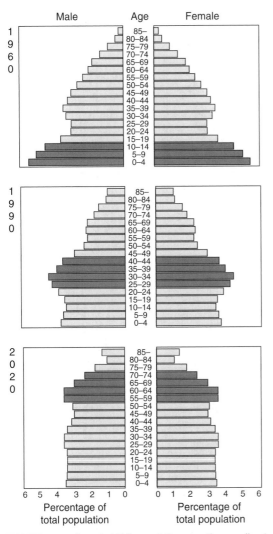

FIGURE 20.1 Expected U.S. population growth according to age through the year 2020. (Source: U.S. Census Bureau.)

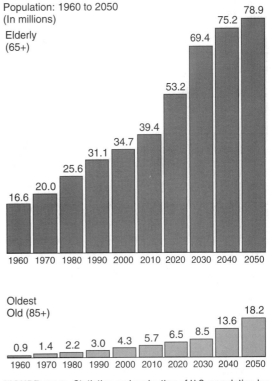

FIGURE 20.2 Statistics and projection of U.S. population by age through 2050. (Source: U.S. Census Bureau.)

Overview/Heritage Domain

The domain *overview/heritage* includes origins, history, life-shaping events, world events, and technological advances and how these affect a person. Consider the rich heritage that Mr. Edmondson in the initial vignette possesses. Someone who has lived to 90 years of age has experienced many major life events individually, within the family, within the community, and globally. Mr. Edmondson remembers the advent of the Model T Ford and the major transformation that ensued in the transportation industry. He witnessed the Wright brothers' first airplane flight, the supersonic jet, the landing of a rocket on the moon, and most recently, the space shuttle. He saw and even participated in the wiring of his community for electricity, which led to advances such as indoor plumbing, heating and air conditioning, and television. In the last 100 years, our society has gone from communicating via telegraph to telephone operators, to touch-tone phones, to cell phones, and finally, to Internet communication. Technological advances have been astounding, and someone who has lived for

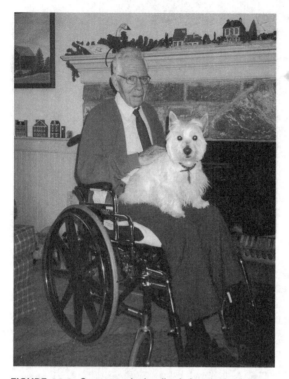

FIGURE 20.3 Someone who has lived almost a century has witnessed and experienced many advances and world events.

90 years brings a perspective that can hardly be understood by the younger generations (Fig. 20-3). Likewise, the older person may be easily overwhelmed by recent advances in technology and find them complicated and intimidating.

In the sphere of politics, Mr. Edmondson has witnessed a number of major world events, including two major world wars, a profound depression, the bombing of Pearl Harbor, the assassination of President Kennedy, the wars in Korea and Vietnam, and most recently, the terrorist attacks of September 11, 2001. All of these events serve to shape his worldview and lend a perspective that only experience can provide. These world events serve as catalysts to challenge one's worldview and reshape values and practices such as work ethics, patriotism, and financial customs. The culturally competent physical therapist considers, appreciates, and even seeks to grow from the wisdom and experience of the older

client. Interaction with the older client brings an opportunity to learn history through the eyes of someone who lived it.

Reflective Exercise

• What major world events and technological advances have you experienced in your lifetime?
• How have they shaped your worldview?

Another consideration within the domain of overview/heritage is *residence*, which encompasses home and community and the concept of stability versus mobility. Many older adults have experienced the stability of marrying and raising their children in the same community where they grew up. They strongly identify with the community where they have lived and labored. Likewise, some may have kept the same job with the same company until retirement. In contrast, their children and grandchildren may have moved from the stability of a single community as recent generations have become much more mobile. Ease of transportation has led to increases in transfers and relocations; job changes are much more common than they were for previous generations.

For older persons, a change of residence, and especially a move out of the community, can be very disruptive and upsetting to their sense of self. Moving to another town or state to live near a caretaking family member requires a traumatic uprooting from the older client's stability of home and community. Elders who emigrate from their home country to live with their children in the United States experience an enormous disruption. An older person may see immigration not as an opportunity but as a necessity to avoid being left behind.[7]

Reflective Exercise

• How do you define community? • How many different geographic communities have you known in your lifetime? • How many different jobs have you held? • What do you know of the history and heritage of older people in your family?

Education and *occupation* are included in the domain of overview/heritage and factor strongly in the culture of an older client. Traditionally, in a physical therapy evaluation, physical therapists inquire about one's occupation, and for the older adult, the answer is "retired." However, the physical therapist should inquire further and learn more about the client's lifework or career. That lifework or career has largely shaped the individual's worldview and may even contribute to the physical impairments the person is currently experiencing. Learning about one's lifework uncovers much about the person's culture and may enable the physical therapist to build important bridges for effective interventions and care.

Figure 20-4 depicts an older client at a younger age in his work uniform. This gentleman came to a physical therapy outpatient clinic after suffering a stroke. Although he presented with only slight impairments, he was very depressed and unmotivated. When the physical therapist began to inquire about his past work, he began to show some enthusiasm and pride as he related his 38 years of service on the local police force. The staff at the clinic began to refer to him as "Chief Mills" out of respect for his career title, and a dramatic transformation occurred in his course of rehabilitation. As the staff recognized and expressed appreciation for his years of service to the community, the client demonstrated greater interest in the program and the staff came to view the client as more than an older person with a disability. Additionally, by allowing older clients to express something of themselves and their lifework, the culturally competent physical therapist helps to negate the negative stereotype within the United States of the unproductive, and therefore unimportant, older person.

Reflective Exercise

• How does your career or lifework shape who you are? • How much do you know about the career or lifework of your older clients?

According to the U.S. Bureau of the Census, the educational level of the older population is increasing. From 1970 to 2001, the percentage of older persons who had completed high school rose from 28% to 70%, and 17% of older persons had a bachelor's degree in 2001. Percentages of those completing high school varied by ethnicity in the following manner: 74% of whites, 63% of Asians and Pacific Islanders, 51% of African Americans, and 35% of Hispanics. The trend toward increased education of older clients will continue as a result of the higher numbers of baby boomers who attended college.[3]

Economics and *politics* factor into the culture of the older client and fall under the domain of overview/heritage. Politics may have had an impact in an older person's decision to opt for early retirement because of incentives or changes in Medicare regulations for health coverage. Currently, older people are part of a political battle regarding the monetary cap on Medicare claims and a prescription drug plan for Medicare

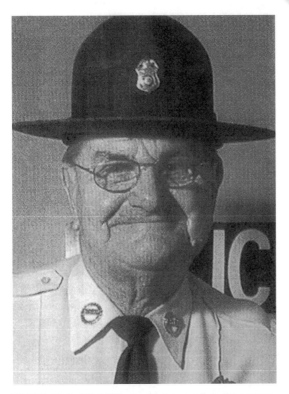

FIGURE 20.4 Chief Mills upon retirement from the community police force. (Photo courtesy of Chief Mills.)

clients. Political challenges will continue in greater magnitude as the population over the age of 65 comes to outnumber the younger generations who are working and paying into the social security system.

Individual economics may change dramatically as one retires or develops chronic impairments that limit one's work productivity and affect one's income. Approximately 10.1% of persons age 65 and higher were below the poverty level in 2001, and 6.5% were classified as "near-poor." Women had a higher poverty rate than men, and the highest poverty rates were among older Hispanic women who lived alone.[3] The Social Security Administration tabulated the major sources of income reported by older persons in the year 2000 as follows: 90% reported social security, 59% reported income from assets, 41% reported public and private assets, and 22% reported earnings.[8] Retirement years may require an adjustment to a different level of income as well as producing insecurity in one's financial future, leading to potential major stress.

The culturally competent physical therapist will recognize and explore the rich heritage of the older client as well as considering the potential stressors and challenges of aging that come with changing residence, economic status, and political factors. By allowing the elder client to reminisce about his or her lifework, life experiences, family, or community, the physical therapist validates the client's experience, increases his or her self-esteem, assists in the resolution of losses, and may improve life satisfaction. Figure 20-5 depicts an older physical therapy client undergoing physical therapy for lymphatic dysfunction (A), with pictures of her out with her girlfriends in New York City (B) and alongside her husband (C), who died 6 years ago. Learning about the client's history not only helps the client to feel validated and understood, but also allows the physical therapist to view the interventions and functional limitations from a broader perspective.

Communication

The domain of *communication* encompasses verbal and nonverbal communication, which also includes the dominant language, volume/tone, touch, name format, and greetings. Additionally, in the older population, physiological changes occur in the neurosensory system, specifically changes involving vision and hearing. The culturally competent physical therapist will be cognizant of these potential changes and will adjust the interaction accordingly to optimize effectiveness of communication.

With age, visual acuity is likely to diminish, particularly with near vision, necessitating the use of bifocals for close reading. The physical therapist should make sure that all forms and paperwork have print large enough for easy reading. Likewise, educational and instructional exercise handouts need to be legible and use larger fonts to accommodate the person who might be experiencing age-related vision changes. Older persons typically experience increased difficulty in adapting to changes in light and dark, requiring some persons to give up driving at night. In general, the physical therapist should ensure that the treatment area is well lit and without obstacles or darkly shadowed corners. When turning the light on or off in a treatment room, the clinician should allow time for the older person's eyes to adjust to the change in light before starting the next activity.[9]

Hearing frequently declines in later years of life. The most common age-related hearing deficiency is a sensorineural hearing loss termed presbycusis. In this condition, sound is transmitted through the external and middle ear, but the inner ear and/or auditory nerve falter or fail in transmission of the sound to the brain. With impaired sound transmission to the brain, the older person has difficulty hearing and discriminating speech, particularly at extremes of frequency. Normal speech contains a variety of frequencies. In presbycusis, the person may hear some of the sounds in the middle frequencies but miss those in the higher and lower frequencies.[9]

To help accommodate sensorineural hearing loss, the physical therapist should speak slowly with a medium pitch and should be positioned so that the client can see the speaker's face. The speaker should not cover his or her mouth with the hands. Sensorineural hearing loss is not helped by a hearing aid.[1] To accommodate an older client's hearing loss, the physical therapist must carefully monitor his or her voice volume

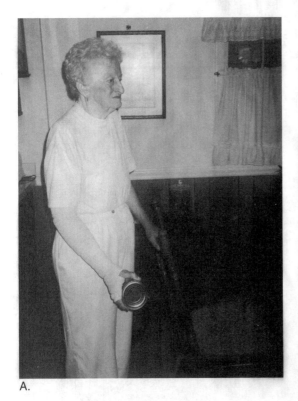

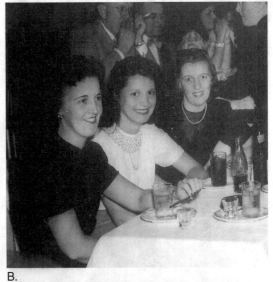

B.

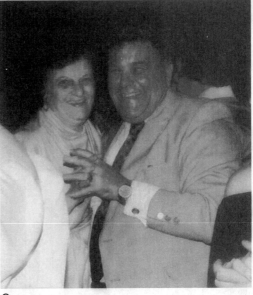

C.

FIGURE 20.5 (*A*) Ms. Fran Sargeant at age 74 undergoing physical therapy in association with cancer-related lymphedema. (*B*) Ms. Sargeant at age 21 at a restaurant in New York with some girlfriends. (*C*) Ms. Sargeant at age 55 dancing with her husband. (Photos for *B* and *C* courtesy of Fran Sargeant.)

A.

and tone so that it is loud enough to be heard but not unnecessarily loud. Do not use exaggerated mouthing when speaking because it changes the tone of the sounds.

Greetings and names comprise another component of the communication domain. Should a physical therapist address the older client by a surname, first name, or title, or should he or she use a more informal nickname? Greetings and names will vary across different ethnic cultures as well (Fig. 20-6). Of utmost importance is demonstrating respect for the client, and beginning with a more formal address is appropriate. The physical therapist should ask for the client's complete name, legal name, and preferred name and note each on the chart for future reference.

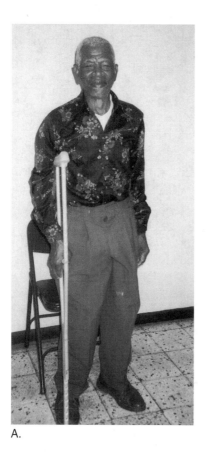

A.

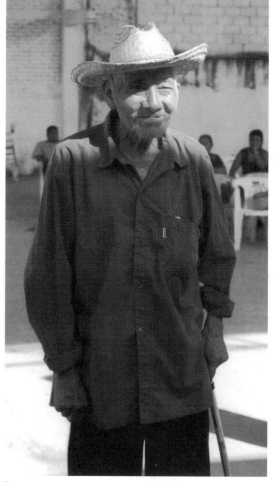

B.

FIGURE 20.6 How the physical therapist addresses these elderly clients will vary across different cultures. (*A*) A gentleman from Jamaica. (*B*) A gentleman from Honduras.

Sense of touch declines with age as well.[1] The physical therapist needs to be aware of potentially diminished sensation when administering modalities or fitting for prosthetics or orthotics. With diminished sensation, there is increased risk of irritation or skin breakdown.

Respectful physical touch communicates powerfully. One must remember that cultural norms for the appropriateness of touch will vary, but also realize that physical touch can be very healing and appropriate, particularly when an older person is socially isolated, with few interactions involving respectful physical touch. The physical therapist might be the one who can encourage

and care for the client with the use of respectful physical touch.

The dominant or preferred language may be a major factor in effective communication. As discussed previously, the United States has experienced various waves of immigration patterns. Many of the European immigrants of the early 1900s are now in the oldest-old group, and while they may have learned some English, their dominant language is that of their mother country. Even those who learned English may find that with age, they lose their second-language skills and rely on the more dominant primary language for communication (Fig. 20-6). Moreover, some recent immigrants may bring their aged parents to the United States. Again, the aged parents may not know English and communication may be a challenge. The physical therapist must be ready to ensure that effective communication occurs across potential language barriers.

Reflective Exercise

- What forms or handouts does your facility use?
- Are they appropriate for communicating effectively with someone who has trouble with vision? • How do you determine what voice volume to use in communication with an older client? • What lighting considerations exist in your facility? • How do you verify that you have communicated effectively with a client? • Have all language barriers been recognized and addressed? • Is your name tag in large print so that the client with a vision impairment can read it?

Family Organization

In collectivist cultures, the group is more highly valued than the individual and most often the family represents the primary group. Family in collectivist cultures includes the extended family, such as aunts, uncles, cousins, and grandparents; older people are highly valued and respected by the group. In the Chinese culture, for example, older people are viewed as very wise, and children have an obligation to care for their aged parents.[10] The Amish build additions to the main farmhouse for their aging parents when the oldest son and his family take over the farm.[9,10] A common sight is an Amish farmhouse with several additions connected to one another housing multiple generations[11] (Fig. 20-7).

In the Arab culture, the oldest sons are expected to care for their aging parents at whatever cost or sacrifice necessary,[12] while in Italian culture, the oldest daughter is expected to fulfill the caretaker role. In the Filipino culture, family structure is well defined to the level of third cousins, and adult children are expected to care for their aged parents in ways that provide for the economic welfare of the entire group.[13]

Conflict may arise when an acculturated child is expected to care for the recently immigrated parent. Jolicoeur and Madden[14] studied the dynamics of informal care of the elderly in Mexican American families and found that the burden for caregiving was high for all levels of acculturation,

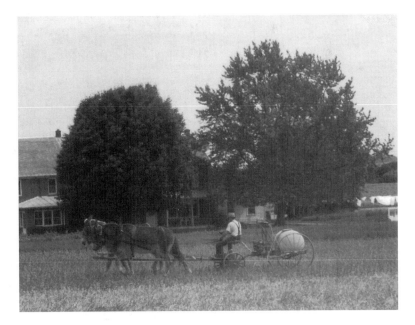

FIGURE 20.7 The Amish care for their elders by building additions onto their farm homes for their aging parents.

particularly for daughters. The degree of satisfaction with the role, however, was reduced for the less acculturated. Others looked at similar issues among Japanese American caregivers and found them to exhibit a significant amount of depression.[15]

Reflective Exercise

• How might the physical therapist involve the family in the plan of care? • What consideration should the physical therapist give to the family dynamics? • How might the physical therapist learn more about the family dynamics? • What responsibility does the physical therapist have for the health and well-being of the caregiver?

In the individualistic culture of the United States, where the nuclear family is the main family unit, older people are not generally integrated into everyday family life and do not command the same respect and elevated position as in collectivist cultures. In fact, in the U.S. culture, where youth, beauty, autonomy, and productivity are core values, older adults struggle for respect and self-worth as they lose their youth, retire from their traditional productive roles, and potentially lose autonomy secondary to disease, chronic illness, or financial loss. Indeed, U.S. society as a whole demonstrates a disregard for older people, as evidenced by television and other forms of media, where youth, beauty, and autonomy are exalted. Butler[16] termed this societal stereotype "ageism," and physical therapists must guard against overtly or covertly validating negative stereotypes or attitudes. One study found that physical therapists routinely set lower goals for their older clients compared with their younger clients.[17] Questionnaires developed around a hypothetical patient scenario were given to 127 physical therapists in clinical settings. Half of the therapists received a scenario where the patient was 28; the other half received the same scenario, but the patient was 78. The physical therapists were significantly less aggressive in their goal setting with the older patient despite the fact that the scenario was the same.[17]

According to U.S. Bureau of the Census data, 4.5% of people age 65 and older lived in nursing homes in 2000. The percentage increases dramatically with age as follows: 1.1% age 65–74 years, 4.7% age 75–84 years, and 18.2% age 85 and older.[4] Of those older persons not living in nursing homes or other institutions, 55% lived with their spouses, with a higher percentage of widowed women versus men.[18,19] Physical therapists will find an increasing number of widowed women living at home alone, with family members, or in nursing homes in the coming years. Some may have migrated from other countries to live with immigrant family members in the United States.

Recent statistics demonstrate that more and more older adults in the United States are active in the care of relatives. In some cases, the older adult is caring for the infirm spouse. In other cases, the older adult is the grandparent caring for the grandchildren.[20]

Reflective Exercise

• Do you identify more with your nuclear family or with your extended family? • What family roles do older people in your family play? • What expectations do you have of your older clients? • Are they appropriate expectations? • Why or why not? • What examples of ageism do you see in U.S. culture?

High-Risk Behaviors

Obesity

The prevalence of obesity in older people negatively affects nearly all body systems as well as overall physical function.[9,21-23] Diabetes, cardiovascular disease, musculoskeletal disorders, cardiopulmonary problems, and cancer have all been proven to worsen in the presence of obesity.[9] As for physical function, Jenkins[23] demonstrated that obesity was an independent variable

Reflection 20.3

Those best qualified to teach geriatric medicine are patients, relatives, neighbors, and caregivers. Use them.[5]

contributing to impaired strength, lower body mobility, and limited activities of daily living among elder patients. Those who were older and obese were more likely to experience the onset of strength impairment and functional immobility. Those who were men or Latino demonstrated fewer strength impairments.[23]

Nutrition

Normal aging results in physiological changes that lead to changes in nutritional requirements. Complications of chronic illness and disease will further alter the older client's nutritional needs. Normal aging causes a decrease in metabolism, although some have noted that this change may be strongly associated with physical inactivity; an increase in physical activity will counter the decrease.[24] Normal aging is also associated with decreased lean body mass and increased fat tissue. An older adult's diet may need to be assessed for adequate protein and caloric intake, particularly when chronic illness is a factor.[25] Recent studies demonstrate significant improvements in muscle strength and physical function with high-intensity strength training, and improved protein turnover even in the older, frail adult.[26,27]

Dehydration is a serious but preventable condition in older adults.[25,27,28] Dehydration can lead to hypotension, constipation, nausea, urinary tract infection, and electrolyte imbalance.[27,28] Signs include loss of skin elasticity, bad taste in one's mouth, drowsiness, and mental confusion.[28] To prevent dehydration, a daily intake of 1500–2000 ml of fluid is recommended (or 6–8 cups of water).[28] The physical therapist must remember that regular rehydration, especially during exercise, is important if the client is not on a fluid restriction for medical reasons.

A decrease in bone mineral density puts the older adult at risk for osteoporosis and the debilitating effects of osteoporotic fractures. Dietary calcium is an important part of the maintenance of strong bones for the older adult, as is a regular exercise program that involves weight-bearing and muscle-strengthening exercises. The physical therapist needs to help clients find and remind them to stick to an acceptable exercise program to improve bone and muscle strength.

"In rehabilitation, food encourages recovery"[28] (p. 45), and all rehabilitation team members should encourage good nutrition for their older clients. Performing a nutritional assessment is beyond the scope of practice for the physical therapist; however, the physical therapist should be aware of the older client's nutritional needs and potential difficulty in meeting those needs. The physical therapist should make the appropriate referrals to the nutritionist or registered dietitian and learn what can be done to encourage adequate nutrition for the patient. Some general tips include (1) eat little and often (every 2–3 hours), (2) have healthy snacks between meals, and (3) incorporate nutritional supplements as appropriate.[28] Physical therapists can encourage patients to eat and should stress the importance of good nutrition in rehabilitation.

The older adult who lives alone without adequate social support may not be consuming a diet with adequate nutrients, and the older client who is ill may not be able to grocery shop or prepare food. The physical therapist should make the appropriate referrals to the nutritionist or registered dietitian and also be aware of community programs such as Meals on Wheels. Additionally, the physical therapist must be aware of the various impacts the physical therapy exercise program has on the older adult's physiological state and plan interventions accordingly.

Death Rituals

Older adults vary in their death rituals and bereavement practices according to their ethnicity and cultural norms. Common to all older adults is the fact that they are likely to face grief and loss as friends and aging family die around them. In a classic work Rees and Lutkins[29] demonstrated a seven-fold increase in mortality within the first year of the death of one's spouse. Zisook and co-workers[30] studied 350 widows and widowers and found that they often manifested significant and disabling depression symptoms 2 years following their loss. Psychology literature often identifies the death of a spouse as one of the most difficult life events. Death of a pet for an older client also rates high.[31] According to Kubler-Ross, Wessler, and Avioli,[32] the stages of bereavement include

(1) distress and shock, (2) denial, (3) anger, (4) feeling low in spirits, (4) resolution, and (5) acceptance. Physical therapists working with older patients who have experienced a great loss can expect their clients to grieve and can provide support for them. If the physical therapist sees that the patient is experiencing an abnormal amount of grief or exhibiting signs of depression, he or she should consult with the family and the appropriate professionals.

Spirituality

Meaning of Life

Eric Erikson[33] is well known for his psychosocial theory of crises or conflicts encountered through the life span. The crisis he equates to later life is that of "integrity versus despair." At this stage, older adults reflect upon their lives and see a life of integrity or despair. If they are relatively happy and satisfied with the decisions they have made in their lives, they will decide upon integrity. In contrast, if they determine they are unhappy because of missed opportunities and poor decisions, they will choose despair.

The older adult is likely to encounter a series of losses that could easily lead to despair. Those losses might include loss of family members and friends to death or relocation, loss of home or community, loss of health or physical function, loss of driving privileges, loss of meaningful employment, and loss of income. The older adult may face several major adjustments in a short period of time, resulting in major stress and potential despair; and within U.S. culture, where the nuclear family is predominant, the older adult may not have strong social support.

Gardiner and colleagues[34] counter that Erikson's theory of development through resolution of crises is rooted in Western culture and cannot be generalized to other cultures. They note that each crisis's successful resolution is dependent upon the cultural lens with which one views the crisis. For instance, a Native American older person may resolve the crisis of integrity versus despair more easily than a European American because the Native American culture commonly embraces the older adult with respect and honor. The Native American older person

may experience a different emotional crisis in his or her later years.

Maslov[35] has identified four basic needs throughout life that are often threatened to some degree for the older adult. The first of the four basic anchorages is the need for an intact body and body image. One's body image becomes threatened with the changes associated with aging. Also, illness and disease might lead to alterations in physical characteristics and function. For example, one who has had to acquire a pacemaker to compensate for a faulty heart rhythm, or undergone an amputation secondary to diabetes, or suffered a stroke from a compromised cardiovascular system must face a less-than-intact body and altered body image.

The second basic anchorage is the need for an acceptable home.[35] Mr. Edmondson in the initial vignette stated clearly that the only acceptable home for him was his present home. Older adults sometimes face the need to make adjustments in their living situation, and much of their psychological health depends on their ability to see their home as acceptable. The physical therapist should consider that recommendations to alter one's home may be met with resistance. For example, a suggestion to add a railing and a ramp to the front entrance of the home may seem like a minor change to the clinician but may be perceived as a major change by the client. The physical therapist should make such suggestions with sensitivity.

Closely related to the need for an acceptable home is the need for socioeconomic stability, Maslov's third basic anchorage.[35] Retirement often means a loss of income. Many older adults transition to a fixed income on social security and rely on pensions and retirement plans to meet the financial needs of the future. The basis of an older person's sense of self-worth must shift from something other than economic productivity, a hard transition to make for someone reared in U.S. culture.

The fourth anchorage described by Maslov[35] is the need for a meaningful identity and purpose in life. With recent retirement, loss of friends and family members through death, and possible change of residence through relocation or migration, the older adult may struggle to find a meaningful identity and purpose in life. Dramatic

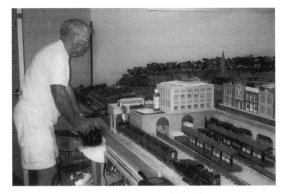

FIGURE 20.8 An older adult can sometimes find meaning and pleasure in hobbies. The physical therapist can structure the physical therapy program toward enabling the patient to pursue his or her hobbies.

changes require adjustment and a reorientation of one's purpose and meaning (Fig. 20-8). Older people in the United States encounter cultural values and messages lauding the importance of youth, productivity, and autonomy. As age-associated declines occur, the older adult struggles to find meaning and identity counter to the prevailing culture.

Reflective Exercise

• What basic anchorages do you hold as important?
• How would you feel if one of those basic anchorages were threatened? • Are the basic anchorages more likely to be threatened in a collectivist culture or in an individualistic culture? • Why?

Recent older immigrants may hold fast to their role and status in the family to make up for their loss of role and position in society, but may experience frustration when their children exhibit values more characteristic of U.S. culture than the culture of their country of origin. A number of studies reveal the intense loneliness and isolation experienced by recent immigrants as their children embrace the fast pace of America, which sometimes keeps them from fulfilling the familial expectations of their parents.[36–38] Studies attribute older immigrants' dissatisfaction to social isolation, lack of social networks, residential and geographic restraints accompanied by potential language barriers, and being left to care for grandchildren because the children are rarely home.[36–38] Treas and Mazumdar[39] conducted a qualitative analysis that identified immigrant elder dissatisfaction. They noted a strong cultural expectation of familial sociability and interdependence. In contrast, U.S. elders typically embraced a balance of intimacy and independence from their children or, as the researchers described it, "intimacy-at-a-distance." Physical therapists may encounter immigrant elders and their families in the midst of a cultural struggle to meet one another's needs and expectations.[39]

Religious Practices

Studies point to the importance of religion in the experience of some ethnic elders. Beyene, Becker, and Mayen[40] interviewed 83 Latino elderly adults and found they identified their sources of strength as family and religion. While they expressed appreciation for the financial and medical care they received in the United States, they voiced concern about the erosion of cultural values such as familial social support and respect for the aged. Likewise, Levin, Markides, and Ray[41] linked religious involvement and psychological well-being in older Mexican Americans. In a population of Jewish elders, religious involvement not only afforded them a sense of well-being but earned them a place of respect and social status.[42]

Reflective Exercise

• Think of an elder whom you respect. What is it about that elder that causes you to respect him or her? • If you were (are) an elder, why would (do) you expect someone younger to respect you?

Healthcare Practices

How many older patients have said, "They say these are the Golden Years … Don't believe it!"? Another popular recommendation from an elder is the directive "Don't grow old!" Senescence, the physical decline that occurs with age, leads to an increase in health problems and in the need to make use of healthcare practices.

Most older adults are familiar with a community-based healthcare system, with their local community family physician at the helm of decision making. Cultural and societal changes along with advances in technology, however, have led to major changes in the healthcare delivery system. The system has moved from a community-based delivery system to an institutionally based system. Patients with an illness enter a system of highly specialized and less personalized healthcare, with many different doctors and healthcare professionals taking part in the care of the client. This can overwhelm older clients and seem far removed from the days of the community family physician who often had a personal history with the client and the client's family. The older client may not trust the new system as readily.

Reimbursement practices have become much more complicated as well. Many older adults did not carry health insurance in their younger years, but costly advances in technology have led to more expensive healthcare. To protect against major financial loss, health insurance has become imperative. Reimbursement becomes complicated, however, and often older and even younger adults become confused and frustrated with trying to understand reimbursement practices and medical bills. The physical therapist might be able to refer the client to a social worker or someone in the business department who can assist the client in understanding the bill and insurance coverage.

Medications also pose a challenge to all clients but may particularly impact the older client. Pharmaceutical considerations include understanding dosages, combinations of drugs, taking medication with food or without food, generic versus brand names, and side effects. Many older clients with complicated medical histories take a number of different pills and can easily become confused or overwhelmed. Pharmaceutical illiteracy and confusion can be very dangerous, and the physical therapist should intervene to make sure the older client is taking the proper medications in the proper manner.

The practice of medicine has shifted from a focus on curative medicine to an emphasis on preventive medicine. Older adults may have trouble appreciating this shift and may find it hard to understand why they should exercise or adhere to a certain diet or medical regimen if they are not experiencing acute illness or symptoms. Some clients, for example, are reluctant to take medicine for their high blood pressure or follow dietary guidelines for diabetes when they do not feel sick. Geissler[43] reports that people of certain cultures are more likely to misunderstand the importance of intervention when they are feeling well. The misunderstanding appears to correlate with an emphasis on curative rather than preventive measures.

Reflective Exercise

• Do you find it difficult to take medicine if you are not experiencing symptoms? • Do you practice preventive medicine through exercise? • Why or why not? • Do your family members?

Physical Rehabilitation

The concept of physical rehabilitation for the elderly is not new, but the means by which we administer physical rehabilitation to the elderly are changing. Fiatarone and colleagues[26,27] conducted landmark studies in the early 1990s that demonstrated significant improvements in muscle strength with high-intensity strength training in adults over 90 years of age. Since then, additional studies have conclusively shown that physical training will improve overall function in areas such as walking, general mobility, and static balance.[44,45] The improved strength and balance are correlated with significant reductions in the risk of falls.[45,46] Even persons with dementia have demonstrated decreased fall risk and overall improvement in functional mobility with a physical training program.[47,48]

One of the challenges in motivating older patients to engage in formal exercise or physical training (Fig. 20-9) is that often the concept is foreign to them. The fitness craze is a relatively

Reflection 20.4

Rehabilitation is complete when the patient can sit on a box of eggs without breaking them.[5]

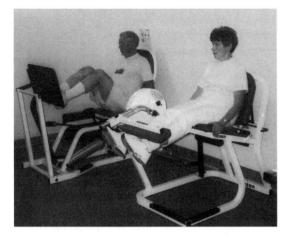

FIGURE 20.9 An older woman and man learn to make exercise a part of their lifestyle at a retirement community fitness center.

new phenomenon in the United States. In 1956, President Dwight D. Eisenhower established the President's Council on Youth Fitness in response to a report indicating that the youth of the United States were less fit than European youth. It was not until 1963 that President John F. Kennedy changed the name and the focus of the organization to include adults.[49] With the shift from the industrial age to the information age, many people have shifted to a sedentary corporate office job. Previously, many jobs consisted of physical labor, and even household tasks were more labor intensive. Some older clients may be accustomed to physical exercise in the context of normal functioning and not as familiar with exercise for the sake of exercise. Older women, in particular, may find a formal exercise program to be a foreign concept.

Crombie and colleagues[50] surveyed individuals between the ages of 65 and 84 to learn their activity level, their beliefs about their activity level, and the deterrents to regular activity. They found that a majority of the sample recognized the many benefits of leisure-time activity, and yet most did not incorporate exercise into their lifestyle. The reasons they gave for this paradox included lack of interest, shortness of breath, joint pain, lack of energy, and fear of overdoing it. Other sources confirm the lack of leisure-time physical activity in people of retirement age de-

---

Reflection 20.5

Sudden death from overactivity is much feared and rarely seen. Gradual death from underactivity is little feared and much seen.[5]

---

spite the additional time retirement affords them.[51,52] Cousins and Janzen[53] identified low self-esteem as a barrier to exercise. Women felt they were too fat or out of shape, and men noted the demoralization of mandatory early retirement and linked their low self-esteem to their loss of identity as a contributor to society. Physical therapists have the opportunity to encourage and motivate older patients to begin to increase their level of physical activity and thus improve their strength, mobility, mental attitude, and quality of life.

Reflective Exercise

• What importance do you place on physical exercise? How committed are you to physical exercise? • How might you help motivate your elder clients to make physical exercise a part of their leisure-time activity? • What barriers might you need to help them overcome?

A number of assessment tools offer the physical therapist a valid means of evaluating patient status and progress; however, often such tools have not been tested across diverse populations and therefore may not always be valid. More research is being done to substantiate the use of specific tools across diverse cultures. For example, the 36-item short-form health survey designed to assess function of elders in eight domains, including physical function and bodily pain, was determined to be valid for a population of Mexican elders.[54] Likewise, the Philadelphia Geriatric Morale Scale proved to be a valid quality-of-life measure in elderly Hong Kong Chinese patients.[55] The physical therapist must consider whether the assessment tool of choice may be biased toward a particular culture before utilizing it with full confidence.

Reflective Exercise

Consider the following excerpt from the 36-item short-form instrument for assessment of bodily pain.[56]
• How much bodily pain have you had during the past 4 weeks?
  None
  Very mild
  Moderate
  Severe
  Very severe
• How do you interpret this item? • Compare your interpretation with another student's or colleague's interpretation. How might cultural differences influence one's response to this question and possibly threaten the validity?

Healthcare Practitioners

Many older adults in the United States grew up with a community-based healthcare system. They had one family physician who knew their ailments and their family's ailments, and had the knowledge and expertise to cure them. A high level of trust and confidence existed between the patient and physician. Some have called this period in medical history the age of paternal medicine. The traditionally male physician spoke with authority, and patients were expected not to question their expertise. Older clients, familiar and comfortable with this approach, may find the present healthcare system frustrating and challenging because individuals are expected to take ownership for their health and raise their own questions.

Societal attitudes have changed as well, influencing healthcare practitioner and client interactions. Rather than accepting the physician's recommendations without question and with full faith, people today seek second opinions and are advocates for their own health. Healthcare providers expect clients to raise questions and to accept responsibility for their health. The older adult might become frustrated and mistrustful of the healthcare practitioner who does not speak with authority and asks many questions of the

client. Much questioning may lead the older adult to question the skill and competence of the healthcare provider, when in fact the healthcare provider is simply seeking to involve the client in the plan of care. The culturally competent physical therapist should be aware that differing expectations and assumptions may exist and should sensitively demonstrate competence and authority while communicating with clients a desire to involve them in their own care.

Reflective Exercise

• What encounters have you had with older clients who may have been confused by different expectations and assumptions regarding healthcare practices?

Reflective Exercise

• What changes have you observed in the healthcare system in your lifetime? • What interactions, positive or negative, have you or your family had with the healthcare system? • What have you learned from these experiences?

Conclusion

Increased life expectancy, the aging baby boom generation, and the fact that physiological aging leads to physical decline and chronic, degenerative illness guarantee that physical therapists will encounter the older adult in their professional practice. The competent physical therapist must be ready to consider the entire culture of the aging adult, recognizing that their worldview and perspective will dictate their compliance and response to intervention. With conscientious consideration of the older adult's culture, the physical

---

Reflection 20.6

Compliance means that the doctor knows best; noncompliance means that the patient knows best.[5]

therapist can successfully bridge cultural barriers and resolve misunderstandings (Fig. 20-10).

Collectivist cultures classically demonstrate a much greater respect toward and an increased commitment to care for and value their older people compared with individualistic societies such as the United States. Physical therapists are likely to encounter more and more older people from collectivist cultures within the United States as the population grows older globally and migration trends continue. Physical therapists must be equipped to consider the needs of the older adult from diverse ethnic cultures as well as their own.

The individualistic culture of the United States, with its valuing of youth, autonomy, and productivity, makes it difficult for one to age gracefully here. Physical therapists must be very aware of negative stereotypes and must guard against their manifestation in their attitudes and practice. By viewing the older adult as a person worthy of respect and taking the time to inquire and make observations about the person's culture, the physical therapist can work to build bridges of care and to counter ageism, remembering that one day he or she will be an older adult.

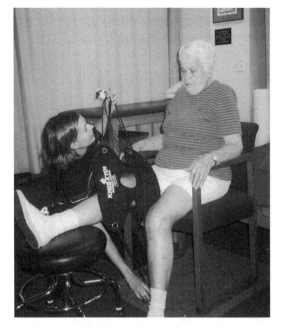

FIGURE 20.10 The physical therapist can successfully bridge potential cultural barriers and resolve misunderstandings with his or her older patient.

CASE STUDY SCENARIO

*M*r. Stu Jenkawich is a 75-year-old man who was admitted to the hospital one week ago to undergo a transtibial amputation of his right lower extremity secondary to a diabetic wound's failure to heal. He completed one week of physical therapy in the hospital and has now been transferred to a rehabilitation hospital. As for his past medical history, he had a myocardial infarction 8 years ago, and he has hypertension and insulin-dependent diabetes mellitus. He had a left total knee replacement (TKR) 10 years ago. He is hard of hearing and wears glasses.

Mr. Jenkawich's wife suffered an aneurysm and died 2 years ago. He has one attentive but very busy son. Mr. Jenkawich was born in Poland and immigrated to the United States with his parents when he was 5 years old. He completed school to the eighth grade and worked for the railroad and later the steel industry. He and his wife raised their two children in a small Polish community in Pittsburgh, Pennsylvania. Although he is accustomed to hard labor, he is not accustomed to formal exercise. He drinks an average of two beers a day and quit smoking 15 years ago.

Mr. Jenkawich's son has made plans to move his father from his home to an assisted living facility, where he will live independently but have access to personal care assistants when needed. The facility is in the town where the son lives, but 3 hours from Mr. Jenkawich's community.

(continued)

Mr. Jenkawich has just been transferred to the rehab hospital to begin rehabilitation services. He is a large man and presents with a bulb-shaped stump. He has not yet been fit for a prosthesis. The acute-care physical therapy notes indicate that Mr. Jenkawich did not advance beyond ambulation in the parallel bars. The acute-care physical therapist's assessment indicates that Mr. Jenkawich has excellent potential to do well with ambulation but lacks motivation.

1. What primary and secondary characteristics (see Chapter 1) of Mr. Jenkawich's culture are known and how might they influence the rehabilitation program?

2. What aspects regarding communication with Mr. Jenkawich should the physical therapist consider?

3. What family dynamics are present and how might they affect Mr. Jenkawich's rehabilitation?

4. What community considerations exist? How might changing the community affect Mr. Jenkawich's outlook?

5. What high-risk behaviors does Mr. Jenkawich exhibit? How might these adversely affect Mr. Jenkawich's rehabilitation?

6. What do you know about Mr. Jenkawich's healthcare practices? What more would you like to know?

REFERENCES

1. Bottomley JM, Lewis CL. *Geriatric Rehabilitation: A Clinical Approach.* 2nd ed. Upper Saddle River, NJ: Prentice-Hall; 2003.
2. Arias E. National vital statistics reports: United States life tables, 2000. Available at: http://www.cdc.gov/nchs/data/nvsr/nvsr51_03.pdf. Accessed July 7, 2003.
3. U.S. Department of Health and Human Services, Administration on Aging. A profile of older Americans. Available at: http://www.aoa.gov/aoa/stats/profile/profile.pdf. Accessed July 7, 2003.
4. Hetzel L, Smith A. The 65 years and over population: 2000. Available at: http://www.census.gov/prod/2001pubs/c2kbr01–10.pdf. Accessed July 7, 2003.
5. Isaacs B. *The Challenge of Geriatric Medicine.* Oxford, UK: Oxford Medical Publications; 1992.
6. Administration on Aging. Fact sheets: Challenges of global aging. Available at: http://www.aoa.gov/press/fact/alpha/fact_global_aging.asp. Accessed July 8, 2003.
7. Gelfand DE. Immigration, aging, and intergenerational relationships. *Gerontologist.* 1989;29:366–371.
8. Administration on Aging. Did you know? 2003 April: Income and poverty among the elderly. Available at: http://www.aoa.gov/press/did_you_know/2003/april.asp. Accessed June 30, 2003.
9. Abrams WB, Berkow R, eds. *The Merck Manual of Geriatrics.* Rahway, NJ: Merck Sharp and Dohme Research Laboratories; 1990.
10. Wang Y. People of Chinese heritage. In: Purnell L, Paulanka B, eds. *Transcultural Health Care: A Culturally Competent Approach.* 2nd ed. Philadelphia, Pa: FA Davis; 2003:106–122.
11. Kraybill D. *The Riddle of the Amish Culture.* Baltimore, Md: Johns Hopkins University Press; 2001.
12. Kulwicki AD. People of Arab heritage. In: Purnell L, Paulanka B, eds. *Transcultural Health Care: A Culturally Competent Approach.* 2nd ed. Philadelphia, Pa: FA Davis; 2003:90–106.
13. Pacquiao, DF. People of Filipino heritage. In: Purnell L, Paulanka B, eds. *Transcultural Health Care: A Culturally Competent Approach.* 2nd ed. Philadelphia, Pa: FA Davis; 2003:138–160.
14. Jolicoeur PJ, Madden T. The good daughters: Acculturation and caregiving among Mexican-American women. *J Aging Stud.* 2002;16:107–120.

15. Morimoto T, Schreiner AS, Asano H. Caregiver burden and health-related quality of life among Japanese stroke caregivers. *Age Ageing.* 2003;32:218–223.

16. Butler RN. *Why Survive? Being Old in America.* New York, NY: Harper & Row; 1975.

17. Barta Kvitek SD, Shaver BJ, Blood H, Shepard KH. Age bias: Physical therapists and older patients. *J Gerontol.* 1986;41:706–709.

18. Smith D. Country's older population profiled by the U.S. Census Bureau, June 1, 2001. Available at: http:// www.census.gov/Press-Release/www/2001/cb01–96.html. Accessed June 30, 2003.

19. Gist YJ, Velkoff VA. Gender and aging: Demographic dimensions. Available at: http://www.census.gov/ipc/prod/ib-9703.pdf. Accessed July 8, 2003.

20. Bryson K, Casper L. Nearly 5.5 million children live with grandparents, Census Bureau reports. Available at: http://www.census.gov/Press-Release/www.1999/cb99–115.html. Accessed July 8, 2003.

21. Himes CL. Obesity, disease, and functional limitation in later life. *Demography.* 2000;37:73–82.

22. Apovian C, Frey C, Wood G, Rogers J, Still C, Jensen G. Body mass index and physical function in older women. *Obes Res.* 2002;10,:740–747.

23. Jenkins KR. Obesity's effects on the onset of functional impairment among older adults. *Gerontologist.* 2004; 44:206–212.

24. Fiatarone MA, O'Neill EF, Ryan ND, et al. Exercise training and nutritional supplementation for physical frailty in very elderly people. *N Engl J Med.* 1994;330: 1769–1775.

25. Chernoff R. Nutritional rehabilitation and the elderly. In: CB Lewis, ed. *Aging: The Healthcare Challenge.* 3rd ed. Philadelphia, Pa: FA Davis; 1996.

26. Fiatarone MA, Marks EC, Ryan ND, Meredith CN, Lipsitz LA, Evans WJ. High-intensity strength training in nonagenarians: Effects on skeletal muscle. *JAMA.* 1990;263:3029–3034.

27. Fiatarone MA, O'Neill EF, Doyle N, et al. The Boston FICSIT study: The effects of resistance training and nutritional supplementation on physical frailty in the oldest old. *J Am Geriatr Soc.* 1993;41:333–337.

28. Copeland J, Hyland K. Nutrition issues in older people. In: Corley G, ed. *Older People and Their Needs.* London: Whurr; 2001.

29. Rees W, Lutkins S. Mortality of bereavement. *Br Med J.* 1967;4:13–16.

30. Zisook S, Schuchter SR, Sledge RA, Pauess M, Judd LJ. The spectrum of depressive symptom phenomena after spousal bereavement. *J Clin Psychiatr.* 1994;55(suppl 4):29–36.

31. Miller RA, Rahe RH. Life changes scaling for the 1990s. *J Psychometr Research.* 1997;43:279–292.

32. Kubler-Ross E, Wessler S, Avioli LV. On death and dying. *JAMA.* 1972;221:174–179.

33. Erikson EH. *The Life Cycle Completed.* New York, NY: WW Norton; 1998.

34. Gardiner HW, Mutter JD, Ksmitzki C. *Lives across Cultures: Cross-Cultural Human Development.* Boston, Mass: Allyn & Bacon; 1998.

35. Maslov AH. *Motivation and Personality.* 2nd ed. New York, NY: Harper & Row; 1970.

36. Kalavar JM. *The Asian Indian Elderly in America: An Examination of Values, Family, and Life Satisfaction.* New York, NY: Garland; 1998.

37. Kritz M, Gurak DT, Chen L. Elderly immigrants: Their composition and living arrangements. *J Sociol Soc Welfare.* 2000;27:85–114.

38. Pyke KD. The micropolitics of care in relationships between aging parents and adult children: Individualism, collectivism, and power. *J Marriage Fam.* 1999; 61:661–672.

39. Treas J, Mazumdar S. Older people in America's immigrant families: Dilemmas of dependence, integration, and isolation. *J Aging Stud.* 2002;16:243–258.

40. Beyene Y, Becker G, Mayen N. Perception of aging and sense of well-being among Latino elderly. *J Cross Cult Gerontol.* 2002;17:155–172.

41. Levin JS, Markides KS, Ray LA. Religious attendance and psychological well-being in Mexican Americans: A panel analysis of three generations. *Gerontologist.* 1996;36:454–463.

42. Shkolnik T, Weiner C, Malek L, Festinger Y. The effect of Jewish religiosity of elderly Israelis on their life satisfaction, health, function and activity. *J Cross Cult Gerontol.* 2001;16:201–219.

43. Geissler EM. *Mosby's Pocket Guide: Cultural Assessment.* 2nd ed. St Louis, Mo: Mosby; 1998.

44. Lazowski DA, Ecclestone NA, Myers AM, et al. A randomized outcome evaluation of group exercise programs in long-term care institutions. *J Gerontol Biol Sci.* 1999;54:M621–M628.

45. Rubenstein ZL, Josephson KR, Thiebold PR, et al. Effects of a group exercise program on strength, mobility, and falls among fall-prone elderly men. *J Gerontol Med Sci.* 2000;55:M317–M321.

46. Perrin PP, Gauchard GC, Perrot C, Jeandel C. Effects of physical and sporting activities on balance control in elderly people. *Br J Sports Med.* 1999;33:121–126.

47. Toulette C, Fabre C, Dangremont B, Lensel G, Thevenon A. Effects of physical training on the physical capacity of frail, demented patients with a history of falling: A randomized controlled trial. *Age Ageing.* 2003; 32:67–83.

48. Binder EF. Implementing a structured exercise program for frail nursing home residents with dementia: Issues and challenges. *J Aging Phys Activ.* 1995;3: 383–395.

49. President's Council on Physical Fitness and Sports. Fact sheet. Available at: http://fitness.gov/pcpfs_fact_sheet.html. Accessed July 8, 2003.

50. Crombie IK, Irvine L, Williams B, et al. Why older people do not participate in leisure time physical activity: A survey of activity levels, beliefs, and deterrents. *Age Ageing.* 2004;33:287–297.

51. Yusuf H, Croft J, Giles W, et al. Leisure-time physical activity among older adults. *Arch Intern Med.* 1996;156:1321–1326.

52. US Department of Health and Human Services. *Healthy People 2010.* Washington, DC: US Government Printing Office; 2000. Available at: http://www.healthypeople.gov/document/. Accessed July 8, 2003.

53. Cousins SO, Janzen W. Older adult beliefs about exercise. In: *Exercise, Aging, and Health: Overcoming Barriers to an Active Old Age.* Philadelphia, Pa: Taylor and Francis; 1998:71–96.

54. Peek MK, Ray L, Patel K, Stoebner-May D, Ottenbauer K. Reliability and validity of the SF-36 among older Mexican Americans. *Gerontologist.* 2004;44:418–425.

55. Wong E, Woo J, Hui E, Ho S. Examination of the Philadelphia Geriatric Morale Scale as a subjective quality-of-life measure in elderly Hong Kong Chinese. *Gerontologist.* 2004;44:408–417.

56. Ware JE, Snow K, Kosinski J, Gandek B. *36-SF Manual and Interpretation Guide.* Lincoln, RI: Quality Metric; 1993.

SECTION 3

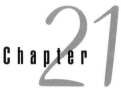

Chapter 21

Establishing a Culturally Competent Practice

● Jill Black Lattanzi, PT, EdD
● Larry D. Purnell, PhD, RN

Dr. Britney Bell is a new graduate from a DPT program and is hired to oversee the start-up of a new, small physical therapy practice in a rural farming community. There are two other established physical therapy practices in town with good reputations. Britney realizes that she is going to have to create a niche that will draw clients if she is to be successful. She learned a lot about the development of cultural competence because her DPT program curriculum had been transformed to reflect cultural considerations. She participated in both a service learning project locally among the homeless and an international immersion experience for 2 weeks in Central America. She took two semesters of conversational medical Spanish as a part of her training as well. Britney does some research on her potential clients and finds that the majority of town members are white, blue-collar workers, with a smaller number of teachers and medical professionals. The community also has a black population who live "on the other side of the railroad tracks" and a migrant worker population from various parts of Central and South America, who work on the local chicken farms and other industries. There is a population of Amish who live and farm in the vicinity as well. Britney decides that one of her niches will be the establishment of a culturally competent practice that will enable her to make a difference in the communities she serves as well as create an environment where all community members feel welcomed and well received.

vignette

(?) How should Britney go about establishing a culturally competent practice?

What is a culturally competent practice?

(?) How might she learn more about the healthcare needs and practices of the various local communities?

Why should one pursue a culturally diverse and competent physical therapy practice? The reasons are numerous and encompass all settings of physical therapy practice. The reasons to have a culturally competent practice are both similar to and different from the reasons for being a culturally competent physical therapist:

1. *To address changing demographics.* As stated over and over in this text, the U.S. population is growing in diversity and is expected to continue to grow. Figure 21-1 includes graphs showing the predicted changes over the next 100 years.[1] Physical therapy clinics will be treating more and more clients of diverse cultures.

2. *To meet regulatory and accreditation standards.* Whether in the inpatient or the outpatient setting, the physical therapy practice is subject to the scrutiny of accrediting bodies and/or regulatory boards. The Joint Commission on the Accreditation of Healthcare Organizations accredits hospitals and similar institutions and mandates cultural and linguistic competence in healthcare. Medicare, a large third-party payer of physical therapy services, mandates that services under Medicare be culturally sensitive and appropriate for all clients. Finally, the U.S. Department of Justice through the Office of Civil Rights dictates that all healthcare providers receiving financial assistance from the U.S. Department of Health and Human Services are prohibited from discriminating on the grounds of race, color, or national origin. The mandate includes discrimination based on ineffective methods of communication between English-speaking providers and people who have limited proficiency in English due to their national origin.[2]

3. *To improve physical therapy outcomes.* Because culture is so closely linked to health beliefs and practices, ignorance of a client's perspective will make the attainment of an effective physical therapy outcome more challenging. The physical therapy practice must be committed to identifying and working within the client's culture to ensure quality service and improve the chances of a positive outcome.[3]

4. *To improve marketing by targeting local communities of diversity.* By gaining the trust of local diverse communities and creating a welcoming atmosphere, the physical therapy practice likely will see an increase in referrals. Word-of-mouth from clients has always been the best marketing strategy. To experience positive interactions with clients from local communities means to have created an excellent marketing source within the larger community.

5. *To decrease the likelihood of malpractice claims.* Physical therapists must make sure that they are obtaining informed consent for treatment. The challenge with informed consent arises when the client speaks or reads a different language. Practitioners must be careful to obtain true informed consent. Second, effective communication is critical to avoid malpractice suits; communication across cultures is subject to unintended miscommunications.[4] A study of malpractice claims demonstrated that lawsuits filed against physicians were most commonly related to complaints regarding communication. On the other hand, physicians who were never sued were described as concerned, accessible, and willing to communicate.[5] Knowing how to communicate effectively across cultures may help decrease the incidence of malpractice claims.

6. *It's the right thing to do.* The ethical code of physical therapy practice for both the physical therapist and the physical therapist assistant mandates that the professional will "respect the rights and dignity of all individuals and shall provide compassionate care"[6] (pp. 693, 698). Implicitly, care must be congruent with the culture of the client.

Projected Resident Population of the United States as of July 1, 2000

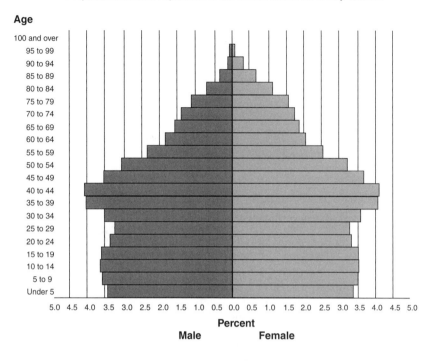

Projected Resident Population of the United States as of July 1, 2100

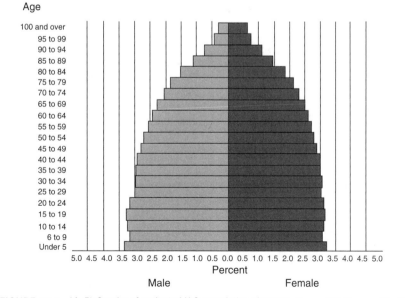

FIGURE 21.1 (*A, B*) Graphs of projected U.S. population changes. (Source: U.S. Bureau of the Census.)

Reflective Exercise

• What reasons exist for you to have a culturally competent practice?

How does a physical therapy practice become culturally competent?

The first step toward establishing a culturally competent practice is a commitment by the owners, managers, and clinicians to embrace the challenge of developing cultural competence as made clear in company mission statements, policies, and procedures.

The second step is to identify the diversity within the community that the clinic serves. The U.S. Bureau of the Census website has numerous resources available to help identify the populations and their demographic characteristics within the geographical scope of practice. The website www.census.gov provides more information.

Once the physical therapy practice has identified the ethnocultural diversity in the community, the following questions should be asked: What are traditional patterns of communication? What is the history of the community? Why did the residents immigrate and under what circumstances? What are the family roles? What are the traditional health practices and beliefs? Is there a folk healer within the community? What type of medicine does the folk healer practice? What is it about the folk healer that has earned him or her the respect of community members?

The answers to these questions can be found by conducting formal research, informal interviews with community members, and consultations with community leaders. Clinic employees familiar with the local communities also serve as excellent resources. In order to promote greater cultural understanding among employees, staff members might be assigned to seek out the information and present it at an in-service. Likewise, community leaders might speak at an in-service and share insights into their respective cultural groups.

Offering in-services and developing a compendium of the cultural beliefs and practices of local communities are practical means of educating employees and ultimately aiding them in their journey toward cultural competency. Box 21-1 lists some of the ways a physical therapy

practice might gain the respect and business of local communities of diversity. Ideas include stocking the waiting room with newspapers and brochures in other languages and participating in community health fairs (Figures 21-2 and 21-3). Box 21-2 identifies how a practice might pursue learning and attempting to meet a diverse community's needs.

Reflective Exercise

• What local communities of diversity does your practice serve? • How might your practice learn more about the local communities and their needs?

Culturally Competent Practice with Various Types of Diversity

Remembering that culture encompasses primary and secondary characteristics of culture (Table 21-1) as well as other subcultures, the culturally

---

BOX 21.1

Ideas for Connecting with Local Community

1. Recognize special holidays.[7]
2. Sponsor community events.
3. Establish a reputation for the provision of culturally competent care.
4. Advertise in local community newspapers or on radio stations.[8]
5. Attempt to learn basic communication skills in the language of the local community.
6. Conduct a healthcare needs assessment survey of the community.
7. Target identified areas of healthcare need for the community.
8. Provide health education information for the identified needs.
9. Participate in community health fairs.
10. Advertise services at bus stops, grocery stores, churches, and other places where diverse populations gather.
11. Provide written instructions in languages and reading levels preferred by clients.

BOX 21.2

Guidelines for Assessing and Meeting Community Needs

Consider and address the following items as appropriate:

1. **Purpose statement**
   What is the purpose of this project?
2. **Target group**
   Who are the target group?
3. **Contacts needed**
   What contacts are needed?
4. **Permissions needed**
   What permissions are needed?
5. **Target group needs assessment**
   What are the target group's needs?
   How will you determine the target group's needs?
   Provide specific method of how you will do this.
6. **Resources needed**
   What resources will you need?
   How do you expect to obtain these resources?
7. **Training needed**
   What training is needed?
   How will you go about getting/giving the training that is needed?
8. **Proposed timeline**
   What is your timeline for completion?
   Set up small deadlines throughout the process.
9. **Follow-up needed**
   What follow-up will be needed?
   How might the program "do harm"?
   How can you ensure that the program "does no harm"?
10. **Program assessment**
    How will you assess the effectiveness of the program?
    What components will you include in the program assessment?

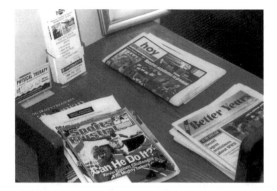

FIGURE 21.2 A physical therapy waiting room with Spanish newspaper.

tude of people and leads to a richness and growth beyond what a homogeneous practice could ever offer.

The Americans with Disabilities Act

In preparing a culturally competent practice for individuals with disabilities, physical therapy practitioners must comply with the Americans with Disabilities Act (ADA) of 1990. The ADA ensures equal opportunity for persons with disabilities. Title I of the ADA requires equal opportunity for employment; Title II prohibits discrimination in state and local government services, programs, and activities, including public education and social service programs; and Title III mandates equal treatment for persons with disabilities in public accommodations and commercial facilities. A public accommodation includes a professional office of a healthcare provider, hospital, or other service establishment.[9,10]

Medical offices have the responsibility of modifying policies and practices to comply with the ADA Accessible Design Standards, which include removing architectural barriers in existing facilities and supplying auxiliary aids to communication as needed[11] (Fig. 21-4). Changes that would result in an "undue burden or in a fundamental alteration in the nature of goods or services"[10] provided by the professional office are not mandated. The cost of furnishing equipment and making changes is borne by the professional office; the employer cannot pass on costs to the employee or client. Questions as to what is reasonable and not reasonable are handled on a

competent practice will also address the needs of people with physical disabilities, including sight and hearing impairments, and explore other dimensions of diversity, such as age, sexual orientation, and more. Diversity encompasses a multi-

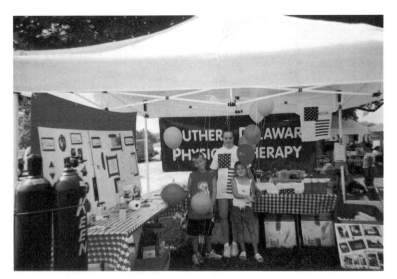

FIGURE 21.3 Physical therapy practice participating in a community health fair.

TABLE 21.1

Primary and Secondary Characteristics of Culture[19]

Primary Characteristics

Nationality
Race
Color
Gender
Age
Religious affiliation

Secondary Characteristics

Educational status
Socioeconomic status
Occupation
Military experience
Political beliefs
Urban versus rural residence
Enclave identity
Marital status
Parental status
Physical characteristics
Sexual orientation
Gender issues
Reason for migration (sojourner, immigrant, or
    undocumented status)
Length of time away from the country of origin

case-by-case basis under section 504 of the Rehabilitation Act.[10] Physical therapy practices should seek input from employees or clients as to how the facility might be more welcoming and accessible.

HIPAA Considerations

In 1996, the United States government passed legislation protecting the privacy of an individual's health information. The Health Insurance Portability and Accountability Act (HIPAA) guarantees clients the right to inspect and amend their health information as well as request a restriction on the disclosure of their health information to others, such as family members.[12] HIPAA aligns with the U.S. values of individualism, autonomy, and privacy. Not all cultures hold these same values; in fact, some may counter HIPAA and prefer that family members receive the medical information and make the decisions. The culturally competent practice will explore this possibility with clients and make arrangements as to who should receive the medical information. Permission should be obtained from the patient in writing.

Terminology Considerations

Physical therapy practices should monitor policies and procedures for respectful verbiage as well as educate staff in the use of appropriate

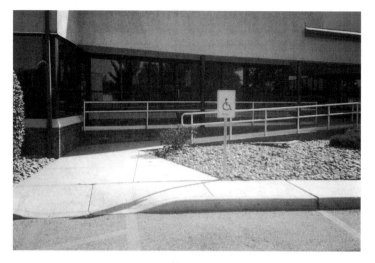

FIGURE 21.4 The ramp in front of this medical clinic has a steeper slope than specified by the ADA, increasing the difficulty for some in wheelchairs to enter independently.

terminology. An important consideration is to always put the person first. For example, say "person with a disability" rather than "the disabled," or "person with quadriplegia" rather than "the quadriplegic." Labels such as "quad" or "para" or "the stroke" or "amputee" used to refer to a person are not acceptable. Avoid outdated terms like "handicapped" or "crippled." Even "physically challenged" or "differently abled" can be offensive. Say "wheelchair user" rather than "confined to a wheelchair" or "wheelchair bound," because the wheelchair does not confine but rather liberates the user. Watch out for negative, disempowering words such as "victim" or "sufferer." Say "person with a stroke" or "person with AIDS" rather than "stroke victim" or "AIDS victim." People who cannot see, hear, or speak are people with visual, hearing, or speech impairments. Avoid referring to them as "deaf and dumb."

Idiomatic expressions are permissible. For example, it is acceptable to say to someone who is blind, "See you later" or to someone in a wheelchair, "Are you going to run to the store?" Such expressions are not usually offensive, and to consciously try to avoid them might put an undue strain on the conversation. Language, terminology, or labels convey powerful messages. The culturally competent physical therapy practitioner will do everything possible to ensure the use of respectful, positive, and empowering language.[13–15]

Wheelchair Etiquette

A wheelchair is part of a person's property and personal space and allows the person freedom of mobility not otherwise possible (Fig. 21-5). Physical therapy practices should have staff knowledgeable in treating people in wheelchairs with respect. Box 21-3 summarizes guidelines for interacting with people in wheelchairs.[13–15]

Accommodations and Considerations for People with Hearing Impairments

Physical therapists should be accustomed to working with people who have physical disabilities related to neuromuscular and musculoskeletal impairments; however, they may not be as experienced in working with individuals with visual and hearing impairments. As with people in wheelchairs, the most important consideration is to demonstrate respect by speaking directly to the person and not to companions or interpreters. The following are some helpful tips for communication:

1. When talking, face the person and make sure that you get his or her attention.
2. Do not obscure you face or lips when talking.
3. Rephrase rather than repeat phrases the person does not understand. A change in sound and pitch may help.
4. Avoid chewing gum when speaking.
5. Don't shout at the person.

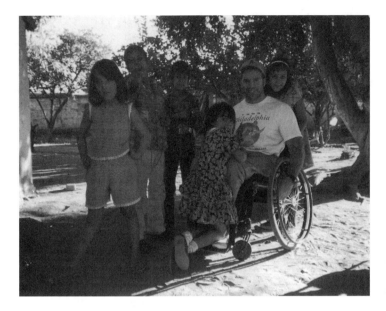

FIGURE 21.5 The wheelchair is considered part of the personal space of the person in the wheelchair. These children should not be climbing on it as they are.

People with hearing impairments may or may not know sign language, and may or may not read lips. Writing messages with paper and pen will suffice for uncomplicated communications such as directions to the cafeteria or completion of admission papers. However, if the exchange is more complicated, such as a discussion of prognosis or instructions for home care, one should summon an appropriate interpreter.

Different types of interpreters will be needed to meet specific communication needs. An oral interpreter is specially trained to articulate speech

BOX 21.3

Wheelchair Etiquette[13–15]

1. Speak directly to the individual in the wheelchair. Don't converse with someone nearby as if the person in the wheelchair does not exist.
2. Relax, make eye contact if culturally appropriate, and converse as you would with anyone else.
3. If the conversation lasts more than a few minutes, consider sitting or kneeling to be on the same level as the person in the wheelchair.
4. If the service counter is too high for a person in a wheelchair to see over, instruct your receptionist to step around it, and to have a clipboard ready if signatures and filling out forms are necessary.
5. Don't pat the person on the head. This is patronizing and demeaning.
6. Be aware of the person's capabilities. Never assume that the person is incapable.
7. Remember that people with disabilities are the best judges of what they can and cannot do.
8. Never assume that the person in a wheelchair needs help. Instead, offer to help if needed and ask the person to tell you how you can help.
9. Never begin pushing the wheelchair without permission from the person.
10. Remember that the wheelchair is not a piece of furniture; it is part of the person's personal space. Don't lean on the wheelchair or set things down on it.
11. When a person using a wheelchair transfers out of it, do not move the wheelchair out of the person's reach.

silently and clearly, sometimes rephrasing words to give additional emphasis to lip movement. Facial expressions and body language also are components of the communication. Oral interpreters serve to enhance communication with someone who can read lips. Sign language interpreters use a combination of hand motions, body language, and facial expressions to convey the message and are useful in communicating with persons who know sign language. Computer-assisted real-time transcription (CART) is helpful if the person does not know sign language and does not read lips. With CART, an operator types what is said into a computer that displays words on a screen.[16]

Physical therapy practices should post signs alerting persons with hearing impairments that services and assistance are available. Practices cannot charge clients extra fees for interpreters or other communication aids. Teletypewriter service (TTY or TDD), a means of exchanging written messages over the telephone, is available through a nationwide relay network by dialing 711. The practice must have a TTY machine on-site to take advantage of this service.

Accommodations and Considerations for People with Visual Impairments

According to the ADA, people with visual impairments are entitled to auxiliary aids to promote effective communication. Examples include taped texts, qualified readers, audio recordings, Braille materials, materials in large print, and service animals. Service animals are animals that are trained to perform specific tasks, such as guiding people with visual impairments and alerting people with hearing impairments (Fig. 21-6). Physical therapy practices must allow people with disabilities to bring their service animals into the clinic unless the animal poses a direct threat to

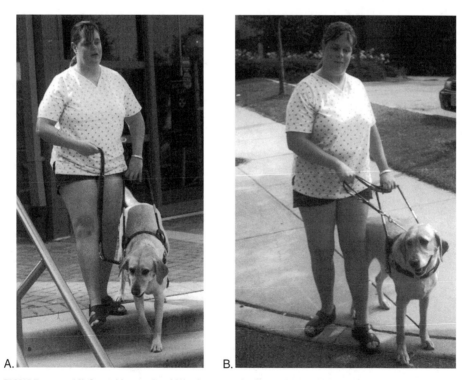

FIGURE 21.6 (*A*) Crystal has a visual impairment and relies on her service dog, Yvonne, to help her down the steps. (*B*) Yvonne is also trained to alert Crystal to upcoming curbs.

BOX 21.4

Tips for Communicating with Someone with a Visual Impairment

1. Identify yourself, your name and your role, before you make physical contact with the person. Be sure to introduce him or her to others in the group.
2. Offer the new client a tour of the facility so he or she can feel more confident of the surroundings.
3. Describe precise locations of bathrooms, water fountains, emergency exits, potential obstacles, and so on.
4. Offer your arm rather than taking the person's. Physical therapists are accustomed to guarding the client by holding on to him or her. It is more appropriate to allow the person with a vision impairment to hold on to you.
5. When giving directions, use specific, nonvisual descriptions.
6. If you must leave a person with a visual impairment, do not leave the individual in the middle of the room. Leave him or her seated alongside a wall or plinth or other landmark. Also inform him or her of the closest exit.

7. If the person has a service dog, walk on the opposite side of the dog so you do not interfere with the animal's working habits.
8. Do not pet a service dog unless the handler gives you permission.
9. Do not feed or water a service dog without the permission of the handler. The service dog is usually on a "park schedule," where intake of food and fluid is scheduled and elimination is predictable.
10. When giving directions to a person with a visual impairment and a service dog, give the directions to the person, not the dog.
11. If the person uses a cane, do not touch the cane or move it. A cane is part of the person's individual space.
12. Labels and signs should use clear lettering and contrasting colors. Have large-print materials available.
13. Keep clients with visual impairments informed of any changes in the layout or new obstacles in the walkway of your practice.

the health and safety of others.[17] Box 21-4 lists some tips for promoting effective communication with people who have visual impairments.

Considerations for Working with People of Different Sexual Orientations

When the physical therapist needs to provide assistance or make a referral for a person who is gay, lesbian, bisexual, or transsexual, a number of options are available. Some referral agencies are local, whereas others are national with local or regional chapters. Many are ethnically or religiously specific. Some national groups that have links to local and regional organizations are listed in Chapter 5.

Degrees of Culturally Competent Practice

The Cultural Competence Continuum developed by Cross and colleagues[18] provides a means of

determining just how culturally competent your practice is. The first level on the continuum is termed *cultural destructiveness.* A culturally destructive practice knowingly or unknowingly constructs barriers to care for certain cultural groups. Perhaps the entrance is inaccessible to people in wheelchairs or translation services are not offered. Visiting hours or clinic hours may fall at times that conflict with a night-shift worker's schedule. Policies and procedures may infringe on the values of certain cultures, such as a visitors policy that restricts a Hispanic client with a large extended family to two visitors for a limited time. Culturally destructive practices are those in which disparities in the treatment of specific cultural groups occur. Again, these practices may be occurring unintentionally and yet result in the disenfranchisement of diverse groups.

Cultural incapacity describes the practice that would like to be more culturally competent but lacks the skills and resources to do so. Translation services are costly, for example, and the size of patient rooms may accommodate only two visitors without interfering with patient care. One must look closely, however, to ensure that cultural incapacity is not just an excuse for cultural destructiveness.

The *culturally blind* practice treats all clients equally, a very common U.S. practice, as equality is a strong U.S. value. This is similar to the person who says that he or she doesn't see black or white skin but treats everyone equally. The problem with this approach is that everyone is not the same. As discussed in this book at length, each person brings his or her own culture to the healthcare interaction, and the culturally competent provider must seek to understand that culture in order to provide culturally appropriate and effective care. By emphasizing cultural blindness, the institution is assuming that each individual should be treated according to the norms and values of the dominant culture, which will fall short of meeting the needs of culturally diverse clients.

Cultural pre-competence defines the fourth stage of cultural practice, where the institution or practice acknowledges the need to move toward a more culturally competent practice and begins to take steps to do so. For instance, administrators may revise mission statements and policies to reflect culturally competent goals. Budgets may be restructured to allow for translation services or other cultural needs. The practice may employ a diverse staff and begin to see them as resources to better understand the local community needs. In other words, the precompetent practice is beginning to pursue items listed on the self-assessment checklist (which follows).

The fifth stage on the continuum is *cultural competence*, where the practice consistently demonstrates respect for cultural differences and actively seeks out resources to expand its knowledge and practice of culturally competent care. The culturally competent practice has many initiatives in place and begins to focus on assessing and re-assessing the effectiveness of those initia-

tives as well as the changing needs of the local community.

The sixth and final stage is termed *cultural proficiency*. The culturally proficient practice not only provides culturally competent care within its walls, but also reaches out into the community to meet its needs in a culturally competent manner. Acting as advocates, employees of the practice might help identify resources to meet needs, lobby for legislation important to the community, or sponsor local charitable events (Fig. 21-7). The culturally proficient practice serves as a model for other practices. The checklist in Box 21-5 provides self-assessment issues to consider, and Box 21-6 presents a list of resources to help your practice move toward greater cultural competence.

Reflective Exercise

- Where does your practice fall on the continuum?
- How many of the items on the self-assessment checklist apply to your practice? • What items might your practice target for change? • What items are not appropriate for your practice and why?

Conclusion

The establishment of a culturally competent practice takes time and commitment and is reflected in several aspects of the practice. To begin with, the organizational mission statement, policies and procedures, and stated goals should demonstrate a commitment to cultural competence. Second, the practices will identify the communities of diversity in the area it serves and will seek to learn more about their culture and healthcare needs. Third, the organization or practice will commit to training staff in culturally competent interactions and physical therapy procedures. By demonstrating respectful interactions with all patients, the physical therapy practice will gain the respect of all whom they serve and will achieve optimal physical therapy program outcomes.

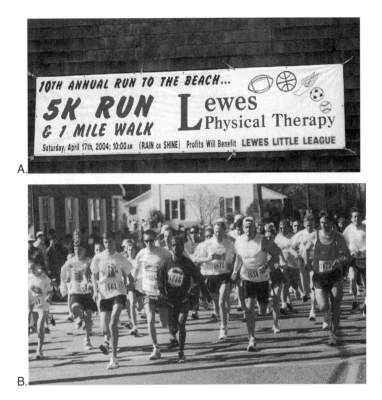

FIGURE 21.7 (*A, B*) A physical therapy practice sponsors an annual 5K race to support a local community charity.

BOX 21.5

Self-Assessment Checklist for the Culturally Competent Practice[19]

1. Written policies are in place that address the needs of non–English-speaking employees, visitors, and patients.
2. Directional and informational signs include translations in local community languages.
3. Forms and written instructions are available in large print or in languages of the diverse populations.
4. Guidelines are in place to address the need for an interpreter.
5. Guidelines exist for interpreters.
6. Orientation and training programs address cultural diversity for the client and employee populations.
7. Community resources are known and made available to diverse communities.
8. Client and staff grievance surveys and procedures are available in languages spoken in the community.
9. Reading materials in waiting areas are available in languages spoken by the community.
10. The organization actively recruits bilingual staff and/or encourages staff to learn a second language.
11. The organization provides English classes for non–English-speaking employees and foreign-language classes for employees working with diverse non–English-speaking clients and visitors.
12. The institution's or practice's library or resources include resources for cultural diversity.
13. The organization attempts to accommodate religious needs into staffing schedules.
14. Patient education materials are in languages of the local communities.
15. The mission statement incorporates the values of cultural diversity.

BOX 21.6

Resources for Establishing a Culturally Competent Practice

1. The National Center for Cultural Competence has resources to help establish culturally competent practice, including a self-assessment checklist and a description of actions and activities to plan, implement, and evaluate the cultural competence of service delivery systems in primary healthcare settings.
   Address and contact information:
   National Center for Cultural Competence
   Georgetown University Child Development Center
   3307 M Street NW Suite 401
   Washington, DC 20007–3935
   Phone: 202–687–5387 or 800–788–2066; Fax: 202–687–8899
   E-mail: cultural@georgetown.edu
   Website: http://www.georgetown.edu/research/gucdc/nccc

2. Obtain map links about your local community from the U.S. Census Bureau website. Go to http://tiger.census.gov. Choose variables you want displayed by clicking on "access tools" at the Census Bureau home page.

3. Contact the appropriate authorities to learn more about the ADA and to obtain the ADA Standards for Accessible Design and the Readily Achievable Checklist for Existing Business Facilities.
   ADA Information Line: 800–514–0301 (voice) 800–514–0383 (TTY)
   Website: http://www.ada.gov

4. *Interpretation Resources and Policy Guidance.* From the Office for Civil Rights, this website provides an extensive description of the Title VI prohibition against national origin discrimination as it affects persons with limited English proficiency.
   http://www.hhs.gov/ocr/lep/guide.html
   Diversity Treatments: Models and Practices, Research and Reports. Provides a website with medical interpretation resources and references.
   http://www.diversityrx.org/HTML/MORES_SMI.htm

5. http://www.hhs.gov/ocr/lep/guide.html

6. http://www.diversityrx.org/HTML/MORES_SMI.htm comes with an assessment tool that may be helpful.

REFERENCES

1. Census Stats
2. Office of Civil Rights Guidelines. Title VI of the Civil Rights Act of 1964: Interpreter services. Available at: http://www.xculture.org/interpreter/overview/civilrights.html. Accessed June 9, 2004.
3. Leavitt R. Developing cultural competence in a multicultural world. *PT Mag.* January 2003:56–69.
4. Ahmann E. Developing cultural competence in health care settings. *Pediatr Nurs.* 2002;28:133–137.
5. Levinson W. Physician-patient communication: A key to malpractice prevention. *JAMA.* 1994;272:1619–1620.
6. American Physical Therapy Association. *Guide to Physical Therapist Practice.* 2nd ed. Alexandria, Va: Author; 2003.
7. Glenn-Vega A. Achieving a more minority-friendly practice. *Fam Pract Manage [serial online].* 2002;9:39–44. Available at: http://www.aafp.org/fpm/20020600/39achi.html. Accessed April 24, 2004.
8. Rust G, Strothers H. Strategies for expanding your patient base in diverse communities. *Fam Pract Manage* [serial online]. 2000;7:31–47. Available at: http://www.aafp.org/fpm/20000500/31stra.html. Accessed April 24, 2004.
9. ADA Business Connection. Introduction to the Americans with Disabilities Act. Available at: http://www.usdoj.gov/crt/ada/adaintro.htm. Accessed May 30, 2004.
10. Johnson LH. The building blocks for helping patients with sight or hearing impairments. *PT Mag.* 2002;10:34–39.
11. ADA Business Connection. The Americans with Disabilities Act. Available at: http://www.usdoj.gov/crt/ada/business.htm. Accessed May 30, 2004.
12. US Department of Health and Human Services. Health Insurance Portability and Accountability Act of 1996. Available at: http://www.hhs.gov/ocr/hipaa/. Accessed June 9, 2004.
13. Tripod. Wheelchair etiquette. Available at: http://members.tripod.com/~imaware/etiquette.html. Accessed May 30, 2004.
14. Independent Living Centre. Wheelchair etiquette.

Available at: http://ilc.asn.au/files/ias_wheelchair_etiquette.pdf. Accessed May 30, 2004.

15. Wheelchairnet. Etiquette. Available at: http://www.wheelchairnet.org/WCN TownHall/Docs/etiquette.html. Accessed May 30, 2004.

16. US Department of Justice. Business brief: Communicating with people who are deaf or hard of hearing in hospital settings. Available at: http://www.ada.gov/hospcombrprt.pdf. Accessed May 30, 2004.

17. US Department of Justice. Business brief: Service animals. Available at: http://www.ada.gov/svcabrs3.pdf. Accessed May 30, 2004.

18. Cross TL, Bazron BJ, Dennis KW, Isaacs MR. *Towards a Culturally Competent System of Care.* Vol I. Washington, DC: Georgetown University Press; 1989.

19. Purnell LD, Paulanka BJ, eds. *Transcultural Health Care: A Culturally Competent Approach.* 2nd ed. Philadelphia, Pa: FA Davis; 2003.

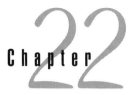

Chapter 22

The Nurturing of Cultural Competence

- Jill Black Lattanzi, PT, EdD
- Larry D. Purnell, PhD, RN

*M*ark Bleacher, a 25-year-old DPT graduate from Des Moines, Iowa, has recently accepted a physical therapist staff position in an urban Chicago hospital. His home community, undergraduate study, and DPT program were largely homogeneous, lacking diversity of culture. Though eager to begin his career in this new position and confident that his schooling has prepared him well, Mark experiences discomfort when he encounters great diversity in colleagues and clients. He quickly recognizes that he is on unfamiliar ground and lacks the skills and knowledge to interact effectively. Mark attended a diversity training workshop as part of his DPT training but feels the need to learn more.

(?) Where might Mark go to get additional training in cultural competency?

(?) How might he nurture cultural competence within his environment?

(?) What resources might be helpful to Mark?

Cultural competence will not come from reading this text or attending a workshop. The development of cultural competence requires time and experience, mistakes and successes. Physical therapists must nurture the development of cultural competence much like a gardener must nurture the growth of a garden. Human beings tend to be ethnocentric, and the notion of considering another's culture and making accommodations to that culture does not occur naturally. The weeds of ethnocentrism tend to choke cultural awareness, sensitivity, and competence. Culturally competent understandings and responses must be nurtured.

This chapter will explore the nurturing of cultural competency through the perspective of the educator and of the physical therapy professional. How does one strive to nurture cultural competence in students, and how does one continue to pursue cultural competence in the professional world? The chapter concludes with a list and description of resources for the nurturing of cultural competence.

Nurturing Cultural Competency from the Perspective of the Educator

The need for physical therapy educators to nurture cultural competency in students is mandated by several physical therapy platforms. First, the *Guide to Physical Therapist Practice*[1] states, "Physical therapists are committed to providing necessary and high-quality services to both patients and clients" (p. 531). High-quality services consist of culturally competent care. Second, Principle 1 of the Code of Ethics requires a phys-

ical therapist to respect the rights and dignity of all individuals, another implication for culturally competent care.[2] Third, the normative models for both physical therapist and physical therapist assistant education articulate professional practice expectations that encompass cultural competence[3,4] (see Tables 22-1 and 22-2). Finally, the Commission on Accreditation in Physical Therapy Education (CAPTE) uses evaluative criteria that require students to "incorporate an understanding of the implications of individual and cultural differences when engaged in physical therapy practice, research, and education"[5]

TABLE 22.1

Professional Practice Expectation 7: Cultural Competence

Definition: *Cultural and linguistic competence* is a set of congruent behaviors, attitudes, and policies that come together in a system, agency, or among professionals that enables effective work in cross-cultural situations.[a]

Culture refers to integrated patterns of human behavior that include the language, thoughts, communications, actions, customs, beliefs, values, and institutions of racial, ethnic, religious, or social groups.[a]

Competence implies having the capacity to function effectively as an individual and an organization within the context of the cultural beliefs, behaviors, and needs presented by consumers and their communities.[a]

7.1 *Identify, respect, and act with consideration for patients'/clients' differences, values, preferences, and expressed needs in all professional activities.*

Educational Outcomes

The graduate:

- Recognizes individual and cultural differences and adapts behavior accordingly in all aspects of physical therapy services.

- Displays sensitivity by considering differences in race/ethnicity, religion, gender, age, national origin, sexual orientation, and disability or health status in making clinical decisions.

- Recognizes aspects of behavior and care affected by individual needs and cultural differences.

- Discovers, respects, and values individual differences, preferences, values, life issues, and emotional needs within and among cultures.

- Promotes representation of individual and cultural differences in practice, research, and education.

- Incorporates an understanding of the implications of individual and cultural differences in the management and delivery of physical therapy services.

- Values the sociocultural, psychological, and economic influences on patients/clients and responds accordingly.

- Is aware of and suspends own social and cultural biases.

- Understands and applies principles of cultural competence.

- Provides care in a nonjudgmental manner when the patients'/clients' beliefs and values conflict with the individual's belief system.

- Demonstrates respect for patient's/client's privacy.

- Values the dignity of patients/clients as individuals.

[a] Working definition adapted from *Assuring Cultural Competence in Health Care: Recommendations for National Standards and an Outcomes-Focused Research Agenda,* Office of Minority Health, Public Health Service, US Department of Health and Human Services; 1999.
From A Normative Model of Physical Therapist Professional Education: Version 2004. American Physical Therapy Association, Alexandria, Va, 2004. Used with Permission.

TABLE 22.2

Performance Expectation Theme 2: Individual and Cultural Differences

2.1 Demonstrates sensitivity to individual and cultural differences in all aspects of physical therapy services.

Educational Outcomes

The graduate will:

• demonstrate an understanding of the major differences between individuals and cultures.

• promote representation of individual and cultural differences in practice, research, and education.

• engage in continuing education opportunities that facilitate and enhance understanding of cultural and individual differences.

• be guided at all times by concern for the dignity and welfare of the patients entrusted to his/her care.

• adapt interactions and services in response to individual and cultural differences.

From A Normative Model of Physical Therapist Assistant Education: Version 99. American Physical Therapy Association, Alexandria, Va, 1999. Used with Permission.

(criterion 3.8.3.1). The mandate for teaching culturally competent care is clearly stated. Additionally, and perhaps most compelling, is the documented lack of cultural understanding on the part of physical therapy students entering the clinical component of their education.[6,7] Physical therapy educators must consider cultural competency training for their students because of the identified need and moral obligation of doing the right thing.

How might the physical therapy educator nurture cultural competence in physical therapist students? Banks[8] has written much regarding multicultural K–12 education and advocates change to and within the curriculum. Table 22-3 depicts various ways of including multicultural education in the curriculum. The additive approach involves simply adding something that touches on multicultural education to a class or unit. The integrative approach describes the infusion of multicultural education through the entire curriculum. Transformation of the curriculum entails complete overhaul of the curriculum such that multicultural education drives all aspects of the education. Finally, social action theory describes the ultimate goal of multicultural education—that students graduate ready to make a positive difference in a diverse world.

PT and PTA Proposed Curriculum Changes

Table 22-3 also proposes curricular manifestations that parallel those of Banks but apply to the DPT, MPT, or PTA curriculum. The first includes a workshop or unit for cultural competency training—the additive approach. Programs may address cultural competence as a unit alongside ethics of practice and psychosocial aspects of patient care or as a separate workshop.[9] Many current texts related to patient care and interactions are structured to allow only a chapter addressing cultural competency.

The integrative approach in PT and PTA

TABLE 22.3

Multicultural Educational Curriculum

K–12	DPT/PTA MANIFESTATIONS
1. Additive approach	1. Workshop or unit
2. Integrative approach	2. Woven throughout curricula
3. Transformative approach	3. Overhaul of policy, mission, and curricula to embrace multicultural education
4. Social action theory	4. Service-learning experiences and international immersion experiences

Source: James A. Banks (1999).[8]

curricula may manifest as cultural training that occurs in several different courses throughout the program. Perhaps the material builds in complexity and scope as it is re-introduced. This is the additive approach repeated and sprinkled throughout the curriculum.

Reflective Exercise

• What examples of additive or integrative multicultural education did you or are you experiencing in your own PT or PTA education? • How helpful was it, or was it not helpful at all? • How might you have learned more?

Medical school, nursing school, occupational therapy school, and physical therapy school educators promote the importance of transforming curricula to reflect cultural competency.[10–15] Bender,[13] a physical therapist and physical therapy educator, identifies the importance of moving cultural competency from "something that is external to our usual behaviors into an internalized core value held by the profession" (p. 8). She advocates for a transformative curriculum at best and recognizes the value of service learning and immersion experiences in giving students firsthand experience in working within the client's natural environment.

Transformative multicultural education in the PT and PTA curricula involves a complete overhaul of the curriculum to make it culturally instructive and culturally congruent throughout. Transformation of the curriculum requires intense and rigorous curricular review and is dependent on total faculty support. Such an overhaul might include transformation such that all client and case scenarios include cultural considerations. Simulated patient experiences might employ trained persons from the local community of diversity. Likewise, the local communities might be asked to review and critique the curricula for authenticity and completeness. Local community leaders might serve as resources for curriculum development.

Other examples of curricular changes toward a stronger multicultural focus include the use of role play to develop cultural competence,[16] culturally competent case scenarios for multicultural

education of health professionals,[17,18] and the inclusion of language training for students who will be working within a large community of persons speaking another language.[19] Competency in conducting a culturally congruent needs assessment history and a culturally appropriate health beliefs assessment are two common skills measured in some curricula.[19,20] One program describes an exercise where a student is assessed on taking a culturally appropriate history of a patient of diversity at a first station. At a second station, the student is assessed on the application of a culturally appropriate intervention and development of a plan of care.[19]

Reflective Exercise

• To what extent is your PT or PTA program transformative in its approach to multicultural education? • How might it be more transformative? • What are the obstacles and difficulties to achieving a transformative curriculum?

Curricular reviewers must look for common errors in curricula that promote cultural bias. A primary error is faulty generalization. This occurs when one specific group is represented and generalized to all groups. Another error is called circular reasoning. This occurs when a norm or ideal defined by the dominant group negates the experience of the nondominant group. Circular reasoning becomes even more of a threat to cultural sensitivity and representation when the norms and values become so embedded that they are accepted and taught without question.[20]

The Byrne Guide for Inclusionary Cultural Content[21] is a tool for reviewing and critiquing curricula. Byrne identifies multiple levels of curricular evaluation, including the examination of instructional materials for cultural bias. She recommends that instructional materials be appraised for six categories of bias identified by Sadker and Sadker.[22] The categories are invisibility or omission, stereotyping, imbalance and selectivity, unreality, fragmentation and isolation, and linguistic bias. Evaluation of instructional materials includes reviewing the representation of examples, pictures and photographs, and terminology.

Service Learning as Social Action

Many PT and PTA programs use volunteer or service-learning experiences to meet the needs of institutional mission statements and accreditation mandates and to enhance student development of cultural competence. Volunteer and service-learning experiences are examples of Banks's[8] social action theory, a fourth curricular approach to addressing multicultural education.

Service learning is a teaching methodology that combines relevant community service experiences with academic coursework defined by specific learning objectives, activities, assessment, and reflection.[23–25] Both the needs of the community and the learning needs of the students are met in service learning. In contrast, volunteerism is defined as "an experience that provides the opportunity to give time and energy to a worthwhile cause"[24] (p. 24). Here the needs of the community or audience are served without formal regard for student learning. Box 22-1 lists components important to consider when establishing a service-learning project requirement.

Village and co-workers[24] have found that 77.3% of PT programs and 60.9% of PTA programs surveyed have used service learning, volunteerism, or pro bono services as part of their curriculum within the last 7 years. The PTA programs were heavier in their use of volunteerism as compared with service learning, most likely because of the availability of fewer faculty members to initiate more involved service learning. The greatest barriers to implementing service-learning projects were identified as time and money; however, another study demonstrated that service-learning projects can be implemented with very little financial commitment and minimal additional time requirements.[25] The Village study[24] identified the development and integration of service-learning activities and goals into the courses as the most time-consuming aspect of service-learning projects.

Several studies have demonstrated conclusively that service-learning experiences develop and nurture civic values and responsibilities within students.[26–28] Likewise, students have exhibited advanced cultural competency skills after participating in service-learning experiences involving diverse communities.[25,29,30] Beling[23] conducted a study on a service-learning project

specific to a geriatric setting and found that the physical therapist students participating in the project demonstrated improved knowledge and more positive attitudes regarding geriatric clients.

Many projects in the literature describe physical therapist students servicing and learning in a

---

BOX 22-1

Community Service Project Guidelines

Consider and address the following items as appropriate:
- Purpose statement
  What is the purpose of this project?
- Target group
  Who is the target group?
- Contacts needed
  What contacts are needed?
- Permissions needed
  What permissions are needed?
- Target group needs assessment
  What are the target group's needs?
  How will you determine the target group's needs?
  Provide specific method of how you will do this.
- Resources needed
  What resources will you need?
  How do you expect to obtain these resources?
- Training needed
  What training is needed?
  How will you go about getting/giving the training needed?
- Proposed timeline
  What is your timeline for completion?
  Set up short deadlines throughout the process.
- Follow-up needed
  What follow-up will be needed?
  How might the program "do harm"?
  How can you ensure that the program "does no harm"?
- Program assessment
  How will you assess the effectiveness of the program?
  What components will you include in the program assessment?

variety of communities and settings, including homeless shelters,[30,31] American Indian reservations,[32] and geriatric care facilities.[23,33] The service-learning projects challenged the students to practice culturally competent patient education, an imperative skill for the physical therapist[34,35] (Fig. 22-1).

One study focused on a service-learning project that was a part of a course titled Health Issues of Ethnic Americans. The course required students to research an ethnic community in their area to learn the impact of history on that community, demographics, traditional beliefs and practices, gender roles, the health status of the community, and barriers to treatment and health services. Students then, with the help of community resources, developed a culturally relevant pamphlet addressing one of the health needs of the community and distributed it within the community in various ways. Qualitative study of this project yielded three major themes. First, the students were found to have developed a greater sense of "ethnic consciousness" or a greater understanding of their own culture and how it differs from others. Second, they not only developed increased sensitivity and awareness but also ex-

perienced applying their knowledge in an action that would help make a change—a type of social action. Third, the project helped to empower students to be citizens contributing to their surrounding communities.[25]

A study of multicultural curricular endeavors in medical schools revealed service-learning projects that were initiated by students. The students saw the need for cultural training when they felt that their faculty demonstrated insensitivity to cultural considerations. As a result, they implemented a program that continues to serve the community and meet academic objectives for student learning.[19,36] Educators must closely examine their own level of cultural awareness and sensitivity and strive for personal cultural competence.

Reflective Exercise

• What experience have you had with service learning? • How valuable was it? • How might you incorporate service learning effectively into the PT or PTA curriculum? • How are you different as a result of the service-learning project?

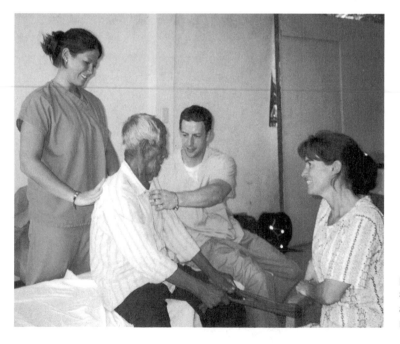

FIGURE 22.1 Service learning provides excellent opportunities for students to hone their skills as well as meet the needs of community members.

Service learning enables students and instructors to move beyond the walls of the campus classroom and the traditional clinics of practice and into the underserved, sometimes misunderstood, and often mismanaged local communities of people. Physical therapists will greatly benefit from exposure to diverse cultures within their local setting, as they will very likely encounter individuals and families from the diverse communities within the walls of the hospital or clinic. Service learning provides the means for the students and instructors to develop and nurture cultural and professional competency in the interaction, evaluation, and design of culturally appropriate plans of care while at the same time serving the needs and learning from local community members of diverse cultures.

International Immersion Experiences as Social Action

International immersion experiences are similar to service learning in that the educational methodology involves both service to the target group as well as educational objectives and defined learning experiences for the student. The literature is growing with examples of international immersion experiences and studies seeking to identify components of student learning.[19,37]

In comparison with the findings regarding service-learning outcomes, international learning experience outcomes speak less of civic duty and more of cultural awareness, cultural sensitivity, and cultural competency development.[38–40] A study of a 1-week physical therapy and occupational therapy learning experience in Belize found that students returned with a heightened awareness of their own culture as well as the cultures of others and were beginning to make applications toward culturally competent practice[41] (Fig. 22-2).

Another study compared the differences in cultural competency development between nursing students who participated in an international learning experience and those who did not. The findings demonstrated that those who had experienced a culture different from their own learned to challenge their own beliefs and values, experienced an increased awareness of self and others, and were better able to recognize their own ethnocentrism than those who had not participated in an international immersion learning experience[42] (Fig. 22-3).

Walsh and DeJoseph[39] explored the experience of nursing students who participated in a short-term learning project in Central America. They identified three emergent themes that directly contribute to student development of cultural competency. The first theme related to "being 'other.'" The students were better able to identify their ethnocentrism when culturally immersed in an environment and community unlike their own. They realized their "otherness" and began to identify ways in which their thinking and clinical practice are ethnocentric. A second and related theme was called "expanding my worldview." The

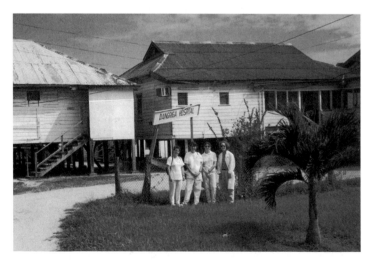

FIGURE 22.2 An international learning experience for nursing and physical therapist students in Belize.

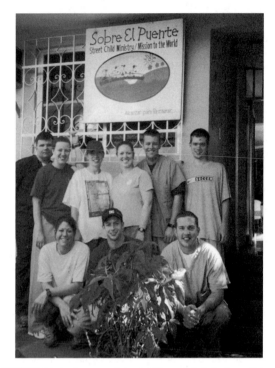

FIGURE 22.3 A group of physical therapist students participate in an international learning experience in Mexico.

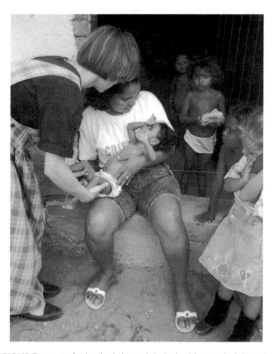

FIGURE 22.4 A physical therapist student learns to interact across cultures as she works with a mother and her child with a developmental disability in Mexico.

students consistently identified ways in which they were challenged to assess and reassess their view of the world. Finally, the authors found that this short-term immersion project was useful in enhancing student awareness of the global society. Students returned reporting heightened awareness of potential conflicts and challenges experienced by minority and immigrant populations in the United States as well as people globally (Fig. 22-4).

Reflective Exercise

• What results have you had with international immersion experiences? • What value do they have?
• What barriers exist to prevent your institution from placing students in international immersion experiences? • Which barriers might be overcome and how?

The institution that sponsored the international immersion experience is also very active in placing students in local service-learning projects. The researchers found that it was not until the students were living and working among their clients in the international immersion experience that they gained greater cultural understandings (Fig. 22-5). The difference was that the immersion experience required them to live and work in a community different from their community of origin and without "a cocoon of inclusion" provided by familiar home, family, and friends. "It is very likely that when individuals leave behind their daily personal and professional relationships and responsibilities to experience immersion in another culture, they are better able to take in the lived experience of another community"[39] (p. 271) and thus move toward greater awareness, sensitivity, and competence across cultures.

Student reflection on the learning experience is a key component of developing knowledge for both service learning and international immersion experiences. Reflection enables the student to consider the interaction in light of ongoing or past experience and is an essential student skill

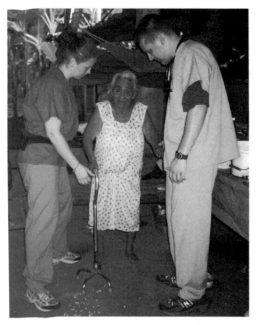

FIGURE 22.5 Physical therapist students visit a woman in her home in Mexico and instruct her in the use of a quad cane. The home visit enables the students to more accurately assess her mobility needs.

for understanding others from diverse cultures.[41] Students may practice reflection in the form of journals, reaction papers, discussion groups, and guided mentorship.[30,33] Reflective journaling is encouraged in numerous physical therapy service-learning projects and may serve as an assessment tool.[23,25,43,44] Physical therapist students participating in a service-learning project involving the homeless learned about the cultural components of the interactions by mentorship from their instructors as well as their more experienced peers.[29,30] Table 22-4 provides an example of an international learning experience incorporated as a course requirement. Box 22-2 lists resources and contacts for pursuing international physical therapy learning experiences.

Reflective Exercise

• How important is self-reflection in physical therapy practice? • In what ways does your current curriculum encourage or incorporate reflective learning? • In what ways do you as a professional clinician practice reflective learning? • How might reflective practice move you or your students toward developing greater cultural competency?

TABLE 22.4

Evaluation Tool for Clinical Elective International Learning Experience

OBJECTIVE	GRADES 1–10
1 The student will independently fit and/or modify adaptive devices to accommodate the individual's needs and environment, and available materials and devices.	
2 The student will independently educate individuals on job and home modification in order to correct body mechanics during daily activities.	
3 The student will score 80% or greater on all quizzes during the independent Spanish educational series of CDs.	
4 The student will effectively set up a physical therapy clinic in a provided space so that clinicians and students have adequate space for treatments and so that patients are triaged in a timely and specific manner.	
5 The student will perform an appropriate physical therapy examination using Spanish as the primary language of communication, either with the patient directly or through a translator into a tribal language.	
6 The student will demonstrate awareness of and sensitivity to cultural situations in interviewing patients and in prescribing physical therapy treatment and adaptive devices.	
Total points	
	Letter grade

(continued)

TABLE 22.4

Evaluation Tool for Clinical Elective International Learning Experience *(continued)*

OBJECTIVE	GRADES 1–10
Grading scale	

Grading scale
10 = performs skills above the level of an entry-level general practitioner
9 = performs skills on the level of an entry-level general practitioner
8 = needs minimal improvement to meet entry-level skill level
7 = needs moderate improvement to meet entry-level skill level
6 = needs additional coursework or clinical experience to meet entry-level skill level
<6 = failing level for any skill
Spanish skills will be graded using quizzes on the educational CDs. The student should obtain a score of >80% for a grade of 9 or a grade of >90% for a grade of 10.
Letter grade: 54–60 points = A
            48–53 points = B
            <47 points = F

—————— ——————
Signature of Student / Signature of Clinical Instructor
Courtesy of Meghan Lee, PT

Conclusion

Whether additive, integrative, transformative, or leading to social action, PT and PTA curricula are moving to embrace a growing diversity of clients in the United States. Physical therapy profession- als must be able to identify their own culture as well as their cultural biases and tendencies to- ward ethnocentrism. Second, they must be ready and willing to learn about the client's culture as well as respect differences. Identification, under-

BOX 22.2

Resources for International Immersion Experiences

1. The APTA Cross-Cultural Special Interest Group has a comprehensive manual of physical therapy international immersion experience opportuni- ties. Contact the CCSIG through the Health Policy & Administration Section of the APTA for a copy.

2. Christian Medical & Dental Society
P.O. Box 7500
Bristol, TN 37621
Phone: (423) 844–1000
Website: www.cmds.org
E-mail: main@cmdsmail.org

3. Doctors without Borders USA
6 East 39th Street, 8th Floor
New York, NY 10016

Phone: (212) 679–6800
Website: www.dwb.org
E-mail: doctors@newyork.msf.org

4. International Medical Corps
11500 West Olympic Blvd., Suite 506
Los Angeles, CA 90064
Phone: (310) 826–7800
Website: www.imc-la.org
E-mail: imc@imc-la.org

5. Health Volunteers Overseas
P.O. Box 65157
Washington, DC 20007
Phone: (202) 296–0928
Website: www.hvouse.org
E-mail: n.kelly@hvousa.org

> The Modified Golden Rule:
> "Treat others as we would like to be treated ourselves, if we were that other person."
>
> *Denise Bender, PT, JD, GCS*

standing, and respect are essential but fall short of culturally competent care. Culturally competent physical therapy care entails the ability to communicate effectively across the culturally diverse client encounter, followed by a culturally valid evaluation, followed by the mutual establishment of culturally congruent goals, and concluding with a culturally appropriate plan of care and interventions.

Nurturing students in the development of cultural competency is aided by a sound curriculum promoting cultural awareness, sensitivity, and competency. The curriculum must be able to adapt and change with the climate and culture of the U.S. population. Ultimately, it is the faculty and instructors who need to embrace cultural competency if culturally competent education of students is to take place. Box 22-3 provides a list of web resources to assist the educator, the stu-

dent, and the professional in the pursuit of cultural competence.

Nurturing Cultural Competency from the Perspective of the PT Student or Professional

While curriculum can provide the framework for learning about the development of cultural competency, ultimately it is the individual who determines to what extent cultural competency learning takes place. Campinha-Bacote[45] has identified a "cultural competence model" that entails cultural awareness, cultural knowledge, cultural skill, and cultural encounters. The center circle of her model that encompasses all of the components is labeled "cultural desire." The clinician must desire to develop cultural competence if cultural competence is to grow. Without desire, clinicians most likely will remain blind to their own ethnocentrism, blind to their own culture, and ignorant of the cultural conflicts and barriers that may exist in their professional practice of medicine.

Perhaps the physical therapist student or professional desires to become more culturally com-

BOX 22.3

Web Resources

http://www.omhrc.gov	Resources for minority health initiatives. Low-cost health education materials available.
http://www.atanet.org	The American Translators Association. Database of over 4,000 accredited translators and interpreters searchable by geographic area.
http://languageline.com	Language Line
http://www.cyracom.net	Cyracom
http://www.onlineinterpreters.com	Online interpreter service
http://erc.msh.org/quality&culture	The Provider's Guide to Quality and Culture
http://ethnomed.org/	Ethnomed: a resource for medical practices of various cultural groups
http://www.georgetown.edu/research/gucdc/nccc	National Center for Cultural Competence (NCCC)
http://www.diversityrx.org	Resources for Cross-Cultural Health Care
http://www.transculturalcare.net/ref_health.htm.	Periodically updated reference and website links to cultural competency in the health field. Put together by Transcultural Care

> "Patients don't care how much you know until they first know how much you care."
>
> *Josephina Campinha-Bacote*[46]

petent but doesn't know where to start. This portion of the chapter will supply some guidance and direction.

Self-Assessment or Reflection

The very first step is for the clinician to identify specific aspects and characteristics of his or her culture. Going back and answering the reflective questions in the first two sections of this text is a good place to start. The authors recommend that the reader write out his or her answers and thoughts for additional reflection at a later time. Taking the time to complete the exercises at the end of the chapters will also lead to greater understanding of the clinician's culture.

Identify and Research Local Communities

Second, the physical therapist should identify the various communities of culture with which he or she works in the professional practice. Are they more rural or urban? Are there different ethnic communities or specific age groups? Are the clients generally of low socioeconomic class, high socioeconomic class, or a mix? Make a list of the various communities of diversity and their primary and secondary characteristics of culture. Learn about each community. Determine the community's history, language, heritage, communication patterns, family roles and organization, and healthcare beliefs and practices, particularly regarding rehabilitation.

In order to learn about the communities, the physical therapist may need to conduct research at the local library or on the Internet. Perhaps a book or a piece of literature on the community will provide insight into the community and its history, heritage, values, norms, and needs.

A second means of acquiring knowledge and understanding about a particular community is to interview one or more community members, remembering that intra-ethnic variations coexist with inter-ethnic variations. The physical therapist could share the findings of his or her research with the community member(s) to confirm the

reliability and validity of the information obtained. He or she should ask members to describe their culture and their experiences living in the community and interacting with the U.S. healthcare system.

A third way of gaining perspective and appreciation for local community cultures is to attend or participate in community events. Perhaps a church service or a holiday celebration will help the clinician to better understand the culture of the local community members.

Negotiating the Practitioner–Client Interaction

Armed with knowledge of his or her own culture, potential biases and tendencies toward ethnocentrism, and some general knowledge of the local communities of diverse culture, the physical therapist is now well prepared to negotiate the interaction with the client. A few rules are important to remember in guiding the cross-cultural interaction.

Rule 1. Do not be afraid to ask questions. The client can be the physical therapist's most valuable resource in attempting to better understand his or her culture. Ask! Use the explanatory model of illness (see Chapter 9) to inquire about clients' beliefs concerning illness or disability causation. Ask them how they prefer to be addressed. Ask with whom they would like you to share medical information and with whom they would not. Ask them what their goals are and if there is anything they are pursuing at home or in their community to cure their condition. Let them know that you are open to understanding them and that you seek to provide physical therapy care that is of high quality and scientifically based but is also in congruence with their cultural practices and understandings as much as possible.

Rule 2. Communicate, communicate, communicate. Invite clients to communicate with you if they are uncomfortable with the program at any time. Be ready to reconfirm their consent to treat repeatedly throughout the program, as some cultures are reluctant to express disagreement with authority. Your clients are your most valuable resource for understanding their culture and identifying potential barriers to effective care. So many barriers can be avoided or overcome with effective communication. Of course, one must remember that communication patterns and styles

> "Do not fear mistakes—fear only the absence of creative, constructive, and corrective responses to those mistakes."
>
> *Rolfe Kerr* [47]

vary cross-culturally, and attention to potential miscommunications is important.

Rule 3. Use your observation skills. Physical therapists are trained to observe—to observe how people move, function, walk, and run. We are taught that observation and history are the two important keys to making a correct physical therapy diagnosis and thus establishing an appropriate plan of care. The physical therapist must apply the same skills to observing patterns of communication and comfort or discomfort with the program. When the physical therapist detects something from observation, he or she should go back to Rule 1 and *ask!* Get clarification on what you are observing and see what might be done to remedy the situation. The worst thing the clinician could do is to plow ahead with the program and continue to erect a barrier to communication and understanding, and ultimately to effective care.

Rule 4. Don't be afraid to make mistakes. The development of cultural competency is all about making mistakes. If a mistake is made, identify it and ask for forgiveness. Rarely will a client refuse a sincere apology. Once again, Rule 2 comes into play. Communicate with the client about the mistake. Both you and the client have an opportunity to learn and grow from the mistake. While serving as a physical therapist in a homeless shelter, one of the authors made the mistake of allowing students to come and palpate a client's lumbar muscles, which were undergoing spasms, without obtaining the client's permission for the students to "poke" at him. The client quickly lost patience and got up from the table and stormed out of the homeless shelter. The author never had an opportunity to get clarification of the problem or ask forgiveness for any mistakes, but did learn to be careful to obtain consent from clients before performing physical touch.

Mistakes and cultural faux pas will happen. The secret is to communicate about them, apologize, and learn from them. The important thing is that you recognize that a mistake was made; how much worse it would be to make mistakes

and be culturally blind so that you do not even recognize them.

Rule 5. Leave your stereotypes at home. The nurturing of cultural competency requires ongoing self-assessment, adaptation, and flexibility. Each encounter is different, with unique challenges and potential barriers. As stated previously, no two cultural groups are alike, and no two people within a cultural group are exactly alike. Intercultural and intracultural variations exist, just as variations in back injuries exist. The culturally competent physical therapist will hone the skills of cultural assessment, remain adaptable, and maintain an open, flexible mindset in order to negotiate each new cultural encounter successfully.

Conclusion

The pursuit of cultural competency is one of the richest, most rewarding and yet challenging endeavors a physical therapist can pursue. Culture influences clinician-client interaction from the moment the physical therapist greets the client to the administration of physical therapy interventions. Every client comes with a culture different to some degree from the culture of the clinician. The clinician's ability or inability to identify and address the cultural element may determine the effectiveness or ineffectiveness of the physical therapy program. The desire to better understand a client's culture along with the goal of designing culturally congruent physical therapy programs is essential for the successful practice of physical therapy. The authors hope that this book will be helpful to the physical therapy professional in his or her pursuit of cultural competence.

R E F E R E N C E S

1. American Physical Therapy Association. *Guide to Physical Therapist Practice.* 2nd ed. Alexandria, Va: Author; 2001.
2. American Physical Therapy Association. *Code of Ethics.* Alexandria, Va: Author; 1999.
3. American Physical Therapy Association. *A Normative Model of Physical Therapist Professional Education: Version 2004.* Alexandria, Va: Author; 2004.
4. American Physical Therapy Association. *A Normative Model of Physical Therapist Assistant Education: Version 99.* Alexandria, Va: Author; 1999.

5. Commission on Accreditation in Physical Therapy Education. *Accreditation Handbook.* Alexandria, Va: American Physical Therapy Association; 2000.

6. Babyar S, Sliwinski M, Krasilovsky G, et al. Survey of inclusion of cultural and gender issues in entry-level physical therapy curricula in New York State. *J Phys Ther Educ.* 1996;10:53–62.

7. Kraemer TJ. Physical therapist students' perceptions regarding preparation for providing clinical cultural congruent cross-cultural care: A qualitative case study. *J Phys Ther Educ.* 2001;15:36–52.

8. Banks JA. *An Introduction to Multicultural Education.* 2nd ed. Boston, Mass: Allyn & Bacon; 1999.

9. Thistlethwaite JE, Ewart BR. Valuing diversity: Helping medical students explore their attitudes and beliefs. *Med Teach.* 2003;25:277–281.

10. Taylor JS. Confronting "culture" in medicine's "culture of no culture." *Acad Med.* 2003;78:555–559.

11. Tervalon M. Components of culture in health for medical students' education. *Acad Med.* 2003;78:570–576.

12. Purnell LD, Paulanka BJ, eds. *Transcultural Health Care: A Culturally Competent Approach.* 2nd ed. Philadelphia, Pa: FA Davis; 2003.

13. Bender GB. Physical therapy education in the new millennium: Patient diversity plays a pivotal role in the shaping of our professional future. *J Phys Ther Educ.* 2002;16:8–13.

14. Black JD, Purnell LD. Cultural competence for the physical therapy professional. *J Phys Ther Educ.* 2002;16:3–10.

15. Leavitt RL. *Cross-Cultural Rehabilitation: An International Perspective.* Philadelphia, Pa: WB Saunders; 1999.

16. Shearer R, Davidhizar R. Educational innovations: Using role play to develop cultural competence. *J Nurs Educ.* 2003;42:273–276.

17. Hadwiger S. Cultural competence case scenarios for critical care nursing education. *Nurs Educ.* 1999;24:47–51.

18. Morell VW, Sharp PC, Crandall SJ. Creating student awareness to improve cultural competence: Creating the critical incident. *Med Teach.* 2002;24:532–534.

19. Loudon RF, Anderson PM, Gill PS, Greenfield SM. Educating medical students for work in culturally diverse societies. *JAMA.* 1999;282:875–880.

20. Lockhart JS, Resick LK. Teaching cultural competence: The value of experiential learning and community resources. *Nurs Educ.* 1997;22:27–31.

21. Byrne M, Weddle C, Davis E, McGinnis P. The Byrne guide for inclusionary cultural content. *J Nurs Educ.* 2003;42:277–281.

22. Sadker M, Sadker D. *Teachers, Schools, and Society.* New York: McGraw-Hill; 1994.

23. Beling J. Impact of service learning on physical therapist students' knowledge and attitudes toward older adults and on their critical thinking ability. *J Phys Ther Educ.* 2004;18:13–21.

24. Village D, Clouten N, Millar A, et al. Comparison of the use of service learning, volunteer, and pro bono activities in physical therapy curricula. *J Phys Ther Educ.* 2004;18:22–28.

25. Flannery D, Ward K. Service learning: A vehicle for developing cultural competence in health education. *Am J Health Behav.* 1999;23:323–331.

26. Waldstein F, Reiher T. Service-learning and students' personal and civic development. *J Exper Educ.* 2001;24:7–14.

27. Morgan W, Streb M. Building citizenship: How students' voice in service-learning develops civic values. *Soc Sci Q.* 2001;82:154–170.

28. Eyler J. Educational innovations—Reflecting on service: Helping nursing students get the most from service-learning. *J Nurs Educ.* 2002;41:453–454.

29. Musolino G, Feehan P. Enhancing diversity through mentorship: The nurturing potential of service learning. *J Phys Ther Educ.* 2004;18:29–42.

30. Black JD. "Hands of Hope": A qualitative investigation of a student physical therapy clinic in a homeless shelter. *J Phys Ther Educ.* 2002;16:32–41.

31. Rose M, Lyons K, Swenson Miller K, Cornman-Levy D. The effect of an interdisciplinary community health project on student attitudes toward community health, people who are indigent and homeless, and team leadership skill development. *J Allied Health.* 2003;32:122–125.

32. Kavanagh K. Summers of no return: Transforming care through a nursing field school. *J Nurs Educ.* 1998; 37:71–79.

33. Village D, Village S. Service learning in geriatric physical therapist education. *J Phys Ther Educ.* 2001;15:42–45.

34. Padilla R, Brown K. Culture and patient education: Challenges and opportunities. *J Phys Ther Educ.* 1999; 13:23–30.

35. Gahimer JE, Morris DM. Community health education: Challenges and opportunities. *J Phys Ther Educ.* 1999; 13:38–48.

36. Tang TS, Bozynski ME, Mitchell JM, Haftel HM, Vanston SA, Anderson RM. Are residents more comfortable than faculty members when addressing sociocultural diversity in medicine? *Acad Med.* 2003;78:629–633.

37. Godkin M, Savageau J. The effect of medical students' international experiences on attitudes toward serving underserved multicultural populations. *Fam Med.* 2003; 35:273–278.

38. Kollar S, Ailinger R. International clinical experiences: Long-term impact on students. *Nurs Educ.* 2002;27:28–31.

39. Walsh L, DeJoseph J. "I saw it in a different light": International learning experiences in baccalaureate nursing education. *J Nurs Educ.* 2003;42:266–272.

40. Haloburdo E, Thompson MA. A comparison of international learning experiences for baccalaureate nursing

students: Developed and developing countries. *J Nurs Educ.* 1998;37:13–21.

41. Ekelman B, Dal Bello-Hass V, Bazyk J, Bazyk S. Developing cultural competence in occupational therapy and physical therapy education. *J Allied Health.* 2003;32:131–137.

42. Barrett K. Facilitating culturally integrated behaviors among allied health students. *J Allied Health.* 2002;31:93–98.

43. Paschal K, Jensen G, Mostrum E. Building portfolios: A means for developing habits of reflective practice in physical therapy education. *J Phys Ther Educ.* 2002; 16:38–53.

44. William R, Sundelin G, Foster-Seargeant E, Norman G. Assessing the reliability of grading reflective journal writing. *J Phys Ther.* 2000;14: 23–26.

45. Campinha-Bacote J. *The Process of Cultural Competence in the Delivery of Healthcare Services: A Culturally Competent Model of Care.* 3rd ed. Cincinnati, Ohio: Transcultural C.A.R.E. Associates; 1998.

46. Campinha-Bacote J. A model of practice to address cultural competence in rehabilitation nursing. *Rehabil Nurs.* 2001;26:8–11.

47. Covey SR. *Seven Habits of Highly Effective People: Restoring the Character Ethic.* New York, NY: Free Press; 2004.

Index

Page numbers followed by "b," "f," and "t" indicate boxed material, figures, and tables, respectively